Cases on Applied and Therapeutic Humor

Michael K. Cundall Jr.
North Carolina A&T State University, USA

Stephanie Kelly
North Carolina A&T State University, USA

IGI Global
PUBLISHER of TIMELY KNOWLEDGE

A volume in the Advances in Medical Diagnosis, Treatment, and Care (AMDTC) Book Series

Published in the United States of America by
IGI Global
Medical Information Science Reference (an imprint of IGI Global)
701 E. Chocolate Avenue
Hershey PA, USA 17033
Tel: 717-533-8845
Fax: 717-533-8661
E-mail: cust@igi-global.com
Web site: http://www.igi-global.com

Library of Congress Cataloging-in-Publication Data

Names: Kelly, Stephanie, 1984- editor. | Cundall, Michael K., 1974- editor.

Title: Cases on applied and therapeutic humor / Stephanie Kelly and Michael K. Cundall, editors.
Description: Hershey, PA : Medical Information Science Reference, [2020] | Includes bibliographical references and index. | Summary: "This book examines on applied and therapeutic humor. It covers topics ranging from propriety, effectiveness, perception, and cultural variables"-- Provided by publisher.
Identifiers: LCCN 2020004637 (print) | LCCN 2020004638 (ebook) | ISBN 9781799845287 (hardcover) | ISBN 9781799845294 (ebook)
Subjects: MESH: Professional-Patient Relations | Delivery of Health Care | Anecdotes | Wit and Humor
Classification: LCC R727.3 (print) | LCC R727.3 (ebook) | NLM WZ 305 | DDC 610.69--dc23
LC record available at https://lccn.loc.gov/2020004637
LC ebook record available at https://lccn.loc.gov/2020004638

This book is published in the IGI Global book series Advances in Medical Diagnosis, Treatment, and Care (AMDTC) (ISSN: 2475-6628; eISSN: 2475-6636)

British Cataloguing in Publication Data
A Cataloguing in Publication record for this book is available from the British Library.

For electronic access to this publication, please contact: eresources@igi-global.com.

Advances in Medical Diagnosis, Treatment, and Care (AMDTC) Book Series

ISSN:2475-6628
EISSN:2475-6636

Mission

Advancements in medicine have prolonged the life expectancy of individuals all over the world. Once life-threatening conditions have become significantly easier to treat and even cure in many cases. Continued research in the medical field will further improve the quality of life, longevity, and wellbeing of individuals.

The **Advances in Medical Diagnosis, Treatment, and Care (AMDTC)** book series seeks to highlight publications on innovative treatment methodologies, diagnosis tools and techniques, and best practices for patient care. Comprised of comprehensive resources aimed to assist professionals in the medical field apply the latest innovations in the identification and management of medical conditions as well as patient care and interaction, the books within the AMDTC series are relevant to the research and practical needs of medical practitioners, researchers, students, and hospital administrators.

Coverage

- Internal Medicine
- Medical Testing
- Medical Procedures
- Chronic Conditions
- Disease Management
- Cancer Treatment
- Disease Prevention
- Diagnostic Medicine
- Experimental Medicine
- Emergency Medicine

IGI Global is currently accepting manuscripts for publication within this series. To submit a proposal for a volume in this series, please contact our Acquisition Editors at Acquisitions@igi-global.com or visit: http://www.igi-global.com/publish/.

The Advances in Medical Diagnosis, Treatment, and Care (AMDTC) Book Series (ISSN 2475-6628) is published by IGI Global, 701 E. Chocolate Avenue, Hershey, PA 17033-1240, USA, www.igi-global.com. This series is composed of titles available for purchase individually; each title is edited to be contextually exclusive from any other title within the series. For pricing and ordering information please visit http://www.igi-global.com/book-series/advances-medical-diagnosis-treatment-care/129618. Postmaster: Send all address changes to above address.

Titles in this Series

For a list of additional titles in this series, please visit:
http://www.igi-global.com/book-series/advances-medical-diagnosis-treatment-care/129618

Diagnostic and Treatment Methods for Ulcerative Colitis and Colitis-Associated Cancer
Ashok Kumar Pandurangan (B. S. Abdur Rahman Crescent Institute of Science and Technolog, India)
Medical Information Science Reference • © 2021 • 309pp • H/C (ISBN: 9781799835806) • US $295.00

Strategies to Overcome Superbug Invasions Emerging Research and Opportunities
Dimple Sethi Chopra (Punjabi University, India)
Medical Information Science Reference • © 2020 • 284pp • H/C (ISBN: 9781799803072) • US $225.00

Enhancing the Therapeutic Efficacy of Herbal Formulations
Rajesh Kumar Kesharwani (Nehru Gram Bharati (Deemed), Prayagraj, India) Raj K. Keservani (Faculty of B. Pharmacy, CSM Group of Institutions, Prayagraj, India) and Anil K. Sharma (GD Goenka University, India)
Medical Information Science Reference • © 2021 • 367pp • H/C (ISBN: 9781799844532) • US $265.00

Exploring the Efficacy and Beneficence of Complementary and Alternative Medicinal Products in Disease Therapy
Etetor Roland Eshiet (Sustainable Energy Environmental and Educational Development (SEEED), USA)
Medical Information Science Reference • © 2021 • 315pp • H/C (ISBN: 9781799841203) • US $295.00

Climate Change and Its Impact on Fertility
Khursheed Ahmad Wani (Goverment Degree College, Bijbehara, India) and Nibedita Naha (ICMR, National Institute of Occupational Health, Ahmedabad, India)
Medical Information Science Reference • © 2021 • 416pp • H/C (ISBN: 9781799844808) • US $265.00

Treating Endocrine and Metabolic Disorders With Herbal Medicines
Arif Hussain (Manipal Academy of Higher Education, UAE) and Shalini Behl (Manipal Academy of Higher Education, UAE)
Medical Information Science Reference • © 2021 • 489pp • H/C (ISBN: 9781799848080) • US $295.00

Handbook of Research on Advancements in Cancer Therapeutics
Sumit Kumar (National Institute of Pathology, New Delhi, India) Moshahid Alam Rizvi (Jamia Millia Islamia, India) and Saurabh Verma (National Institute of Pathology, India)
Medical Information Science Reference • © 2021 • 913pp • H/C (ISBN: 9781799865308) • US $465.00

IGI Global
PUBLISHER of TIMELY KNOWLEDGE

701 East Chocolate Avenue, Hershey, PA 17033, USA
Tel: 717-533-8845 x100 • Fax: 717-533-8661
E-Mail: cust@igi-global.com • www.igi-global.com

This text is dedicated to all the medical care professionals, front-line workers, and others across the globe *that were so important in the fight against COVID-19. We could think of no better group of people who* deserve the dedication. We hope this text helps provide more smiles and laughs.

Table of Contents

Preface

PURPOSE OF THE ANTHOLOGY

The idea behind the creation of this text starts, as many good ideas do, with two colleagues having a conversation. One of us is a communication scholar and the other a philosopher. We both have an interest in humor. After some conversations and working through various ideas, we came upon an approach of working on a project on humor and medical care in a way that fairly treated issues (e.g. when can you use humor in medical care, does it help?) related to humor and medical care, but did so in a novel way. We also wanted to show the different perspectives of our disciplines and how this broader appreciation could be helpful to readers.

We noticed there was often just an article or two out there discussing the use of humor in medical care, broadly conceived, that one could find in a journal, or as a special edition, but the pickings were slim. What made matters worse is that while there were these discussions on humor based on the general idea that humor was helpful for health and in health care settings, much of the available content was limiting for a variety of reasons. Firstly, it was sporadic and made tracking down specific cases difficult. Secondly, the content available was either a short story relating the outcomes of humor's use in a specific situation, or it was a deeper theoretical treatment by researchers on the issues of humor, but the application of the theoretical issues wasn't detailed in a way that people might use later on. The latter sort of content isn't terribly helpful for the practicing healthcare professional as it can get bogged down in the minutiae, thus making it difficult to draw conclusions from. The former might not do any more than promote common sense ideas like "you shouldn't make fun of people" or "don't joke about politics." These platitudes will not get you very far if you want to know how, when, and why you can and should use humor in medical care settings in an effective way.

As a result, we set out to create an anthology that provided not only appropriate discussions of humor and the issues that arise in its use within a healthcare setting, but also one that provided usable materials for people to then apply. We thought this last part important because, to our knowledge, there isn't a text out there that does this. It's all well and good to discuss the theoretical issues related to humor in healthcare settings, but it's often difficult for non-specialists to leave more theoretical discussions with a clear sense of how they might apply these theoretical considerations. With all this in mind, plus the joy of reading about humor and laughter, we set out to create this anthology.

Our goal with this text is to provide practicing healthcare workers, medical students, or anyone interested in knowing the role of humor in healthcare, with an introduction to the ideas and issues that can arise when and where we find humor within the healthcare environment. We also wanted to make sure that the content of the anthology was informed and guided by practicing researchers who have expertise in humor or health. In short, we wanted to provide an anthology that wasn't too heavily weighted with academic jargon and research, and tied directly to actual cases of humor as related by practicing healthcare professionals.

Some of the cases clearly show the usefulness of humor while others show where the humor can create unintended tension. While most of the cases are friendly to the use of humor, and we are clearly apologists when it comes to humor, it shouldn't simply be assumed that humor only ever has beneficial outcomes. It isn't always thus. Part of providing a fair and encompassing presentation of humor in healthcare means addressing when it has gone wrong, and how one can learn from those cases and work to use humor more effectively.

Humor and Health

One might think that some sort of argument should be made to support the view that humor is important for healthcare. That is, we should provide evidence that would convince a healthcare practitioner that they need to be using humor in their interactions with patients. While we will provide a brief summary of evidence to that effect, the truth is, the question isn't, "Why should you be adding humor to your interactions with patients?" Rather the real question is why aren't more healthcare professionals intentionally practicing humor in their care?" The available evidence, of which we can only provide a snapshot, is clear. Humor is important for our health and as such, deserves a space in the toolbox of techniques that healthcare professionals use.

Let's begin with the psychological benefits of humor. Beyond the commonsense notion that we tend to feel good when we laugh and enjoy jokes, there have been a number of studies investigating the benefits that laughter and health have. Cann and Collette (2014) found that self-enhancing humor led to greater resilience and overall better psychological health. Houston et al. (1998) found that older individuals of residential communities had reduced anxiety levels and depression if they participated in a humorous activity than those who did not. Finally, researcher Martin (2019) has spent over three decades investigating humor and recently found that certain types of humor called "adaptive humor styles" are important to well-being.

The salutary effects of humor and psychological well-being can also be seen in the workplace. The presence and use of humor in these situations is also beneficial. Campbell et al. (2001) identified positive correlations between humor orientation and employee satisfaction, managerial responsiveness, and approach strategies. Later research found supervisor humor to have a positive influence on employee empowerment (Gkorezis et al., 2011).

Researchers like Savage et al. (2017) find that the reason that psychological well-being and health are improved through laughter and humor relates to the way in which we experience laughter and humor, that is in social contexts. The sharing of laughter and humor helps strengthen the bonds with those we laugh and joke with. Thus the case for humor as helpful for psychological well-being is strong. Let's turn now to the effects that humor and laughter have been shown to have on our physical health.

The study of the effects of humor and laughter on physical health is largely a recent phenomenon. This is largely due to the work of Norman Cousins in his groundbreaking book *Anatomy of an Illness* (Cousins, 1979). This book helped usher in much research into the effects that laughter and humor have on a variety of physical traits. Following Cousins' (1979) work, Berk et al. (2001) has shown that mirthful laughter helped patients increase helpful neuroimmune factors like leukocytes, T- Cells, and natural killer cells. Cancer patients have also shown a positive correlation between humor and comfort levels when humor is present (Christie & Moore, 2005). One of the reasons that people report feeling better when laughing or experience humor, is that the mesolimbic reward center of the brain is active during experiences of humor (Mobbs et al., 2003).

An introduction is not the best place to get an in-depth review of all the literature on humor and laughter and their effects and relations to physical and psychological health. However, it is not unreasonable, based on this evidence, to realize that humor and laughter play an important role in health and well-being.

Structure of the Anthology

There are 40 chapters in this anthology. The chapters come in pairs. The first paper of each pair of chapter will feature a case written by a healthcare provider or patient describing a time they experienced humor at play in the healthcare setting. Some of these cases describe humor that was successful and additive to the healthcare environment. Others describe instances in which the humor was detrimental.

The second paper within each pair is a response to the case wherein an academic with expertise relevant to the case, and in regard to humor, breaks down the variables involved in the case and makes recommendations for humor in the healthcare setting based upon that case. More specifically, each response is broken into three primary sections:

1. A review of academic literature relevant to the case
2. An application of that literature explaining its role in the case
3. Lessons that healthcare providers can take from the case

Each response author has attempted to write their paper so that the academic analysis can be followed by anyone, making this book accessible to audiences without an expertise in the represented academic fields. Response authors hold degrees in a variety of academic disciplines, but most come from communication or philosophy. For a full overview of respondent credentials please see Appendix A.

A final note about the authors included in this anthology. We have individuals who are members of the Asian-American, Latinx, LGBTQ, African-American communities. We have contributors who identify as men and women. We also have contributors from two disciplines as well as people from various ranges within the academy, from undergraduate and graduate students, to professors. Case authors provide narratives from a variety of contexts including, but not limited to, primary care visits, nursing, emergency room visits, EMT rescues, psychiatric sessions, phlebotomy sessions, dentist visits, and even homeopathic care treatment.

Concluding Remarks

While a plethora of research exists on the connection between health and humor, what is lacking so far has been practical instructions for how healthcare providers can effectively integrate humor into their care. This text seeks to be a first step in filling that gap.

We leave it to you, the readers, to let us know how well we've reached our goals. Ahead lie 40 chapters each with a unique case of humor and a response from an academic. We can assure you that we learned as much as we expect you will from the cases and the responses. Putting this anthology together has been a wonderful challenge. We invite you to dig into these chapters and enjoy.

REFERENCES

Berk, L., Felten, D., Tan, S., Bittman, B., & Westengard, J. (2001). Modulation of Neuroimmune parameters during the eustress of humor-associated mirthful laughter. *The Journal of Alternative Therapies*, *7*(2), 62–75.

Campbell, K. L., Martin, M. M., & Wanzer, M. B. (2001). Employee perceptions of manager humor orientation, assertiveness, responsiveness, approach/avoidance strategies, and satisfaction. *Communication Research Reports*, *18*(1), 67–74. doi:10.1080/08824090109384783

Cann, A., & Colette, C. (2014). Sense of humor, stable affect, and psychological well-being. *Europe's Journal of Psychology*, *10*(3), 464–479. doi:10.5964/ejop.v10i3.746

Christie, W., & Moore, C. (2005). The impact of humor on patients with cancer. *Clinical Journal of Oncology Nursing*, *9*(2), 211–218. doi:10.1188/05.CJON.211-218

Cousins, N. (1979). *Anatomy of an illness: As perceived by a patient*. W.W. Norton Company.

Gkorezis, P., Hatzithomas, L., & Petridou, E. (2011). The impact of leader's humor on employee psychological empowerment: The moderating role of tenure. *Journal of Managerial Issues*, *23*(1), 83–95.

Houston, D. M., McKee, K. J., Carroll, L., & Marsh, H. (1998). Using humor to promote psychological well-being in residential homes for older people. *Aging & Mental Health*, *2*(4), 328–332. doi:10.1080/13607869856588

Martin, R. A. (2019). Humor. In M. W. Gallagher & S. J. Lopez (Eds.), *Positive psychological assessment: A handbook of models and measures* (pp. 305–316). American Psychological Association., doi:10.1037/0000138-019

Mobbs, D., Greicus, M., Abdel-Azim, E., Menon, V., & Reiss, A. (2003). Humor modulates the mesolimbic reward centers of the brain. *Neuron*, *40*(4), 1041–1048. doi:10.1016/S0896-6273(03)00751-7

Savage, B., Lujan, H., Raghavendar, R. T., & DiCarlo, S. (2017). Humor laughter, learning and health! A brief review. *Advances in Physiology Education*, *41*(3), 341–347. doi:10.1152/advan.00030.2017

Acknowledgment

Thank you to our reviewers!

Allison Noyes

Andrea Meluch

Amy Werner

Candy Noltensmeyer

Chris Kramer

Elizabeth Sills

Elizabeth Spradley

Elizabeth Victor

Florian Fisher

Ian Stark

Kenneth T. Rocker

Laura Miller

Nick Innarino

Ryan Goke

Scott Christen

Scott Eldgredge

Steve Cox

Susan Weiczorek

Suzy Prentiss

Ty Spradley

Warren Bariess

Chapter 1
You Dropped Your Butter

Monalisa M. Tailor
Norton Healthcare, USA

Dolly Parton has many memorable songs, but arguably her most famous song is *Jolene*. In this song, Dolly has a conversation with a woman named Jolene, who she thinks very highly of, so highly that she is afraid her husband might like Jolene more than her. In 2019, Parton explained to her fans that *Jolene* became so popular not because it is catchy, not because it had a novel storyline, but because it was a song about feeling insecure...making it a song about something everyone could relate to. It is true, everyone feels insecure at times, and truthfully, there are not many places in this world designed to make a person feel more insecure than hospital.

Yes, hospitals are places of healing. Yes, hospitals are places of discovery. Yes, hospitals can be places that bring families together. Yes, many healthcare professionals work very hard to communicate skillfully so that their patients do not feel insecure.

However, hospitals are also places where a team of professionals point out things that are wrong with you. They find your flaws and document them, put your flaws on record to be shared with other professionals and to make sure that they themselves remember what exactly is wrong with you. In this process of identifying flaws for the sake of improving one's health, it is inevitable that the process of becoming healthier will lead some patients to feel insecure. Those insecurities often lead to anxiety.

This particular humorous event took place with a woman who was feeling quite insecure, particularly about her physical appearance. For the sake of ease, we will call this patient *Lisa*. At the time of this appointment, Lisa had been struggling with chronic weight gain for quite some time. She was determined to get to a healthy weight and was being extremely careful about her eating behaviors. Gone were greasy foods, sugars, and beloved bread with butter. She had also been taking medication to help manage her weight, but the medications were not successful.

One day, Lisa came to see me for her appointment. She was a bundle of nerves as she was prone to be when she came to see me for appointments in which her weight was going to be discussed. All of her insecurities were rising up to the surface, manifesting in visible signs of anxiety. She was getting sweaty, she was fidgety, and her heart rate had risen.

DOI: 10.4018/978-1-7998-4528-7.ch001

At the check-in desk, Lisa was second in line. Before her stood another woman rummaging through a large shoulder bag. Lisa noticed that something fell out of the woman's bag and tried to catch it before it hit the floor. The object that had fallen out of the bag was an entire stick of butter.

Oh the irony...here was Lisa constantly worried about her weight, avoiding unhealthy foods at all cost...and she comes into the doctor's office to have a whole stick of butter literally flung in her direction.

The irony broke through her anxiety and turned into laughter. By the time she got back to my office, she was visibly in a better mood. When she told me the story about the butter at the check-in desk we both laughed. In fact, we laughed on and off for 30 minutes about the incident. Through the laughter, Lisa found her way to honesty, and she was able to discuss the fact that her own anxieties were most likely what was preventing her from losing weight. The humor was essential to dispelling the anxiety and all the nervousness. Had Lisa come back to the office as a bundle of nerves, we would not have likely made as much progress as we did. When we experience anxiety, our body believes we are in a fight or flight mode. As a result, our heart races, our breathing becomes shallow, it's hard to focus, and our goal is to get away from danger. In terms of weight, this triggers our adrenal glands to help keep us going, and also releases cortisol which causes weight gain. So thanks to a stick of butter and a pinch of laughter, Lisa was able to find the real source of her weight battle.

REFERENCES

Smith, P. S., Parton, D. (Writers) & Fleming, A. (Director). (2019). Jolene [Netflix series episode]. In S. Haskell (Producer), Dolly Parton's Heartstrings. Los Gatos, CA: Netflix Studios.

Chapter 2
Response: "You Dropped Your Butter" – Laughing the Pain Away: The Cathartic Value of Relief Humor in Health Communication

Ian Stark
https://orcid.org/0000-0002-9357-215X
Texas Tech University, USA

CONCEPTUAL REVIEW

Researchers have long debated the exact functions and mechanisms of humor, with most scholars aligning with one of three large theoretical propositions (Meyer, 2017). Perhaps the most popular of these propositions is the idea that humor is a function of situational incongruity, in which things are funny because they are unexpected (Berger, 1976; Clarke, 2008; Deckers & Divine, 1981; McGhee, 1979). Less popular is the idea that humor arises from positions of perceived superiority, in that things are funny because they enforce social hierarchies (Feinberg, 1978; Gruner, 1997; Lintott, 2016; Morreall, 1983). Least popular is the idea that humor exists as a function of psychophysiological stress relief – and so goes the general academic wisdom.

Notably, the relief theory of humor operates in essentially the opposite mindset of the other two. Specifically, instead of identifying funny things because of the way they *make us feel* (e.g., superior, surprised), this theory posits that things are funny because of *how we are feeling* (e.g., tense, nervous) and how they bring those feelings to resolution (Berlyne, 1972; Meyer, 2000; Morreall, 1983). Put differently, according to relief theory, this release of tension is psychologically perceived through humor and physiologically expressed through laughter.

DOI: 10.4018/978-1-7998-4528-7.ch002

The academic disputes about these three theories are infamous, even sparking attempts to create "atheoretical" research evading them (Martin, 1996). It is a debate that will not likely be ended by any proclamations of this text. However, from the perspective of a humor practitioner, it is also a debate that is not, in and of itself, especially relevant (Baisley & Grunberg, 2019). Arguably, from a strictly practical point of view, it is decidedly counterproductive to attempt to assess the definitive strength or weakness of the three primary theories in a vacuum.

Instead, by taking a theory-agnostic approach, each of these individual conceptualizations of humor can be useful in providing different approaches to examining and eliciting humorous responses in specific situations. In toolbox fashion, these different ideas may be applied in particular communication situations, allowing them to serve as informative heuristics rather than empirical rules. From this frame of reference, any theory can be impactful – even the unusual and occasionally maligned relief theory. This chapter explores how relief theory may be an ideal model for humor in health communication, inasmuch that this context can be reliably framed through the theory of catharsis (Scheff & Bushnell, 1984).

In a nutshell, catharsis is a psychological concept that posits that an individual's built-up negative feelings (e.g., anger, sadness) can be processed effectively and safely through the use of purging activities (Jackson, 1994). Such activities might include any courses of action that actively engage with and then subsequently dispel these negative feelings. For example, one person's binge of sad movies on Hulu may be another person's afternoon of angry video games on Steam, or yet another person's dive into raunchy comedy specials on Netflix. The main idea here is that the activity is impactful to the individual and relatable to their emotional state.

Ideally, catharsis serves to provide a "lighter" outlet (Jaffee, 1996) for feelings that might, in absence of their purgation, otherwise be left to fester and be acted upon in an undesirable manner, such as lashing out at others or self-harming. Perhaps one of the simplest and most promising cathartic exercises is the act of laughing at one's self and/or one's situation – becoming, in effect, one's own jester – in order to defuse any tensions entangled within (Warner, 1991). This lesson of laughing at one's self has been applied quite broadly for purposes ranging from the management of one's own personal mental health status to the diplomatic dance of avoiding large-scale international conflicts (Steele, 2020).

Though cathartic events are usually conceived as individualized experiences, some circumstances have the potential to bring individuals together through shared emotional distress (Pennebaker & Harber, 1993). Most commonly, these are big, socially destructive events like natural disasters or terrorist attacks, but they can just as well be states of living and being in a particular culture or community. Regardless of the specific reason, when cathartic moments involve multiple individuals in shared states of experience, they are referred to as collective catharsis. The concept of collective catharsis sheds light on why, of the three main humor theories, relief humor is most uniquely beneficial to healthcare.

At some level, this is because medical spaces, by their very nature, are characterized by a collective sense of tension (Dieser et al., 2017). Whether it be sitting in the waiting room of an urgent care center or laying on the archetypal counselor's couch, the people in these spaces experience a shared state of tension informed by their experiences of unwellness. For that matter, the same can be said for the very healthcare providers working in those spaces! After all, being surrounded by death and disease all day doesn't exactly lend itself to a cheery disposition, and healthcare workers have been known to become decidedly macabre as a result of these experiences in their profession (Watson, 2011).

In addition to the signals from the medical space itself, patients are inundated with pre-existing notions of what healthcare spaces and experiences should be through the propagation of reductive media images (Seale, 2003), with the television medical dramas (*House*, *Scrubs, Grey's Anatomy*, etc.) being particularly prominent. These images even create parasocial expectations of what actual interactions with healthcare providers should entail (Fadenrecht, 2015). While this dramatic form probably creates more interesting stories, it does so at the expense of engendering an association and, indeed, expectation of distress with medical care.

Bearing this combination of personal experiences and social influences in mind, it's clear that healthcare patients are thoroughly primed for emotional tension. It follows, then, that releasing this tension through humor can have a therapeutic effect, reducing the stress associated with healthcare experiences (Bast & Berry, 2014) and creating a mindset more suitable for making a recovery. Though laughter probably isn't the *best* medicine, per se, the mindset shift it brings can actually have a significant positive impact on a patient's actual recovery outcomes (Hasan & Hasan, 2009). If nothing else, releasing these emotions through laughter is generally preferable to letting them ferment and explode outward through destructive actions.

Pennebaker and Harber (1993) identify three distinct stages of collective catharsis: (1) the emergency stage in which tension spikes, (2) the plateau stage in which tension is maintained, and (3) the extinction stage in which tension is dissolved. Ostensibly, a person or group should progress through these stages in that order, but, in practice, individual members of a group may well be operating at different stages of catharsis at the same time. Nonetheless, these stages may serve as a useful framework for identifying the presence and potential of catharsis in a humorous situation.

The following case analysis employs Pennebaker and Harber's (1993) stages as a rhetorical lens through which to understand the relieving humor of the dropped butter incident. First, the plateau stage will be explored as a period of protracted tension buildup associated with a topic of stress – in this case, the medical visit about the patient's weight. Then, the emergency stage will be articulated in terms of a specific event – the dropped butter – that throws these built-up feelings into sharp relief. Finally, the extinction stage will be visualized as the steady dissipation of tension – the adjusted treatment regimen and clearer path toward health recovery – following its sudden release.

APPLYING THE LENS

Stage 1. Plateau

Lisa is quite tense at the prospect of visiting the doctor about her weight issue. At the end of the day, there are essentially only three potential outcomes to that conversation: (1) she is still overweight, (2) she is more overweight, and (3) she is less overweight than she used to be. Options 1 and 2 are horrible, dominating the mind with their anxious worries and long-term health consequences. That being said, Option 3 is not great either, in that it offers only the validation of short-term change at the continued expense of long-term responsibility. Even if she's doing well, the prospect of sustaining it can be exhausting.

Unfortunately, Lisa's situation is far from unusual. Oftentimes, healthcare patients will experience considerable distress at the idea of visiting the doctor for any number of conceivable reasons. For example, is that weird-looking bump a mole or melanoma? Alternatively, are these intrusive thoughts due to stress or schizophrenia? Oh man, is it actually all in the head – and if so, is that worse? The fact is, one does not generally go to the doctor's office because one is doing *well.* Even if one is just getting a simple annual check-up, the fact that they *have to check* to make sure their body is not failing on them can be painfully anxiety-inducing.

Not to mention, this explanation is not even considering the non-diagnostic reasons why Lisa and other patients like her may be experiencing distress. Doctor's offices, counseling centers, hospitals, and all manner of healthcare facilities are intimidating locations with overhanging concerns like the possibility of acquired infectious diseases, the financial stress over the billing process, the professional challenge of missing time off from work, and the list goes on. All of these factors contribute to the creation of a plateaued state of tension that Lisa likely experienced before even receiving care.

Stage 2. Emergency

Enter the infamous dropped butter. Society may never know the circumstances that led to this individual having a bar of butter in their bag – perhaps it is a comfort item, or a compulsive carry-on, or simply the unfortunate result of mis-scheduling a doctor's appointment with a grocery shopping trip. Regardless of the cause for which it fell, in falling, the butter captured the essence of many of Lisa's concerns about weight, health, image, etc. and threw them on the ground for the world to see. And how did she react in this situation? Did she curse the universe for its unusual twist of fate? Did she break down in tears at the overwhelmingness of it all? Did she sigh heavily with the weight of existence on her shoulders?

No, she did not. Quite the opposite, in fact: she laughed, and from a cathartic lens, it is easy to see why. Due to the circumstances surrounding her doctor's visit, she was full of tension. However, when the butter hit the floor, it exposed that tension – a cathartic purge of all of her health-related anxieties exemplified by congealed fat. In other words, when the butter was released from its bag, it also released Lisa's built-up dietary anxieties from her body without her ever picking up a spoon.

In this moment, the unique suitability of the relief theory of humor for health communication contexts is most visible. It was not the unexpectedness of the falling object that made it funny, as incongruity theorists may argue; it was the fact that the object just happened to be butter (symbolizing Lisa's weight issue). Likewise, it was not the fact that the butter fumbling was publicly embarrassing, as superiority theorists may argue, but rather it was that there was butter in the situation at all. Yes, it was specifically the appearance of butter that created the emergence of humor, which was only able to be activated because of Lisa's pre-existing psychological state.

Stage 3. Extinction

When Lisa entered her physician's office and regaled her of the butter story, there was suddenly an important decision to be made: How should she respond? On the one hand, Lisa was a returning patient and she likely already had a plan for how this meeting was supposed to play out. So, she could choose to play a normalizing role and bring the situation back home to that comfort zone. On the other hand, Lisa seemed genuinely happy and motivated, which is something that her physician had not observed from her in a great while. If she wanted, she could embrace this surge of emotion and see where it takes her.

In this case, Lisa's physician chose to embrace the humor, which presented yet another question of how to proceed: Which type of humor is happening here? If she took an incongruity approach, she might interpret the falling butter as a funny coincidence, which, while not wrong, is an incomplete picture of what is happening. If she were actively bad at her job, she might have even taken a superiority approach – perhaps joking that the butter is the universe giving Lisa a sign and/or making fun of her for being overweight. Thankfully, she did neither of those things, and instead intuitively responded in the mode of relief humor – albeit probably without knowing any of these choices by name.

Ultimately, Lisa's physician made the right call by accepting Lisa's sense of humor and validating her emergent feelings of cathartic relief. In doing so, Lisa's physician enabled her to move beyond the isolated emergence of humor – incorporating it into the rest of the consultation and adjusted treatment regimen – and creating a longer-term coping mechanism for the associated stressors that spawned it. She effectively guided Lisa through the emergency stage of catharsis and allowed her to make progress toward extinction of the original distress about her medical visit.

PRACTICAL APPLICATIONS

The remainder of this chapter will be dedicated to actionable takeaways that can be derived from the preceding content, including recommendations informed by relief humor and catharsis more generally, as well as recommendations informed specifically from the case of Lisa and the butter. In both instances, these are intended to serve as general guidelines for consideration in medical practice – not hard rules per se. At the end of the day, the objective of this text is not to override the physician's best judgment in otherwise clear-cut cases, but rather to provide a set of conceptual tools from which to approach appropriate unusual situations.

Recommendation #1 is to Validate Emergences of Humor

Even if you do not necessarily find them amusing. If your patient is laughing, it is important to show them that your office is a safe space to express themselves in this manner. This is especially applicable if the patient is laughing nervously and/or looking to you for approval of their joke, as these signs may indicate tension needing to be released. If you do not validate them, you may prevent them from accessing the relief function of humor, or, even worse, you may pervert their relief humor into a case of superiority humor at their expense. Of course, you certainly would not intend to do that, but humor is largely the realm of perception, not intent.

How Do I Implement This Recommendation?

Where possible, show genuine emotional connection to the humorous attempts made by your patients. Where not possible, fake it till you make it; pretending to laugh at someone else's jokes is a social skill like any other, and one that will improve with time. The easiest way to get started with this is to recognize the expression of your patient when an attempt at humor is being made and respond accordingly. If they are guffawing, guffaw back. If they are deadpan snarkers, give them a satisfying chuckle. Even if you do not nail the exact intensity of expression, the main idea is to display that you "get it."

Recommendation #2 Is To Be Aware of Pre-Existing Plateaus

Understand that the medical interaction begins far before your patient actually sees you. In Lisa's case, this was made obvious by her experience at the check-in desk, but the interaction does not necessarily begin at that desk, either. Did they have difficulty getting a spot in the parking lot? Maybe they heard an advertisement about their medication on the radio? Ooh, maybe a politician said something controversial about the healthcare industry on television! Whatever the cause, patients come in with a wide variety of pre-existing expectations and anxieties, which, though central to the success of relief humor in medicine, also contribute an unfathomable number of unknowns.

How Do I Implement This Recommendation?

This application is twofold: (1) observing factors local to your healthcare setting and (2) observing factors in the broad societal setting. For the former case, take stock of the environments immediately preceding your provider-patient interaction. What was their wait time like? Did they have a conversation with the receptionist? Was there a lot of noise in the lobby? For the latter case, try to keep a pulse on the social discourse around healthcare (broadly speaking) and your specific discipline (be that general practice, psychiatry, dentistry, etc.). What are people saying about it? Is there any misinformation going around? How might that affect your patient?

Recommendation #3 Is To Embrace Momentum Toward Extinction

Recognize the value of unexpected yet impactful patient interactions. In all likelihood, Lisa's physician did not learn anything in medical school about how to handle spontaneous dairy-based epiphanies; all the same, she handled this situation with aplomb. Lisa was in a state of mind that her physician most likely did not anticipate, but one that nonetheless held great potential for treatment. So, while Lisa's physician may have stepped into that office with a distinct, entirely different treatment plan, she adapted and overcame the situation which led to a better outcome.

How Do I Implement This Recommendation?

Avoid seeing your patients as "patients" or, worse, as "diagnoses," and instead, try to conceptualize them as "people." Otherwise, you will quickly realize that medical language can easily lend itself to prescribed and rigid sequences of cause and effect (i.e., apply "X" treatment in "Y" amount to "Z" condition) which leave little room for pattern deviance and situational interpretation. Thus, instead of relying exclusively on the familiar, be prepared to accept new information and adjust to the personality of your patient – should it present itself – even if it means throwing out everything you had in mind when you first walked through the door.

Recommendation #4 Is To Laugh With Your Patient, Not At Your Patient's Expense

This sounds obvious, and perhaps it should be, but it bears mention all the same. Yes, this chapter has spent the majority of its content exploring how humor can be beneficial in a healthcare setting. No, this beneficence is not going to be the case in every conceivable instance. Quite to the contrary, in many situations, introducing humor into a medical case where it is unwanted and/or unwarranted is a terribly counterproductive idea. Not only will this likely strain the professional relationship between the physician and their patient, but it may even worsen the patient's prognosis for their condition.

How Do I Implement This Recommendation?

Like many social situations, this is a case best navigated by *listening* and *evaluating* before you even begin to think about *speaking*. In general, the person introducing humor into the medical interaction, if it is indeed introduced at all, should be the patient, not the physician. By situating the patient's sense of humor as the conversational point of origin, you minimize the risk of inadvertently harming them with your humor. Likewise, by maintaining the patient as the center of discussion, you can observe if their humorous demeanor changes, as it may well do, throughout your meeting.

REFERENCES

Baisley, M. C., & Grunberg, N. E. (2019). Bringing humor theory into practice: An interdisciplinary approach to online humor training. *New Ideas in Psychology, 55*, 24–34. doi:10.1016/j.newideapsych.2019.04.006

Bast, E. S., & Berry, E. M. (2014). Laugh away the fat? Therapeutic humor in the control of stress-induced emotional eating. *Rambam Maimonides Medical Journal, 5*(1), e0007. doi:10.5041/RMMJ.10141 PMID:24498514

Berger, A. A. (1976). Anatomy of the joke. *Journal of Communication, 26*(3), 113–115. doi:10.1111/j.1460-2466.1976.tb01913.x

Berlyne, D. E. (1972). Humor and its kin. In J. H. Goldstein & P. E. McGhee (Eds.), *The psychology of humor: Theoretical perspectives and empirical issues* (pp. 43–60). Academic Press. doi:10.1016/B978-0-12-288950-9.50008-0

Clarke, A. (2008). *The pattern recognition theory of humour*. Pyrrhic House.

Deckers, L., & Devine, J. (1981). Humor by violating an existing expectancy. *The Journal of Psychology, 108*(1), 107–110. doi:10.1080/00223980.1981.9915251

Dieser, R. B., Edginton, C. R., & Ziemer, R. (2017). Decreasing patient stress and physician/medical workforce burnout through health care environments: Uncovering the serious leisure perspective at Mayo Clinic's campus in Rochester, Minnesota. *Mayo Clinic Proceedings, 92*(7), 1080–1087. doi:10.1016/j.mayocp.2017.03.017 PMID:28624118

Fadenrecht, K. M. (2015). *The influence of medical dramas on patient expectations of physician communication* (Master's thesis). University of Montana.

Feinberg, L. (1978). *The secret of humor*. Rodopi.

Gruner, C. R. (1997). *The game of humor: A comprehensive theory of why we laugh*. Transaction Publishers.

Hasan, H., & Hasan, T. F. (2009). Laugh yourself into a healthier person: A cross cultural analysis of the effects of varying levels of laughter on health. *International Journal of Medical Sciences, 6*(4), 200–211. doi:10.7150/ijms.6.200 PMID:19652724

Jackson, S. W. (1994). Catharsis and abreaction in the history of psychological healing. *The Psychiatric Clinics of North America, 17*(3), 471–491. doi:10.1016/S0193-953X(18)30094-7 PMID:7824376

Jaffee, B.-J. (1996). Using laughter as a cathartic process in grief counseling. In J. D. Morgan (Ed.), *Ethical issues in the care of the dying and bereaved aged* (pp. 283–296). Routledge.

Lintott, S. (2016). Superiority in humor theory. *The Journal of Aesthetics and Art Criticism, 74*(4), 347–358. doi:10.1111/jaac.12321

Martin, R. A. (1996). The situational humor response questionnaire (SHRQ) and coping humor scale (CHS): A decade of research findings. *Humor: International Journal of Humor Research, 9*(3-4), 251–272. doi:10.1515/humr.1996.9.3-4.251

McGhee, P. E. (1979). *Humor: Its origin and development.* W. H. Freeman.

Meyer, J. (2017). *Understanding humor through communication: Why be funny, anyway?* Lexington Books.

Meyer, J. C. (2000). Humor as a double-edged sword: Four functions of humor in communication. *Communication Theory, 10*(3), 310–331. doi:10.1111/j.1468-2885.2000.tb00194.x

Morreall, J. (1983). *Taking laughter seriously*. State University of New York Press.

Pennebaker, J. W., & Harber, K. D. (1993). A social stage model of collective coping: The Loma Prieta earthquake and the Persian Gulf War. *The Journal of Social Issues, 49*(4), 125–145. doi:10.1111/j.1540-4560.1993.tb01184.x

Scheff, T. J., & Bushnell, D. D. (1984). A theory of catharsis. *Journal of Research in Personality, 18*(2), 238–264. doi:10.1016/0092-6566(84)90032-1

Seale, C. (2003). Health and media: An overview. *Sociology of Health & Illness, 25*(6), 513–531. doi:10.1111/1467-9566.t01-1-00356 PMID:12919443

Steele, B. (2020). "A catharsis for anxieties": Insights from Goffman on the politics of humor. *Global Society,* 1-15. doi:10.1080/13600826.2020.1828296

Warner, S. L. (1991). Humor: A coping response for student nurses. *Archives of Psychiatric Nursing, 5*(1), 10–16. doi:10.1016/0883-9417(91)90004-O PMID:2039275

Watson, K. (2011). Gallows humor in medicine. *The Hastings Center Report, 41*(5), 37–45. doi:10.1002/j.1552-146X.2011.tb00139.x PMID:21980898

Chapter 3
Infusions and Explosions:
Reframing Through Belly Laughs

Joy Todd
Enloe Medical Center, USA

Susan Avanzino
California State University, Chico, USA

A little over 20 years ago, while working at a hospital in Northern California in the field of pediatric oncology, I was giving a 10 year old boy, "Johnny," an infusion of platelets. This had become a regular occurrence since he fell out of remission nearly a year after receiving a bone marrow transplant. He had a form of leukemia (Philadelphia Cell) that has significantly poor outcomes and we were buying him a little more time. He had been my patient for that entire year, and I had grown close with him and his family.

As with many children with cancer, Johnny had wisdom beyond his years and an intermittent seriousness usually reserved for adults. He worried about how his parents would fare after he died, and he made them promise that they would never divorce. He had a cherub like look, partly because of the prednisone that he regularly took which gave fullness to his cheeks and beyond. He also had a playful personality and a coy twinkle in his eye.

This particular infusion was taking place in a ward for outpatient infusions and GI procedures (mostly diagnostic) on the first floor of the hospital. About halfway into the infusion, a loud noise erupted. We both looked to the source of the noise, which was a closed door about 6 feet from Johnny's bed. I quickly realized that we were located close to the wall of bathrooms and an unfortunate GI patient was having an explosion of gas. We had been here numerous times before but had not been located so close to the bathrooms, nor had we experienced such an outburst.

This explosion interrupted my small patient who was just talking about what he wanted to be when he grew up and then shifted to talking about his understanding of what death would be like. As soon as we both looked at the closed door, we looked at each other, not knowing how to react. He tightened his lips and he tried not to laugh, but he lost the battle of control and broke into uncontrolled laughter, which was contagious and led to my own laughter. Just when we thought we could catch our breath, new

DOI: 10.4018/978-1-7998-4528-7.ch003

explosions of gas erupted and continued for several minutes. Johnny laughed so hard that he cried. As the poor person kept passing more and more gas, we both continued to laugh full body-shaking belly laughs. Johnny had gone back to being a normal 10 year old boy, just for a few minutes. When we would try to stop laughing, we would look at each other and just start laughing again.

Eventually the poor person emerged from the bathroom and we both tried to stifle our laughter while averting our eyes. There were a few more infusions before Johnny succumbed to the cancer; with each infusion, we would giggle a little at the memory. What could have been a somber and scary time had become a time of human connection and even shared joy. Johnny's parents did struggle after his death as he had anticipated, but because of their promise to him, they overcame their struggles and their marriage survived. They credit Johnny with that and were amazed in his insight.

While just a moment in time, what made this exchange impactful was the deep sense of letting go and experiencing a moment of freedom that transcended the primary context of the appointment. This was true for me and Johnny; we formed a deeper human connection with a shared belly laugh. That experience carried into our remaining time together, where a smile could trigger the memory even as time was waning. It strengthened my underlying presupposition that laugher can reframe an experience. It can give us a new lens to see the same situation in a new, less stressful light. In this case these infusions could have been a time of fear and trepidation. Instead, they became a time of joyful human connection, a time that we actually looked forward to. The dismal prognosis didn't change, but our lived moments were fuller.

It's one of my most precious memories. His smile and infectious laugh will always be etched in my memory.

Chapter 4
Response: "Infusions and Explosions: Reframing Through Belly Laughter"

Vanessa Voss
Lone Star College, University Park, USA

LITERATURE REVIEW

Incongruity Theory of Humor

This theory of humor proposes that the essence of all humorous states involves something which deviates from the norm. Let's take for example one of my favorite Far Side cartoons. In this comic, a portly young man in a shop looks up to a shelf full of food goods far out of his reach. Underneath this comic, the caption reads "Inconvenience Store" (Larson, 1990, p. 66) What is found funny here are the variety of unexpected details that do not follow everyday patterns. We are used to the norm "convenience store," but this norm has been subverted by the prefix "in" to negate it. The concept of a convenience store has deviated from what it is expected to be (It is a place to grab something easily) to a place which is its opposite. One may even find the incongruity in the cartoonish shape of the put-upon customer looking up, as it is not the normal shape of a person to be this stout, round, and neckless. This is why humor is often achieved through cartoons since they can be like us but at the same time be divergent from the normal "human look" enough to arouse humor. Schopenhauer writes, "[t]he case of laughter in every case is simply the sudden perception of the incongruity between a concept and the real objects which have been thought through it in some relation, and laughter itself is just the expression of this incongruity" (Morreall, p. 52). Concept: convenience store, easy and quick access to goods for real people. Image: difficult to get goods posing as convenient and human-looking beings posing as real humans.

Humor might be things seen as congruent incongruences: seeing both the connection and the disconnect at the same time. This is the nature of puns or wordplay humor. Recall George Carlin's response to the phrase "near miss." It is a strange congruent-incongruence, and it makes him irate (VoxTalk, 2014).

DOI: 10.4018/978-1-7998-4528-7.ch004

The audience laughs at the joke because all at once they know what "near miss" means in everyday English. It means something almost was hit or crashed into but did not get hit or crash into in the end. They know this, they are aware of this truth. However, they also now know the opposite: that this word *literally* does not mean that at all, as Carlin deftly points out. The phrase really should be "near hit," for "near miss" literally means they almost DID hit or crash, but IN FACT, did not. They hold these two contrary ideas at once, knowing both to be true.

This is the very heart of the incongruity theory of humor, this fundamental holding of two contrary truths at the same time. It answers the question of *what* it is that makes something funny. Nevertheless, it does not finish the story of humor. Some incongruencies are funny; some are not. Puns like "near miss" or "the meaning of opaque is very unclear" are benign: harmless little linguistic violations, as many jokes, are. The incongruity theory of humor can do a lot of explanatory work in showing us why something arouses amusement, but what distinguishes not funny versus funny violations of the norm? McGraw (n.d) says we laugh at incongruities that are not only surprising, but also ones that are benign violations. An angry bear busting to a crowded lecture hall is incongruous with the norm, but hardly funny, as many will be mauled and injured. It is not benign, though it is a violation of the norm. But a streaker dashing at full speed into a crowded academic setting and then exiting is funny, because we know a streaker to typically not be threatening, but yet is still a violation of the norm. And not an extreme violation either. A streaker who does not dash but lingers for all to see in great detail? That would be too great a violation and therefore not funny in most scenarios. For an incongruity to be funny, it must not be a threat, and this does seem to be somewhat context-dependent. Perhaps it might even involve presupposing a comic distance of time or space, which would allow things that seem a bit of a violation or threat appear less ominous and thus could be framed as a joke.

Stoicism

For this section, we will be focusing on the Stoic idea of eudaimonic virtue ethics, especially in relation to the link between the good life and the human struggle with "indifferents", as well the most excellent of virtue's byproducts, *ataraxia* (ἀταραξία), translated as tranquility or as freedom from pain or trouble. (Pigliucci, n.d). This section will explain these ideas in more detail, using the foundational writings of Epictetus, Seneca, and a modern scholar of Stoicism, Pigliucci.

Pigliucci (2017) writes that, "...Stoic ethics isn't just about what we do-our actions-but more broadly about how our character is equipped to navigate real life" (p. 72). The ethical focus for the Stoic is on having the right character in order to live the good life. Their idea of proper virtue is a golden mean between those focused solely on virtue alone for a good life (c.f., Socrates, Cynics) and those who focused on the good life as awarded by virtue in relation to good fortune and circumstance (c.f., Aristotle). For Socratic and Cynical thinkers, virtue alone was enough for the good life. Poverty, ugliness, and discomfort mattered little in the quest for virtue (just think of the life of the Cynic Diogenes, famous for living an indigent lifestyle on the streets, living in a ceramic jar and mocking Alexander the Great). For Aristotle, virtue was the key to the good life, but the good life would be hard to achieve if one was born to bad parents, into poverty or slavery, and ugly. To quote Aristotle (1934),

[n]evertheless it is manifest that happiness also requires external goods in addition, as we said; for it is impossible, or at least not easy, to play a noble part unless furnished with the necessary equipment... For many noble actions require instruments for their performance, in the shape of friends or wealth or political power; [16] also there are certain external advantages, the lack of which sullies supreme felic-

ity, such as good birth, satisfactory children, and personal beauty: a man of very ugly appearance or low birth, or childless and alone in the world, is not our idea of a happy man… (p. 15-16).

One may develop a good character, which shows a life of the habits of virtue, but alas, the overall goal of a good life, the happy life, will be tough to achieve for ugly and low born persons.

The genius of Stoicism is bridging these two views. Stoics say that there are things indeed outside of our control, some being good to us and others not. Those things outside of our control which are to our benefit, such as good parents, money, and good looks, are called "preferred indifferents" (Pigliucci, 2017, p. 75) and do help with living a good life. But these goods should not have the power over our ability to live well, say the Stoics. They are indifferent in the end; they are a boon, but nothing more (thus the term "indifferent"). Stoics also recognize we must contend with things they call "dispreferred indifferents" (p. 75), the things that bad fortune brings us which we also have no control over, like poverty, exile, abusive parents, and ugliness. But these things also do not exclude us from living a virtuous (and therefore tranquil) life. It is worth considering for a moment the situation of Epictetus: Epictetus spent a good part of his life as a slave. His name, ἐπίκτητος, means "acquired" (Perseus, n.d). Historians do not even know what name his birth parents gave him. His state of slavery counts as a "dispreferred indifferent," a state that is out of his control and not one of good fortune, yet a state that does not stop one from achieving a good life. For Stoics, either indifferent could not ultimately stop one's chances at achieving a virtuous, thus good, and therefore tranquil, happy life.

The purpose of a Stoic life is not to be an armchair thinker and ponder ceaselessly about virtue, but to live it. One should use their rational faculties in order to fulfill their lives as a social being, which is an essential part of our nature. To live in accordance with nature was key to living well, and that nature was social and rational, and both aspects of humanity were clearly aspects we could begin cultivating from a young age to make these aspects shine like a polished gem in adulthood.

Stoic ethics consist of four cardinal virtues: courage, temperance, justice, and practical wisdom. "Justice can be conceptualized as practical wisdom applied to social living; courage as wisdom concerning endurance; and temperance as wisdom with regard to matters of choice." (Pigliucci, n.d., pp. 59). Courage in the Stoic sense is about facing the harsh reality of the world and facing the "indifferents" (good or bad) that are immovable and out of one's control. de Botton (2000), writing about Seneca's Stoic wisdom in his popular book, *The Consolations of Philosophy*, says Stoic courage is facing the "collusion of a wish with an unyielding reality" (p. 80). Temperance is associated with the restraint of our desires considering what is and is not possible in the external world which is often beyond our control. In contemporary usage, the term Stoic is often used to describe someone who expresses no emotion. But for the true Stoic, emotion is not the enemy to be destroyed entirely, but the inability to control emotion and let it get the best (and thus the worst) of us. A Stoic should not avoid feeling the emotions of loss, but feel the emotions relevant to the amount required of the situation and respond to them in a rational manner. In chapter 23 in Seneca's work *On the Happy Life* (1882), he writes about how to handle the sorrow felt when one loses a dear friend: "To lament the death of a friend is both natural and just; a sigh or a tear I would allow to his memory: but no profuse or obstinate sorrow" (Seneca, p. 194). In his letter "On Consolation to Marcia" (1910), Seneca advises a woman who has lost her son to cease grieving. He tells her that the death of a child, while tragic, is not uncommon and not unnatural. Deaths like this happen, and while it seems unjust to her that other sons live while her's does not, it's a part of human life that Fortune is indifferent to. While Seneca advises Marcia to stop actively grieving, he only advises her to do it since the sorrow overwhelms all aspects of her life.

Seneca is not arguing it is wrong to feel sorrow. In fact, it is very much appropriate to the Stoic life. It is when sorrow takes over one's rational mind causes a person to lose their emotional moderation that the proper virtue of temperance has been lost. The third Stoic virtue of justice is concerned with how we should be fair and treat others with dignity and practicing good citizenship. We must always think of how our actions will come to affect others, not only ourselves. And the fourth virtue, practical wisdom, which can be equated to a sort of mindfulness, one which "tells us how to react to situations," (Pigliucci, p. 25). This is the skill to know what act to take when situations arise in the world. Stoics thought that this virtue required the study of logic, as well as reflection and study. These were essential in developing cognitive strength in order to meet whatever Fortune might have in store for you, your loved ones, and your community.

While virtue itself is good and should be practiced for that very reason, virtue does offer a very excellent side-effect that is important to the good life: *ataraxia* (ἀταραξία). *Ataraxia*, as mentioned earlier, is often translated as tranquility or as freedom from pain or trouble. *Ataraxia* is often associated with the writings of Epicurus who sought out the happy life of philosophy in practice. Epicurus was a hedonist, meaning he thought the ultimate good for mankind was pleasure. Unlike the way the word hedonism is used today, Epicurean hedonism means the seeking of the reduction of pain and the pain caused by desiring unnecessary things, like luxury goods. (de Botton, p. 60). For the Stoics, *ataraxia* was also a good thing to achieve, but unlike the Epicureans, it was not the end goal in life to be sought, but a by-product of living with the four cardinal virtues. By living in accordance with the four cardinal virtues, one's desires would be kept in order and thus one could avoid pain caused by one's lack of control. For example, if we are temperate, we won't eat more ice cream than what makes us pleasantly satiated. We will eat the right amount relative to our hunger, not the amount that our taste buds demand, which will cause us to be ill. *Ataraxia* is achieved when we have eaten the right amount. For the Stoic, the pleasure is not inherently a bad experience to have, but only in so far as it is in balance with what is needed. Much like our passions must be under control, so much our experiences of pleasure as well. Neither passion nor pleasure should be holding the reigns, but our virtuous character. Otherwise, we fail to live a good life, and thus fail to gain the secondary benefits of virtue: *ataraxia* as happiness.

Practical Application

Johnny, the young cancer patient, has the weight of adulthood placed on his shoulders. He knows he is going to die; he knows he will not experience adult life and knows his family will mourn his loss. He has the concerns that usually occur to us later in our adult life to contend with as a child. Yet, Johnny approaches his situation as a Stoic, and though it might seem odd to say he acts as a Stoic when he laughs, he truly does. At the beginning of the case, the nurse and Johnny are discussing what "his understanding of death would be like." This is a moment of serious reflection and reasonably seen as a somber moment. But as they begin their discussion, they hear the noise of flatulence from a nearby bathroom. This, of course, is followed by Johnny and then the nurse's laughter. This is very much in line with what makes something funny under the incongruity theory of humor. When we are in situations in which a somber attitude and seriousness is normal protocol, we do not expect certain events to occur. When we speak of death, especially one involving a young child, no one would predict that toilet sounds would be involved. Our expectation is thwarted by a fart. A fart does not jive with the grave nature of discussions of death and causes an "incongruity": seriousness, death, sorrow.

Laughing at a fart in this situation is part of a Stoic lifestyle. Nothing embodies facing the reality of a situation out of one's control (death) with laughter more than a Stoic attitude, which can include the act of laughing. In Morreall's book *Taking Laughter Seriously* (1983), he discusses the relation of laughter to freedom in the way that laughter can take a person out of a painful moment to allow a uniquely objective and sometimes aesthetic moment. The example Morreall gives is of a man pouring his morning coffee on his breakfast cereal instead of milk. For that moment, the man looks at his actions outside of himself, sees the error, and finds the humor within it. Without seeing it outside of oneself, the other option is to remain attached to the personal experience. Morreall says the emotion of anger or frustration will occur, since you have not seen the error as humorous any longer, but something that is painful to you- the loss of coffee and Fruit Loops.

Of course, Johnny is not discussing the loss of his breakfast with the nurse, but the loss of his life. Morreall (1983) also addresses situations too heavy for most to bear and when they sometimes lead us to laughter. He uses a quote from psychologist and Holocaust survivor Viktor Frankl on the subject of using humor to face horror:

Unexpectedly most of us were overcome by a grim sense of humor," (during the Holocaust) "...Humor was another of the soul's weapons in the fight for self-preservation...Humor more than anything else in the human make up can afford an aloofness and an ability to rise above any situation, if only for a few seconds (Morreall, 1983, p. 104).

Morreall then applies this very thinking to the experience of being in a hospital, where humorous names are given to various, sometimes life threatening, diseases, and jokes will be made between healthcare professionals and between healthcare professionals and patients. Morreall writes if humor involves a distancing from life's troubles, then perhaps the highest form of this 'stepping back' is gallows humor, in which a person is able to achieve enough distance from his own situation of impending death to joke about it (p.92). What makes something funny is an incongruity, but the way to make the variety of painful experiences funny is to create some distances by viewing the situation as coolly and objectively as possible, even when you are the one with the inoperable cancer. Humor allows a moment of aesthetic distance, and with that, a moment of relief for the suffering the situation brings.

Let us now apply this framing of incongruous humor to the good life of a Stoic. Recall that the good life of a Stoic is achieved by living virtuously, especially in practicing the four cardinal virtues: courage, temperance, justice, and practical wisdom. The excellent byproduct of living a good life of virtue is a state of *ataraxia*: freedom from pain, or tranquility. As the nurse stated, "[t]he dismal prognosis didn't change, but our lived moments were fuller." By laughing during a period of difficulty, of facing an impending untimely death with giggles, both the nurse and Johnny are living the Stoic virtue of courage. They are facing harsh reality, of which they can do nothing to change, as it is. They are still living as if a tranquil and joyful life is available, regardless of bad fortune. When Epictetus speaks in *Discourses* on dealing with things that are in our control and things that are not, he states, "[21] What should we have ready at hand in a situation like this? The knowledge of...what I can and cannot do. [22] I must die. But must I die bawling?" (Epictetus, 2008, p. 7). To apply it to our case, "I must die. But must I die bawling? *No, you may choose to laugh.*" Granted, Johnny is not facing death at this very moment, but Epictetus (2008) writes that to live with virtue, you must act appropriately during each event at that moment. He says that when it is time to dine, you dine, but when it is time to die, then you will die. The virtue of temperance is found in living appropriately at the right time; do not worry about things when it is not the time for them. To apply this to our case, "When it is time to laugh, we laugh."

The Stoic virtue of justice is concerned with good citizenship and our proper reverence to others. Johnny and his nurse do not wish to laugh directly at the gentleman having gastric troubles, but rather laugh at the sounds they hear when he is not facing them directly. The humor they found in the event is not at the expense of the gentleman, but laughter considering the incongruity itself, as well as the cultural norm of finding toilet noises funny. If they did not care for the feelings of the gentleman, they would laugh even when he exited the bathroom. Stoic citizenship is also expressed in the care that the nurse gives to Johnny when he laughs. She does not scold Johnny or lecture him about medical issues concerning bowels. Instead, she recognizes the youthful joy children find in toilet jokes and shares in a proper giggle. The fourth and final virtue, practical wisdom, is the skill of knowing what act to take in different situations. Clearly, the nurse and Johnny know when it is the right time to break from a discussion of death to engage in a shared laugh.

These virtues, as expressed by Johnny and the nurse, show the noble strength needed in order to meet Fortune, and to face her with the tranquility bestowed upon you by acting virtuously, in this case, the ray of light in the form of a reasonable momentary giggle during cancer treatment. Laughter as a break from the seriousness of childhood death due to cancer is an ethical path to take when practiced at the right moment and place and with the right moderation.

When Johnny and his nurse laugh during Johnny's cancer treatment, for a moment they both master a painful reality of the impending death of a child. It is an unpleasant situation, indeed, but by practicing Stoic virtues and realizing and reflecting on the moments of incongruity in life, the unexpected can become a moment of freedom from suffering. A sudden fart can create a moment of tranquility; a giggle can create the good life, even if it only be a short one.

Recommendations

When you are with a patient, make sure to be a Stoic, not a "stoic". Remember that being a virtuous healthcare provider doesn't mean holding back all emotion; being a virtuous healthcare provider is being a Stoic who knows that having the correct amount of emotions at the correct time leads to a good medical practice. Medicine is not just about healing the body but creating virtuous relationships between provider and patient.

Pigliucci writes, "[t]reat every human being-regardless of his or her stature in life-with fairness and kindness," (2017, p. 205). When your patient cries, empathize with them but with temperance. Make sure to treat all patients who cry with equal consideration, regardless of their situation or social standing. For some patients, they will be devastated at hearing a cancer diagnosis, while others will express the same devastation at hearing that they have a minor fraction of a pinky toe bone. Listen to all your patients and their needs equally, with temperance and kindness. And of course, when they laugh, journey with them in their mirth. If they want to joke about their situation, let them lead the way down that path and join in when prudent.

Part of treating patients with a true Stoic attitude and with fairness requires that you listen first to what their needs will be. Epictetus writes, "…let silence be the general rule, or let only what is necessary be said and in few words," (Epictetus, 2008, p. 118), meaning speak when is necessary, but also make sure you leave yourself open to hear what needs to be heard. Your patients do want to know your medical diagnosis and advice, but do not let your position of authority and expertise stop you from truly hearing and being silent when it is necessary to listen to your patients. Epictetus does go on in the same passage, "[l]et not your laughter be much, nor on many occasions, nor excessive," (p. 118). But of course, do laugh at the right time.

Sometimes the best way to deal with things like death is through the lens of humor. Nothing says "dispreferred indifferent" than illness and death. But it's ok to laugh at it. Sometimes a shared laugh at the pain is the best route to *ataraxia*. Also, you may practice creating incongruity in certain patient settings. Perhaps intentionally spoofing your own expertise (wearing a stethoscope wrong and correcting it) could make a child laugh. You will not have harmed the child (it is benign), but in fact, made the child better off in a stressful situation. But the best route to follow is to listen to what the required action should be in relation to your patient. Laugh when they laugh, suffer with them in solidarity when they suffer. Listen and they will let you know what they require.

REFERENCES

Aristotle. (1934). *Nicomachean ethics* (H. Rackham Trans). Harvard University Press, Perseus Digital Library. (Original work published 350 B.C.E.)

de Botton, A. (2000). *The consolations of philosophy*. Pantheon Books.

Epictetus. (2008). *Discourses and selected writings* (R. Dobbin, Trans.). Penguin Classics. (Original work published in 108)

Larson, G. (1990). *Weiner dog art: A Far Side collection* (Vol. 15). FarWorks.

McGraw, P. (n.d.). *Humor research lab (HuRl)*. http://humorresearchlab.org

Morreall, J. (1983). *Taking laughter seriously*. State University of New York Press.

Morreall, J. (1986). *The philosophy of laughter and humor (SUNY Series in Philosophy)*. State University of New York Press.

Perseus Greek Word Study Tool. (n.d.). Retrieved January 15, 2021, from http://www.perseus.tufts.edu/hopper/morph?l=%E1%BC%90%CF%80%CE%AF%CE%BA%CF%84%CE%B7%CF%84%CE%BF%CF%82&la=greek#lexicon

Pigliucci, M. (2017). *How to be a stoic*. Basic Books.

Pigliucci, M. (n.d.). Stoicism. *Internet encyclopedia of philosophy*. https://iep.utm.edu/stoicism/

Seneca, L. A. (1882). *On the happy life* (R. L'Estrange Trans). Independently Published. (Original work published in 58)

Seneca, L. A. (1910). *Minor dialogs together with the dialog "On Clemency"* (A. Stewart, Trans.). George Bell and Sons. (Original work published in 40)

VoxTalk. (2014). *George Carlin near miss*. YouTube. https://www.youtube.com/watch?v=zDKdvTecYAM

WisemanR. (n.d.). *LaughLab*. https://richardwiseman.wordpress.com/2018/04/17/laughlab/

Chapter 5
A Unit of Blood and a Pinch of Humor

Joshua Tovey
Independent Researcher, USA

"There is a thin line that separates laughter and pain, comedy and tragedy, humor and hurt."

- Erma Bombeck

Humor is a language. In the medical field it is spoken in a wide variety of "dialects" and is very often used for the same reasons, sympathy, empathy, and distraction. As a phlebotomist working at a blood bank, opportunities for using humor to my advantage were never in short supply. To help understand my thoughts, feelings, and actions, as well as set the stage for this case, first I shed some light on where I was in my medical career as a phlebotomist as well as a little about the blood donation process. Then, I provide a detailed case of my use of humor during an autologous blood donation with a scared but brave young donor and her parents.

To kick off my path in the medical field, I completed a nursing assistant certificate program and then immediately acquired certification as a phlebotomist. I very quickly started my first job at Medic Regional Blood Center, in Knoxville, Tennessee, where I began job-specific training that would only vaguely resemble what I had learned thus far. For instance, when someone goes to donate their blood at a blood bank, the first part of the donation process is a very personal and somewhat lengthy screening questionnaire. As the trained phlebotomist, nurse, or screening technician very clearly asks each question, a kind of basic health assessment is performed with their eyes and ears above and beyond the Q&A. Signs of anything potentially disqualifying, from a sinus infection, all the way to alcohol consumption, are extremely important and they must be identified and assessed to ensure safe blood supply. Sometimes a particular medication might be disqualifying, other times, what it was prescribed for might be the issue. We aim to uncover factors that would or could negatively impact a unit of blood or negatively react with anticoagulants.

DOI: 10.4018/978-1-7998-4528-7.ch005

The donor very rarely has any clear idea whether or not their blood is safe at the time of donation due to the vastness of disqualifying factors; hence, this laborious process. Even traveling to particular elevations in some parts of the world at certain times of year are factors that must be documented and then compared with the most recent data from the CDC in order for a judgment to be made by our medical director. This is because of parasites like plasmodium, which is responsible for malaria in humans. All of these "factors" are only portions of the initial screening process. I've touched on them mostly to describe how personal this process is and how interpersonal you really must be in order to get a donor from point A to point D as painlessly as possible. They are doing this for free – they've chosen to do it – so it becomes even more paramount that they feel comfortable and befriended, not bewildered, or worse.

After being screened, the donor will be moved into the donor room to a chair and will soon be approached by a nurse or phlebotomist. It is in this moment, as a phlebotomist, I begin to pay attention to and evaluate the emotional state of the donor after being screened. Some of our veteran donors have fun with us through the brief physical and screening process because they know everyone there and all the questions. New or newer donors have varying results but tend to have many similarities as well. As they lay there in a medical chair, their minds will begin to wander, and not typically very far from the room. The patients are thinking about all the people in white lab-coats, the big needle, losing 450mls of blood, and all for what!? For most patients this is when the stress will begin.

It is so important to talk to them, to mindfully use humor, or to ask them a question in order to rein in their attention and distract them from the inevitable. Nervous donors have elevated heart rates and will bleed quite fast, often resulting in a bad experience in some capacity for the donor. Humor very often seems to be the best possible solution in my experience. Conversation, unless done very well and with a bit of luck, is only an intermittent solution here as it doesn't always evoke the emotion required in order to redirect someone's attention. Of course, laughing releases endorphins like dopamine into your blood from the pituitary gland, which means you're using science, which I quite like!

After becoming proficient, or better, at my craft, the more seasoned staff began "allowing" me to perform some of the more important and often quite difficult sticks or venipunctures. These were patients sent over by their surgeons to have an autologous unit of blood (meaning they were giving blood to use for themselves) drawn for a large surgery usually only a few weeks away. A lot of these patients were older and receiving knee or hip replacement surgeries, while another large portion were children who are inching closer to a spinal fusion. It would be these patients that truly made me recognize what a tool humor was: attention spans a little shorter, a little more curiosity, and certainly more fear of whatever all this stuff is going on around them. The patient's emotions as well as the parents', who are usually standing directly behind the patient, seem to show a little more. It becomes a little easier to read the situation and improvise for a better result. After building on all of these observations and realizations, I had an experience that sealed the deal for me, targeting humor and interpersonal savvy as my newest skills to unearth, dust off, and master.

A fairly normal day had occurred for several hours until a 9 year old girl in a wheelchair, due for a spinal fusion in a few weeks, came rolling through our front entrance. Slouched almost unreasonably to the side of her wheelchair, tightly clung to a stuffed animal that looked to have been recently passed down by a young, very nervous Hercules (yes, the Demi-God – Otherwise, how did it appear so particularly "squeezed"?). All of this painted a picture for me. My first instinct was to try to get the parents to loosen up a little because they were giving off a bit of that "terror" vibe. You know the one, where you're waiting for your 9-year-old to have a spinal fusion, and only a couple weeks prior you're there to watch her lose roughly one eighth of her blood – on purpose, for medical reasons.

Displaying confidence is crucial here, but I find that humor can trump anything. Being fun or funny in these situations seemed to naturally convey confidence anyway. Being aware that the parents and the child feed off each other emotionally, it was important for me to occupy their minds in that moment. I remember scrubbing the girl's arm with a povidone-iodine scrub, which has a fun reddish/yellowish sort of color. I asked her, jokingly, "Do any of your friends have tattoos?" As she looked up at me silently questioning why or what I was really asking, I said, "This color on your arm is permanent. Something like a tattoo! I'm trying super hard to make it pretty but I'm just not much of an artist."

Instant shock! After a silent look to her parents, to confirm it was just a joke and not something permanent, she began to giggle briefly. Both parents' moods seemed to lift. They drew in closer around her and started talking more and even joking amongst each other – almost as if they had gotten comfortable. Needless to say, by this time, I've made quite a display with my "tattooing" all over this poor girl's arm for a little more than 30 seconds. For those that are concerned, I stayed well within my "aseptic-technique" guidelines to ensure an uneventful recovery from the stick I would be performing with a 16-gauge needle very shortly. Steering away from lengthy pauses was top priority here as they provide space for the inevitable stress to flood back into the light, for both parents and patient!

I began preparing the blood bag and kit which comes pre-assembled and hermetically sealed, equipped with that very large needle I referred to only a moment ago. As I was setting up, I placed the blood-bag on a scale for keeping weight, and she spoke to me on her own for the first time! She asked, "Is it going to hurt?" For some reason I answered very speedily and said, "YES! It hurts! But not for long. Has anyone ever pinched you?" To which she quickly answered with a fairly engaged, "Yes."

"Well," I said, "I'm gonna pinch ya!" "And when I do, I want you to continue to lay very still, ok"? She gave just enough of a nod of the head to let me know she understood. I grabbed a warmed blanket and placed it on her and had both parents hold it to block any view of the needle. I uncapped the needle and situated her arm just where I needed it.

Then, I pinched her, right on the shoulder! I used just enough pressure that it could be briefly construed as pain, and then very quickly advanced the needle. I taped the needle down with Dora the Explorer Band-Aids (to sweeten the deal) and had previously asked a nurse to deliver a cold orange juice right after the stick. The young patient nervously smiled and giggled just a little as one or perhaps two tears rolled down her face, and voila, success! As she sipped some of her orange juice she paused, turned to me, and said, "Hey! You pinched me!" I nodded my head to confirm that indeed, I kept my word and I really did pinch her. Her parents and I had a chuckle about my throwing in a pinch of humor into the equation. As waves of relief came over me, I could see that this "production" had gone well, and it was all smooth sailing from here. Both her mother and father thanked me and said they were relieved that they encountered someone who cared enough to transform the blood collection process for their little girl. They told me she was quite nervous leading up to this and she had already been through so much.

Funny, I had never thought of it as a "production" until now. As I reflect on the experience, I realize that a great deal of things had to take place to get this patient from A to D. I have a feeling now that doing all of this for her also helped me to remain confident so I could do my job well when I was faced with these circumstances. It would have been far too easy for me to think a little too much and conjure up just enough anxiety to affect my performance. Using humor to fulfill her needs seemed to suppress any trace of anxiety I might have experienced otherwise. In the end, humor came to all of our aid, helping the patient, the parents, and even myself to have a smoother experience.

Chapter 6
Response: "A Unit of Blood and a Pinch of Humor"

Allison Leigh Noyes
Loyola Marymount University, USA

REVIEW OF RELEVANT RESEARCH

Communication is the process through which the individual motivations for using humor can be linked to the social functions of humor. From a communication perspective, humor is a message sent by an individual with particular motivations, but that message is also interpreted by another individual or a group within a particular social context (Lynch, 2002). Both the other individual and the context play as important of a role in the humor exchange as the individual making the joke. One element of context that is particularly relevant to the interpretation of humor is the play cue. Cundall (2007) explained that "play is indicated through nonlinguistic cues that we naturally perceive" (p. 209). Play cues serve as a kind of "invitation for the hearer to come closer to my outlook or take on a situation" or "to share an understanding of the world" (Cundall, 2007, p. 208). A communication perspective that accounts for sender motivation, social context, and receiver interpretation can be valuable for understanding humorous exchanges between patients and caregivers. Empirical research on humor and communication provides additional insight into these exchanges that can help us to understand the use of humor in this case study.

Humor, Anxiety, and Distraction

Research has found that humor can lessen patients' pre-procedure anxiety in provider-patient health encounters and identified distraction as the mechanism through which humor has this effect. Berger et al. (2014) conducted a quasi-experimental study involving a "Wacky Wednesday" intervention that transformed the surgical admission experience using humorous staff attire as well as gifts and costumes for the pediatric patients and their parents. At admission, they found significantly lower anxiety scores among children in the Wacky Wednesday group than the control group; they also found that both children and parents in the intervention group had significantly less anxiety right before the surgical procedure

DOI: 10.4018/978-1-7998-4528-7.ch006

as well. A series of experiments done by Strick et al. (2009, 2010) concluded that distraction is the mechanism through which humor attenuates negative emotions and specifically distraction resulting from the cognitive demands required to process and resolve incongruity-based humor—rather than the positive emotion brought about by the humor.

Distraction may also be the mechanism through which humor enables patients to better cope with pain, especially because findings that look at humor as well as other distracting stimuli have sometimes found that humor is not the only distraction that improves patients' coping abilities. In an experimental study, Zillmann et al. (1993) found that while exposure to humorous content significantly increased participants' tolerance of physical discomfort, so too did content in the genre of tragedy. The researchers concluded that it was not necessarily the positive feeling evoked by the humorous content that produced the effect but rather the level of absorption in the content. In that study, the humorous content was delivered before the painful stimuli, so it did not test the extent to which humor can distract from pain when delivered simultaneously, but other research has examined this effect.

In one lab study, researchers had participants submerge their hand in very cold water while watching different types of engaging content—humorous, repulsive, or neutral (Weisenberg et al., 1995). Participants rated all content conditions as equally engaging, but participants in the neutral content group exhibited no increase in pain tolerance while participants in both the humorous and repulsive content groups demonstrated a significant increase in pain tolerance. Clearly humor did not uniquely distract participants from their pain as repulsion had the same effect, but the high level of engagement participants experienced in the content from the neutral condition also suggested that it may not be distraction alone that increased participants' pain tolerance. The researchers proposed the idea that it was actually a combination of distraction and emotional arousal, humorous or other, that increased pain tolerance.

More recent quasi-experimental field research has found that the usefulness of humor for coping with pain resulting from a medical intervention may depend largely on the patient's coping style. Findings from one study indicated that humor may prove more useful for coping with pain if patients have a direct problem-focused coping style and less useful if they have an avoidant emotion-focused coping style (Goodenough & Ford, 2005). There is also evidence that humor therapy can reduce perceptions of pain for patients dealing not just with acute pain but with chronic pain as well (Tse et al., 2010).

From a communication perspective, the use of incongruity-based humor to create a cognitively demanding distraction in provider-patient interactions can be understood through expectancy violations theory (EVT; Burgoon & Hale, 1988). This theory basically suggests that we typically have expectations for how others will behave in interpersonal encounters due to social norms. When people violate our expectations, we experience emotional arousal, which stimulates us to positively or negatively evaluate the violator and ultimately to accept and make sense of the violation by developing a rationale for it or to reject and be troubled by the violation. Some researchers have argued that the best way to define a humorous incongruity is as a benign violation "that threatens a person's . . . normative belief structure but that simultaneously seems okay" (Warren & McGraw, 2015, p. 1). This definition raises the question of how to go about violating someone's expectations in a way that threatens their normative belief structure while simultaneously seeming "okay" in order to elicit an interpretation of the violation as humorous instead of inappropriate.

One important factor in how an expectancy violation is interpreted is how the receiver feels about the violator. A study examining college instructors' inappropriate communication in the classroom found that if the instructor's other behaviors created an enjoyable classroom environment for students, this created a positive perception of the instructor that neutralized students' dissatisfaction with the inappropriate communication (Sidelinger, 2014). Another important factor is the context in which the violation takes place, which can be shaped to some degree by nonverbal play cues sent by the violator (Cundall, 2007). A final key factor in the interpretation of a violation as humorous is individual differences in the receiver's personality and emotion regulation (Papousek et al., 2014). In a health setting, clinicians may not have much influence over the last factor, but they do have some ability to shape how patients feel about them as well as the playfulness of the context in which their patient interactions take place. While the use of incongruity-based humor as a distraction from anxiety and pain is perhaps most relevant to this case study, humor also functions in some other important ways in this patient interaction as well.

Humor, Relationships, and Coping With Job Stress

Humor can also be used by clinicians to develop, maintain, and shape relationships with their patients. Clinicians in this situation might use humor to signal confidence, competence, or credibility. One study found a positive relationship between perceived physician humor orientation, which is one's predisposition to use humor in social situations, and perceived physician credibility as well as patient satisfaction (Wrench & Booth-Butterfield, 2003). In another study, findings indicated that humor of any kind signaled confidence; however, there was a distinction between appropriate and inappropriate humor in signaling competence (Bitterly et al., 2017). While appropriate humor signaled high confidence and high competence and had the effect of increasing the humorous person's status, inappropriate humor signaled high confidence and low competence, which decreased their status. Other research has also emphasized the importance of caution given the potential for humor to harm the patient provider relationship if used incorrectly or in the wrong situation (Chapple & Ziebland, 2004; Pinna et al., 2018).

In addition to the usefulness of humor for patients in a healthcare setting, there is evidence that humor may be useful for clinicians as well as they cope with job demands and stress, which is common in health organizations. In a study that looked at physician humor, patient satisfaction, and self-reported patient compliance, a relationship was found between physician humor and patient satisfaction and between patient satisfaction and patient compliance suggesting that there may be some indirect relationship between physician humor and patient compliance with medical advice (Wrench & Booth-Butterfield, 2003). Humor may help caregivers to cope with stress. Survey studies within the health context as well as in other organizational contexts have directly linked the variables of humor orientation, coping ability, and job satisfaction. Findings were similar for a group of employed college students as they were for nurses working in a health setting; higher humor orientation resulted in higher job satisfaction due at least in part to higher coping efficacy (Booth-Butterfield et al., 2007; Wanzer et al., 2005). Finally, an additional factor that may be relevant to clinicians' use of humor in managing the demands of their job is that of persistence. Experimental research has found evidence that humor can increase task-related persistence, especially in people who generally have a more humorous outlook on life (Cheng & Wang, 2015). Increased task-related persistence in the healthcare setting may alleviate job-related stress or even prevent it to some degree. Taken together, the research on humor demonstrates just how useful a comedic approach to provider-patient interactions can be for managing patient anxiety through distraction, developing and maintaining relationships with patients, and managing job stress.

Humor Use In The Case Study

The case study described a phlebotomist's use of humor in his job at a blood donation center. It included the general process of conducting a blood draw as well as a specific and somewhat complex situation that involved an encounter with a very sick pediatric patient and her parents. We learned that the blood draw process typically begins with a lengthy and very personal questionnaire to ensure that the blood is safe for donation. Although there is no clear use of humor in the case study in this part of the patient encounter, it is important to remember that at the end of the case, the author describes the whole process as a "production." If we think about the use of humor as a whole production that involves much more than just the actual instances where humor is deployed, then this screening process becomes important to the use of humor because it serves as the first opportunity to begin creating a playful or positive context that opens the possibility for using humor later as a distraction. It also serves as an opportunity to assess more than just the factors that could disqualify the donor's blood. The research on humor use suggests that while it can be highly effective in the health setting, it can also be risky. If the humor is perceived as hurtful or humiliating it can actually damage the patient-provider relationship (Chapple & Ziebland, 2004). Similarly, although the use of appropriate humor can increase the user's status by signaling confidence and competence, the use of inappropriate humor can decrease the user's status by signaling incompetence (Bitterly et al., 2017). The screening process offers an opportunity to assess the patient and the situation in advance—before the critical moment when humor might be most useful—while also enabling the screener to begin creating a context that feels playful or positive so that the later use of a humorous incongruity as a distraction has a better chance of being interpreted as humorous rather than inappropriate.

The next opportunity for assessment and perhaps even a "test run" for using some humor came once the patient had completed the questionnaire and moved to a chair in the donor room. The phlebotomist noted that this is the time when anxiety and stress will typically ramp up, especially for first time donors because they are just lying in the chair, anticipating the big needle and all the blood they are going to lose. The case author explains that this is the point when it is crucially important to mindfully use humor to distract the patient by turning her attention away from her nervous thoughts; if they begin the blood draw on a nervous patient with an elevated heart rate, she will bleed very fast resulting in a negative experience, so distraction is the key. Asking questions or engaging in conversation are other possible options for distraction, but the phlebotomist notes that these are inferior to humor because a distraction without the emotional element of humor or laughter may not redirect the patient's attention for very long. The research on humor and pain tolerance supports this conclusion finding that it may actually be a combination of distraction *and* emotional arousal that increases patients' tolerance of pain (Weisenberg et al., 1995).

The specific patient encounter described in the case was a particularly challenging one because it was a pediatric patient, just 9 years old, who was giving blood for herself to be used a few weeks later when she had spinal fusion surgery. These kinds of cases are apparently considered "difficult sticks" because they often involve patients with shorter attention spans and more curiosity and fear—as well as the added element of concerned parents. The case author recalls the initial encounter with the family as they came through the entrance; his wise assessment found the parents as well as the patient looking terrified. Recognizing the impact of the parents' fear on the child, he understood the need to engage them as well, not just the patient.

Once he had the family in the donor room, he took advantage of the opportunity for spontaneous, context-based humor that could serve multiple purposes during the blood draw preparations. He seemed to intuitively understand what we know is true from research—that humor could help him to build a relationship with mom and dad by displaying confidence and competence (Bitterly et al., 2017) while simultaneously distracting his young patient (Berger et al., 2014). This use of humor in the preparatory phase of the encounter also allowed him to do a "test run" under less risky circumstances than the needle stick itself to see how the family would react. His question about whether any of the patient's friends have tattoos came out of nowhere and caught the patient's attention. While he scrubbed the patient's arm with the tinted povidone-iodine solution, he told the patient very seriously that the color would be permanent like a tattoo, and this had exactly the intended effect of "instant shock."

The type of humor used here is very important; the phlebotomist did not simply tell a traditional joke but instead created a cognitively demanding incongruity in the existing situation that required the patient's mental resources to process thus effectively distracting her from her anxiety (Strick et al., 2009). He followed the shocking statement—that the color from the solution was permanent—with a self-deprecating one ("I'm trying super hard to make it pretty, but I'm just not much of an artist"), which reinforced the incongruity and then silently looked at mom and dad to confirm that he was joking. This silent look played an important role in the humor situation because it served as a nonlinguistic play cue. Cundall (2007) suggests that an incongruous message alone is not humorous unless it is interpreted as such, and a key factor in that interpretation is an appropriately playful context. In that simple silent look to mom and dad, the phlebotomist invited them, as well as the patient who clearly saw the look, to share his playful outlook on the situation. Upon seeing the silent look, the patient understood the humor and giggled causing a chain reaction in which the parents' moods improved, and their behavior toward their daughter changed; it became more playful as well.

Next came the main event—the actual needle stick. While the phlebotomist had already carefully assessed the situation to ensure his use of humor was appropriate and engaged in a successful "test run" that had helped him to build a relationship with the family while simultaneously distracting them from their anxiety, the next phase would require him to distract them from the patient's actual physical pain. The initial humor encounter developed his relationship with the patient enough that the patient felt comfortable asking if the needle was going to hurt. He responded truthfully that it would hurt briefly but then quickly stepped back into the world of play by asking if anyone had ever pinched her. When the patient responded that they had, he told her that he was also going to pinch her. This is a common comparison that phlebotomists use—that the needle may feel like a pinch. However, in this case, once the patient was ready with a blanket blocking her view of the needle, the phlebotomist actually pinched the patient on her shoulder just *before* he advanced the needle into her arm. The patient clearly felt the needle because a few tears slid down her face, but she was also so surprised that she smiled and giggled nervously as she processed another incongruity in the situation—that the clinician had *actually* pinched her! Perhaps she became so absorbed in the playful situation (Cundall, 2007; Zillmann et al., 1993) and so distracted and emotionally aroused by the surprise (Weisenberg et al., 1995) that she barely noticed the pain from the needle. The laughter shared by the phlebotomist and the parents and the gratitude they expressed to him was evidence that he had earned their trust in that brief time while also putting the patient at ease and successfully carrying out his job. Given all that their daughter had been through and how nervous she had been for the blood draw, mom and dad were so appreciative that the phlebotomist had "cared enough to transform the blood collection process for their little girl"—another indication that his use of humor had served as an invitation to leave the world of seriousness, anxiety, pain, and needles and to enter a world of silliness and play (Cundall, 2007).

At the end of the case study, the phlebotomist explains that humor served another important purpose in the situation—to reduce his own anxiety and give him the confidence necessary to do his work. He acknowledged the complexity of the situation with the emotions of the whole family impacting the experience and the success of the blood draw on the line. If he were to overthink the situation and get anxious, the patient and parents would likely sense his anxiety and become more anxious themselves making the job so much more challenging. Research has found that humor use by clinicians is linked to better mental health and emotional well-being and may be linked to better coping efficacy, which results in higher job satisfaction (Wanzer et al., 2005). In this case, humor clearly helped the phlebotomist to cope with job stress; it certainly makes sense that better mental health and emotional well-being would be linked to one's ability to cope with job stress and ultimately one's job satisfaction. Considering that a phlebotomist may encounter many similarly complex situations in a single day, the regular use of humor with different patients may also improve persistence—enabling him to perform the same challenging routine over and over again (Cheng & Wang, 2015).

Key Takeaways From The Case Study

This case study highlights one clinician's successful use of humor to accomplish multiple goals at once—including the primary goal of drawing blood from a very sick and very nervous pediatric patient with concerned parents. The encounter highlights some important lessons about using humor in interactions with patients. First, humor can be a useful tool for clinicians working with patients who are anxiously anticipating a difficult or painful procedure. Although the research findings are a bit mixed on the use of humor to help patients cope with anxiety and physical discomfort, there is enough evidence to indicate that the phlebotomist's successful use of humor in the case study was not a mere fluke. Experimental and quasi experimental humor interventions have resulted in less anxiety for patients and in the case of pediatric patients for their parents as well (Berger et al., 2014; Yovetich et al., 1990). Lab research has found that it is actually the distraction resulting from the cognitive demands of incongruency resolution—rather than the positive emotion—that lessens anxiety (Strick et al., 2010). While humor is not the only distraction that can increase patients' tolerance of pain, it can also be effectively used for this purpose (Tse et al., 2010; Weisenberg et al., 1995; Zillmann et al., 1993).

The case study really highlighted the use of situational incongruity to draw the patient's attention away from her anxiety and pain. The just-serious-enough talk of 9-year-olds having permanent tattoos resulted in a reaction of "pure shock" by the patient that may have jolted her out of her anxious thoughts, and the pinch to her shoulder right before the needle advanced again forced her to process the fact that this medical professional had *actually* pinched her at a moment when she might otherwise have been anticipating pain. The incongruities that the phlebotomist created in the situation were accompanied by play cues, like the silent look to mom and dad, that served as invitations to briefly enter this world of humor and play and forget about the needles and blood draws and upcoming surgeries (Cundall, 2007). Humor is one form of distraction that can really absorb patients' attention while also arousing their emotions. Of course, there are other forms of distraction that may accomplish these specific goals, but humor can serve a secondary purpose of helping the clinician to build a relationship with the patient. The phlebotomist noted the importance of displaying confidence in a situation like the one he faced in the case study with terrified parents and a seemingly overwhelmed pediatric patient. Research has found that humor, when used appropriately, can signal confidence as well as competence and credibility (Bitterly et al., 2017; Wrench & Booth-Butterfield, 2003). While humor may not be the only effective form of distraction from anxiety and pain, it has other relational benefits that allow it to serve many different purposes at once.

In addition to the clear usefulness of humor as a tool for clinicians in interacting with anxious patients, another lesson we can learn from the case as well as the research on humor is that it should be used only with great care. One important feature of the case study is the pediatric patient. While the patient's age made the case situation more complex in some ways because of the additional variable of the parents' anxiety and concern and the potential fragility of a sick child, it also created just the right context for the phlebotomist to use playful situational incongruities as a calming distraction. Some of the research on humor and distraction from anxiety has also focused on pediatric patients; the interventions that worked in this research (e.g., Wacky Wednesday dress up) would probably not work in the same way with adult patients (Berger et al., 2014). The type of humor used must appeal to the patient or it could be interpreted as inappropriate, which may then actually decrease the patient's perception of the clinician's competence and status and fail to create the intended distraction and positive effect. In one study of humor use in interactions with adult men who had testicular cancer, researchers found that while humor use could facilitate uncomfortable or difficult interactions, the patients were sometimes upset by jokes or were afraid that jokes would be embarrassing to them; the researchers recommended looking to the patient for a cue that humor use would be appropriate (Chapple & Ziebland, 2004).

The research on incongruities and expectancy violations provides suggestions for improving the likelihood that this type of humor will be interpreted as intended, and the case study reinforces these suggestions by framing the use of humor as a "production." Clinicians hoping to use humor as a distraction should think about the entire patient encounter as part of the "humor production." While actual instances of humorous incongruity may only be used in one or two specific moments to distract the patient, the entire interaction between the clinician and the patient could determine whether the clinician is able to successfully use humor as a distraction in those key moments. From the beginning of the patient encounter, clinicians should try to establish a positive relationship with the patient; this improves the chances that the patient will make sense of an expectancy violation as humorous rather than inappropriate. Second, clinicians should begin to assess the patient's emotional state and potential receptiveness to humor from the beginning of the encounter and use all interactions with the patient as an opportunity to begin creating a playful context. In this case, the phlebotomist assessed the patient's and her parents' level of anxiety when they first arrived and then eased into his use of humor prior to the actual blood draw as he disinfected the patient's skin. This gave him the opportunity to test whether his use of humor would be viewed as appropriate before there were needles involved. Finally, clinicians relying on humorous expectancy violations to distract patients should ensure that they are prepared to use nonverbal play cues—like a silent look, a wink, or a smile—to indicate the use of humor and help the patient to resolve the incongruity in a way that results in positive affect.

Certainly, some of the benefit from humor use comes from the fact that it simply makes the job easier by facilitating relational development with the patient or decreasing patient anxiety and increasing pain tolerance allowing clinicians to meet their instrumental goals. However, there may be additional benefits of humor use for a clinician's well-being that extend above and beyond the facilitation of instrumental goals, and this is what makes the use of humor so unique in encounters with anxious patients. While there are likely other ways to accomplish each individual goal that humor facilitates, humor may be uniquely suited to accomplish all of these goals simultaneously, which the phlebotomist illustrates in his case study, noting that "in the end, humor came to all of our aid, helping the patient, the parents, and even myself to have a smoother experience."

REFERENCES

Berger, J., Wilson, D., Potts, L., & Polivka, B. (2014). Wacky Wednesday: Use of distraction through humor to reduce preoperative anxiety in children and their parents. *Journal of Perianesthesia Nursing*, *29*(4), 285–291. doi:10.1016/j.jopan.2013.06.003 PMID:25062572

Bitterly, T. B., Brooks, A. W., & Schweitzer, M. E. (2017). Risky business: When humor increases and decreases status. *Journal of Personality and Social Psychology*, *112*(3), 431–455. doi:10.1037/pspi0000079 PMID:27831701

Booth-Butterfield, M., Booth-Butterfield, S., & Wanzer, M. (2007). Funny students cope better: Patterns of humor enactment and coping effectiveness. *Communication Quarterly*, *55*(3), 299–315. doi:10.1080/01463370701490232

Burgoon, J. K., & Hale, J. L. (1988). Nonverbal expectancy violations: Model elaboration and application to immediacy behaviors. *Communication Monographs*, *55*(1), 58–79. doi:10.1080/03637758809376158

Chapple, A., & Ziebland, S. (2004). The role of humor for men with testicular cancer. *Qualitative Health Research*, *14*(8), 1123–1139. doi:10.1177/1049732304267455 PMID:15359047

Cheng, D., & Wang, L. (2015). Examining the energizing effects of humor: The influence of humor on persistence behavior. *Journal of Business and Psychology*, *30*(4), 759–772. doi:10.100710869-014-9396-z

Cundall, M. K. Jr. (2007). Humor and the limits of incongruity. *Creativity Research Journal*, *19*(2–3), 203–211. doi:10.1080/10400410701397263

Goodenough, B., & Ford, J. (2005). Self-reported use of humor by hospitalized pre-adolescent children to cope with pain-related distress from a medical intervention. *Humor: International Journal of Humor Research*, *18*(3), 279–298. doi:10.1515/humr.2005.18.3.279

Lynch, O. H. (2002). Humorous communication: Finding a place for humor in communication research. *Communication Theory*, *12*(4), 423–445. doi:10.1111/j.1468-2885.2002.tb00277.x

Papousek, I., Schulter, G., Lackner, H. K., Samson, A., & Freudenthaler, H. H. (2014). Experimentally observed responses to humor are related to individual differences in emotion perception and regulation in everyday life. *Humor: International Journal of Humor Research*, *27*(2), 271–286. doi:10.1515/humor-2014-0018

Pinna, M. Á. C., Mahtani-Chugani, V., Sánchez Correas, M. Á., & Sanz Rubiales, A. (2018). The use of humor in palliative care: A systematic literature review. *The American Journal of Hospice & Palliative Care*, *35*(10), 1342–1354. doi:10.1177/1049909118764414 PMID:29587520

Sidelinger, R. J. (2014). Using relevant humor to moderate inappropriate conversations: Maintaining student communication satisfaction in the classroom. *Communication Research Reports*, *31*(3), 292–301. doi:10.1080/08824096.2014.924339

Strick, M., Holland, R. W., Van Baaren, R. B., & Van Knippenberg, A. D. (2009). Finding comfort in a joke: Consolatory effects of humor through cognitive distraction. *Emotion (Washington, D.C.), 9*(4), 574–578. doi:10.1037/a0015951 PMID:19653782

Strick, M., Holland, R. W., Van Baaren, R. B., & Van Knippenberg, A. D. (2010). The puzzle of joking: Disentangling the cognitive and affective components of humorous distraction. *European Journal of Social Psychology, 40*(1), 43–51. doi:10.1002/ejsp.720

Tse, M. M., Lo, A. P., Cheng, T. L., Chan, E. K., Chan, A. H., & Chung, H. S. (2010). Humor therapy: Relieving chronic pain and enhancing happiness for older adults. *Journal of Aging Research, 2010*, 1–9. Advance online publication. doi:10.4061/2010/343574 PMID:21151506

Wanzer, M., Booth-Butterfield, M., & Booth-Butterfield, S. (2005). "If we didn't use humor, we'd cry": Humorous coping communication in health care settings. *Journal of Health Communication, 10*(2), 105–125. doi:10.1080/10810730590915092 PMID:15804903

Warren, C., & McGraw, A. P. (2015). Differentiating what is humorous from what is not. *Journal of Personality and Social Psychology, 110*(3), 407–430. doi:10.1037/pspi0000041 PMID:26692355

Weisenberg, M., Tepper, I., & Schwarzwald, J. (1995). Humor as a cognitive technique for increasing pain tolerance. *Pain, 63*(2), 207–212. doi:10.1016/0304-3959(95)00046-U PMID:8628586

Wrench, J. S., & Booth-Butterfield, M. (2003). Increasing patient satisfaction and compliance: An examination of physician humor orientation, compliance-gaining strategies, and perceived credibility. *Communication Quarterly, 51*(4), 482–503. doi:10.1080/01463370309370169

Yovetich, N. A., Dale, J. A., & Hudak, M. A. (1990). Benefits of humor in reduction of threat-induced anxiety. *Psychological Reports, 66*(1), 51–58. doi:10.2466/pr0.1990.66.1.51 PMID:2326429

Zillmann, D., Rockwell, S., Schweitzer, K., & Sundar, S. S. (1993). Does humor facilitate coping with physical discomfort? *Motivation and Emotion, 17*(1), 1–21. doi:10.1007/BF00995204

Chapter 7
A Trip to the "Filling" Station

Kenneth T. Rocker
Massey University, New Zealand

For many people, going to the dentist can be traumatizing. However, from a dentist's point of view the experience can be very "refilling." This is one of the various dry jokes my dental surgeon likes to use frequently when greeting his customers. After a warm welcome, you enter the "filling station," which is just the office in which he operates. After a preliminary round of x-rays, he will look at the results and explain that dentists can solve problems well because it is easy to get to the "root" of the problem. As a kid, I had many visits where he would discover new cavities because of my love for sweets. He would always say, "I'm not sure if you golf, but you sure do have a hole in one today." Whenever I needed a tooth removed, he would joke that his wife wanted to take him out for lunch that day but he "already had a tooth to take out," referring to my tooth. General jokes that he uses after every visit include, "you only have to brush the teeth you want to keep," and "You brush your teeth at night to keep them. You brush your teeth in the morning to keep your friends happy."

I have never found my dentist to be funny; mixing dental practices with comedy usually turns out to be an awkward exchange for me. I am sympathetic to my dentist and his staff because I understand that to run a successful business, dealing with people of different personalities, it is important from both an ethical and business standpoint to cater to their needs to create a satisfying experience. Clearly, my dentist believes that humor is the gateway between himself and the client, so perhaps there are lots of patients who do appreciate his jokes. I am curious how he would even know whether they thought the jokes funny or not.

For me, the never-ending murmur while he operates with my mouth pried wide open has always made me wonder how he could actually expect anyone to respond to his humor at all. I am almost certain that the patients' responses do not influence his decisions to keep using the same type of humor. The humor itself is an element of his personality and what you expect to receive if you primarily use him for your dental needs. My whole life he has insisted on using the same jokes during every visit. It would not be a visit to Dr. XXX's office if you did not hear a dental joke you have heard before. It is inevitable that instead of leaving the room to look at my X-rays, he will insist on leaving to review my "Tooth-Pic's."

DOI: 10.4018/978-1-7998-4528-7.ch007

If I did not think it was funny the first time, the probability was low that I would find it funny the 20th time. Yet, I have grown to appreciate him for trying to make me laugh in the first place.

Because I can feel the effort behind the humor is for my benefit, I have grown to overlook his lack of good jokes by accepting him for who he is. As a result, I find myself using the same type of cues that I use when other people I like tell me dry or non-humorous jokes. I do not directly tell people their jokes are bad, I just respond as if the humor was neither good nor bad by staying quiet, acting as though I missed what was said, or at most giving a small "fake" smile. Of course, this is aided by the fact that my dentist's jokes are typically delivered when I cannot speak anyway. Even if I wanted to respond verbally, it would be in my best interest to keep my mouth steady to avoid any social mistakes during the visit. Telling somebody they are not funny could in some cases be interpreted as a sign of disrespect. The last thing I want to do is develop a bad rapport with someone I trust to operate on my body.

There have been times though when I especially did not care to hear any jokes during my appointment simply because I was having a bad day. It is on those days that I notice that even the dental assistants and other staff are also unamused by his jokes. I would often see his colleagues use body language that led me to believe the people he worked with felt the same way about his jokes as I did. I could sense the faintness in their laughs and lack of enthusiasm in their smiles when they attended to his orders. Most of the staff have been there for as long as I can remember. I am sure they probably also get tired of hearing repetitive jokes in the office on a daily basis. There are times when they try to seem amused, but for the most part they casually carry on their duties without acknowledging the jokes at all.

My family has always believed in retaining the same healthcare professionals over a lifetime. We believe in supporting businesses that not only cater to the quality of work we expect, but also those who make the effort to treat us like we matter to them as a family. So, although Dr. XXX's bad jokes are not enough of a detriment to make me consider an out-of-network dentist, it certainly makes the appointments more arduous, even if I do consider him to be "family." His jokes simultaneously manage to make me feel as though he cares because he is trying to build a rapport and lessen my anxiety, but also as though he is oblivious because he never pays attention to anyone's response, or lack thereof, to his jokes.

Building loyalty between a well-executed service and the client is something I personally believe to be the foundation of a good business. Although my dentist unintentionally annoys me, I believe that his humor has truly benefited him in the long run by creating an environment where individuals like myself can be comfortable knowing what to expect. Also, by using humor in the first place, he creates a warm environment where patients at least know he is trying to be kind to them. I can certainly remember appreciating his jokes more as a child. So, although the humor is not beneficial to me and I wish he would notice my days when the bad jokes are not improving my mood, I think that overall the humor is probably beneficial for the majority of his patients who also feel his efforts to comfort us through humor.

Chapter 8
Response: "A Trip to the *Filling* Station"

Steven Gimbel
Gettysburg College, USA

HEALTHCARE, SELF-CARE, PERSONHOOD, LANGUAGE, AND HUMOR

Healthcare is a peculiar line of work in that it is both work and care. Work is where you sell your labor to someone else to acquire money for yourself. Care is where you give of yourself for the wellbeing of someone else. Feminist writers have long noted the contrast between these two types of human relationships. Healthcare is a peculiar sort of relationship that involves both and also requires a delicate balancing act between work and care. Patients pay for the care they receive, but that does not make them customers in the normal sense. The healthcare relationship is one that clearly requires the healthcare provider to consider the best interest of the patient; but, as with all relationships, that concern needs to go both ways. Healthcare providers have to remain cognizant of the need to maintain their own humanity while giving to others.

Since the relationship involves work there are some relevant ideas from Marx (1844) that will help to clarify some of the issues that arise in any work setting. Marx argues that workers in a capitalist society become alienated in four ways:

1. Workers lose their identity to their career, (e.g., someone who paints is painter).
2. Workers become alienated from the products of their labor (e.g., while a painter may be able to hold their own painting, a laborer cannot touch their labor).
3. People become viewed as "human resources" rather than individuals.
4. People become alienated from their "species being" (Marx, 1844, p. 75), their ability to construct their own identity.

The first three sorts of alienation mentioned combine to rob us of our ability to be who we want to be. Since that is the essential property of being human, we are robbed of our humanity. This alienation

DOI: 10.4018/978-1-7998-4528-7.ch008

creates situations where workers can become divorced from their work and lead to unhealthy work conditions (Marx, 1844).

When it comes to human relationships, Gilligan (1982) argues that there are two very different sorts of structures for human relationships: contractual and care-based. A contractual relation is one in which each party enters the relationship out of self-interest. The relationship is based on an agreement and when each acts, he frees himself from the relationship. When you fulfill your part of the contract, you are no longer bound by the contract. On the other hand, a care-based relationship is based on concern not for oneself, but for the other in the relationship. When you act in such a relationship, you do not extricate yourself from the relationship, but embed yourself deeper within it. A medical care relationship is thus one where these areas of care and contract overlap. While there is clearly a contractual aspect, any good medical care provider is engaged in a care relationship that doesn't end when the bill is paid.

Further developing aspects of care, Noddings (1984) constructs an ethic based on this notion of care. Care is offered by the one-caring and received by the one-cared-for. An act is genuine caring if it is completed for the benefit of the other. An act is good if it is an act of genuine caring designed to strengthen the relationship in which it occurs. In addition to having moral obligations to those other people you care about, Noddings (1984) argues that you also have a care-based relationship with yourself. You create an achievable ideal self, and you owe it to yourself to do what you can to achieve it. While you must care for others, you must always care for yourself.

While the above ideas are important to understand the particulars of this case, there is research into language use that is also important to present. We not only need these social and ethical tools, but a couple that relate to humor and language more generally.

Raskin (1985) differentiates between two types of speech acts. Some utterances are bona-fide communication. These are sentences that are intended to convey information. "Your pants are on fire!" is meant to tell you something that is likely to be relevant to you. Other utterances are non-bona-fide communication, these are not meant to convey information. If I tell you, "So, a priest, a rabbi, and Michael Cundall walk into a bar," I do not want to construe this as a claim about the world. Not all speech is meant to be informative.

This is an idea that was further developed by Austin (1962), who extends the view that language is a tool. We do things with words. We promise. We bet. We marry. We don't just use words to express things, we actually use words to do things. In understanding what we are doing when we are speaking, Austin distinguishes between three aspects of an utterance. You commit a "locutionary act" when you say something to be understood. If I were to say the sentence to you, "The barn door is open," then I have engaged in a locutionary act. If I simply cleared my throat, I would have uttered something non-locutionary. With the utterance, I will have committed an "illocutionary act" if I was trying to do something with the locution. The same locutionary act might have a whole range of illocutionary acts associated with it. The uttered sentence "The barn door is open" might be uttered in order to answer the question, "Is the barn door open?" or it might be a warning that the bull is about to escape, or it might be a description expressed cryptically to alert you that the fly on your pants is open without proclaiming the embarrassing fact, so everyone knows it. In all three cases, the same locution was spoken, but in each case, it was intended to do a completely different thing: answer, warn, and describe. The speech act is "perlocutionary" if there was a goal it was designed to achieve. In the first case, the perlocutionary force is getting you the answer to your question. In the second case, it was to keep you from being gored by the bull. And in the third case, it was to spare you the humiliation of accepting your "physician of the year" award with your trophy exposed and getting gored by a bull of a different sort.

This understanding of language use and function was later extended by Grice (1975). He points out that conversation is a cooperative endeavor. If you have ever tried to talk to someone who had no interest in talking to you, you know that the conversation doesn't take off, doesn't flow, doesn't evolve normally. There are, Grice (1975) argued, rules that are followed by people who do choose to engage in conversation together. Conversation is a rule-based activity. Grice (1975) formulated four "conversational maxims" which he contended form the framework for conversational activity. The Maxim of Quantity implores you to "Make your contribution as informative as is required (for the current purposes of the exchange)." According to the Maxim of Quality one ought to, "Try to make your contribution one that is true." By the Maxim of Relation, we must "Be relevant." And finally, the Maxim of Manner demands that you "Be perspicuous." To be a responsible conversant, one should follow the rules because they will allow the conversation to be maximally successful and efficient.

Usually, we follow those rules in conversation. But sometimes we don't. Violating a conversational maxim is what Grice (1975) terms an "infelicity." When you find your co-conversant to have been infelicitous, you could think one of two things about the faux pas. On the one hand, you might think that your partner was careless and lost track of themselves in the passion of the discourse, or perhaps is of lesser breeding and simply was not properly schooled in conversational etiquette, but either way it was an innocent mistake and should be overlooked. But on the other hand, you might think that your conversational partner is fully in control of their conversational faculties which you know to be as well-honed as your own. In this case, the infelicity must have been intentional. Why would such a thoughtful, cooperative individual intentionally commit such an error? Surely, it is a signal alerting me to something that ought not be said aloud.

Perhaps you were discussing the details of the personal affairs of a colleague that border on the scandalous. Suddenly, your conversational partner ends a sentence in the middle and begins discussing the weather. This is a clear violation of the Maxim of Relation. The new utterance is in no way germane to whether his wife knows about the aforementioned expenditures. Taking your co-conversant to be a strict adherent of the Principle of Conversational Cooperation, you quickly infer what he must have been signaling: the colleague is approaching and will overhear us and that must be quickly addressed. So, you follow the turn and continue to engage about the weather. This sort of inference from a violated maxim is what Grice (1975) terms a "conversational implicature." When someone says something that seems like a violation of the rules of conversation, we make a logical move to what they really meant to say without saying it.

Finally, we will have to consider some work specifically in the philosophy of humor. Gimbel (2017) may not be the smartest philosopher writing about humor today, but he is widely regarded as the best looking – at least he was in 2017. Gimbel (2017) argues against the obvious, seemingly common-sense view that the purpose of a joke is to be funny. He argues that while the most common purpose of joke telling is to generate comic amusement in your audience, jokes may, in fact, be used for an incredibly wide range of purposes. You can make a joke to draw attention to yourself. You can tell a joke to excuse yourself from the attention drawn to you. You can tell a joke to ingratiate yourself with someone. You can tell a joke to insult someone. There are so many reasons we tell jokes that have nothing to do with comic amusement. I am a dad. I love to tell dad jokes to embarrass my teenagers in front of their friends. The dad jokes I use are not funny…that's the point. But they are jokes. Jokes have all sorts of perlocutionary functions, getting laughs may be the most common, but it is far from the only one.

Healthcare Providers Are People, Too

The reciprocity of the health-care relationship given current societal conditions is obscured in two ways. One is the capitalist exchange model of healthcare. But the other comes from the fact that there is a hierarchical difference between the members of the relationship. In the case of doctors or dentists and patients, there is often a difference in education and class wherein the patient, on the one hand, has the power of being the customer, but less power from social status. In the case of nurses' assistants or dental hygienists, often both hierarchical indicators favor the patient. This unevenness, whichever way it points, creates a barrier to seeing the relationship between the patient and the provider.

Given the above there are a variety of issues that become apparent in this case. There's the fact that the healthcare relationship has aspects of both a contractual relationship and a care relationship. That includes the self-care aspect of any relationship. There is also the fact that we can and often do use language to do a variety of communicative tasks. In fact, jokes are a way to play with language to do a variety of things, cause amusement in others, yourself, or make your children feel embarrassment.

As with all the cases in this anthology, there is a care element present. The dentist owes to his patient a certain level of care. But the dentist also owes himself a level of self-care. Perhaps the dentist isn't using the humor to amuse the patient, but rather does so because he enjoys telling the jokes no matter how shopworn they may be. As a result, any patient would do well to remember that healthcare providers are people who are working hard for the patient's well-being and needs, in any small way they can, to reciprocate. Maybe that means something as simple as letting the dentist have his cheesy little jokes as he takes good care of your mouth.

As this is a case study and we don't know exactly the intentions of the dentist, there might be ways in which these jokes are coded bona-fide communication. Let's assume that there is a difference between normal conversation and humorous conversation. Grice (1975) is correct that both are cooperative endeavors governed by rules, but their difference will require different rules. Instead of the usual Maxim of Quantity, we would have the Maxim of Humorous Quantity, which might be something like "Make your jokes only as long as they need to be." Extended shaggy dog stories, for example, would not be a good idea when someone has a 50-minute appointment (it would be fine to make passing puns, but to use up the majority of the patient's time for your own amusement is rude). The Maxim of Quality would be replaced with The Maxim of Humorous Quality that would demand that you "Try to make your contribution one that is funny." The Maxim of Humorous Relation, would have you "Only make jokes about something relevant to the situation." Don't tell random jokes. If you are going to joke around, it should be about what is at issue. And finally, the Maxim of Humorous Manner demands that you "Only make jokes that are fitting with the dignity of your professional position." Even routine medical treatment is a big deal to those to whom it is being done. It might be thoroughly routine to the practitioner, but not so to the patient who wants to make sure you are fully present and taking their situation seriously. These rules are good to follow in most professional humorous engagements.

When a medical professional breaks a rule, just as in the Gricean (1975) type case, the patient must make a decision. Our dentist is clearly violating the Maxim of Humorous Quality. He is telling jokes that he has to know are not terribly funny. And even if they were, he knows that the patient has heard them many, many times and therefore, any amusement will wear off after a while.

So, the question is whether the doctor is making a mistake in violation of the principle of humorous cooperation or whether it is an intentional error designed to send a signal. If it is intentional, what is the humorous implicature that one ought to make from it? What is the signal the dentist, in this case, is trying to send? Might Gimbel (2017) be right that jokes have lots of different possible purposes and maybe the purpose here is something other than generating amusement on the part of the patient?

To unpack the meaning behind the jokes, let us start with the form of the joke. All of the examples contained in the narrative of the case study are pun-based. Who enjoys puns? People who are fascinated by words. Those drawn to words are likely big readers. People who read a lot are generally well-educated. So, one implicature that the dentist is leading his patient to draw with his barrage of dental puns is that the doctor is a well-educated person. Yes, the diploma on the wall conveys that, too, as does the white coat and having to call him by the honorific "doctor," but the implicature from the joke can be unpacked in such a fashion that it gives the nervous patient who is worried about pain reassurance that he is in the hands of someone smart and thereby competent.

Further, they are not random jokes. These are all jokes relevant to the professional context. They are bad jokes, yes, but they are bad dental jokes. The constant flow of them signals that the dentist has been collecting them over a long period of time. To have this many bad dental jokes means that he has been committed to dentistry for a long time. Experience and commitment are correlated with competence. So, again, we have an implicature that should lead the patient to have a standard fear obviated to some degree.

Finally, that the dentist feels comfortable joking tells the patient that the routine exam is not viewed by the dentist as a matter of the utmost gravity. If something were terribly wrong, the jokes would stop. The constancy reassures the patient that while this may be the most exciting element of your day, it is nothing that a professional is overly concerned about. This is routine. It will get taken care of. You will be fine.

Now we consider that the purpose of a joke is not always to be funny, but rather sometimes to self-sooth the joke teller (Gimble, 2017), we consider what that could mean for this case. Consider for a moment the possibility that the jokes told by this dentist are not told at all for the sake of the patient, but rather the dentist himself. In this capitalist culture where human services are treated as commodities (Marx, 1844), people are burnt out, left feeling dehumanized. They are exhausted. Sometimes they need to engage in behaviors to invigorate themselves. If this dentist tells these jokes to meet his own psychological needs, allowing him to provide his best healthcare, then the jokes are quite possibly a necessity.

One sees one's dentist every six months for a cleaning and a check-up. The dentist knows your mouth, your problems, and, frankly, your breath. He works as quickly and painlessly as possible having you rinse as often as he can without slowing down the process so you are in the chair as little as possible while still getting the highest quality care he can give. Doesn't the patient then have some obligation to the dentist other than having his insurance company cover the bill? Is there not a reciprocal obligation in a care-based relationship of the sort we see in Noddings (1984)? Care is a richer relationship than a commodity-based relationship. We get to know our healthcare providers, especially providers like a dentist. For all of the work the dentist puts into caring for his patients, he may need them to allow his little jokes to give their own form of care back. The question most critical to this point is: How are the patients to know that their doctor needs this form of care from patients to continue providing optimal healthcare?

Self-Care and The Awareness

Humor in healthcare usually focuses on the patient. Can humor be used to ease stress, to communicate more effectively, or to connect more deeply? Absolutely. But, as Gimbel (2017) shows, humor is used for a wide range of purposes. It is a Swiss Army knife that can accomplish many ends. One of which concerns the healthcare provider and not the patient. To avoid the sort of alienation that Marx (1844) outlines and to practice a Noddings (1984) style self-care, you need to make your workplace joyful.

Humor is one effective way of doing that. Jokes can lift your spirits, not only the patients, and get you through days of facing people who would rather be anywhere else.

You have a relationship with your patients. You need to think of them as people who need your help. They are not machines on an assembly line. They are human beings and to be good at your job, you need to think of them as such.

But when you do so, you are establishing a care-based relationship. That sort of relationship is reciprocal. You are caring for them, and so they owe you care as well. This reciprocity will not be symmetric. As with a parent and a child, one side can care for the other in ways the other could never care for the first. But such asymmetry does not mean that there is not some level of care-based obligation that is present. As a healthcare worker, you are not just a worker; you are also a person, a person who is a part of this relationship. And as such, you deserve a level of care and respect from the patients as well.

This can be expressed through the humor in the sort of extension of Grice (1975) that we sketch. Again, as Gimbel (2017) points out, humor is incredibly useful for a wide range of uses. The risk, however, is that when you communicate indirectly in the way that Grice (1975) discusses, you cannot be guaranteed that the listener will draw the implicature you intended. You may set out the dots and the listener may connect them in a direction completely different from your intention.

What seems to exist now in this case is a patient who may be unaware of the objective of the humor. Would the patient change his perception if the doctor had indicated that his use of the same old jokes is a way he deals with the stress of his job? It makes him enjoy his day and thus be a better dentist. The answer seems to be yes. But as humor and language can be used to accomplish a variety of reasons and uses, a medical care provider should realize that some may not take their humor as such. The negative feelings could have been avoided if the dentist had advertised that he tends to use this sort of humor, over and over again, because he enjoys it. If it bothers the patient, let him know, but understand that this is a coping mechanism for him. It's an act of both patient and self-care if the dentist were to make this known. Since communication can, even in the best of situations, get muddled and we as patients and caregivers want our providers and patients, this extra step in the communication chain could have avoided the situation exemplified in this case.

This does not mean that humor is inappropriate, but there is always a risk of being misunderstood and since humor tends to violate normal practice in order to work, there is more opportunity for an interpretation to go awry. For the medical professional, be careful. But, also, be funny. For any would-be patient, and anyone reading has likely been a recipient of medical care and treatment, remember that the relationship is more, thankfully so, than a commodity being sold.

REFERENCES

Austin, J. L. (1962). *How to do things with words*. Oxford University Press.

Gilligan, C. (1982). *In a different voice: psychological theory and women's development*. Harvard.

Gimbel, S. (2017). *Isn't that clever: A philosophy of humor and comedy*. Routledge. doi:10.4324/9781315112633

Grice, H. P. (1975). Logic and conversation. In P. Cole & J. Morgan (Eds.), Syntax and semantics (Vol. 3, pp. 41–58). Academic Press.

Marx, K. (1844). *Economic and philosophical manuscripts of 1844*. Prometheus.

Noddings, N. (1984). *Caring: A feminine approach to ethics and moral obligation*. University of California Press.

Chapter 9
Humor in Family Therapy

Isaac Evans
Tennessee Technological University, USA

In-home family therapy can be one of the most unpredictable ways to do therapy. In fact, sometimes it's hard to consider it therapeutic at all. At times I am an iconoclast, there to dismantle their every way of life. These are times when I am the villain and the family just wants me out of their lives. Then at other times I am the public eye, allowed into their home to see how great they are and to see the beautiful masks they have adorned. After I leave, those masks come off, and they return to the chaos that is normal for them. Humor is often absent when I am the villain and when I am the public eye. The families hide their use of humor which is another way to make themselves look "right" to outsiders.

But sometimes I have a family who doesn't dare to change at all. They allow authenticity to reign supreme. They hide nothing and they put on no masks. It is in these homes that humor isn't used as a tool intentionally, but rather humor is laid out in the open like an unavoidable bomb to the therapeutic process. Calling it a bomb is intentional because it can truly shake up a session in ways that are difficult to predict. Some would view it as damaging the session, counselor client relationship, and possibly the entire treatment plan. However, unforeseen humor, like anything that makes human beings human, can be used by the therapist to create a space where there might not be one. Let me give you a real-life example.

There was one family in particular that took on this viewpoint of "hide nothing, we aren't going to stop being us just because you are here." I am placed in the home due to a teenager acquiring an aggravated assault charge and his brother acquiring an assault charge himself. The home is being run by a single mom since the father ended his own life over a decade ago. There's not much humor to be found in a story like that, but like most life situations, humor is going to find its way to wiggle and worm its way in, whether it is welcome in or not.

One of my first sessions with the family takes place at the dinner table like it's a family meeting. One of the first tasks is to sweep the home and see if there are any weapons or any safety hazards. Lots of times the family is hesitant to allow a stranger to walk into all their bedrooms, likening it to a S.W.A.T. officer busting in and relinquishing them of all their rights. But not this family. These two brothers were more than happy to show off their ninja stars, nunchucks, knife collection, samurai swords, spears, and shuriken: 40-50 dangerous weapons in the hands of two kids with a history of physical aggression. I

DOI: 10.4018/978-1-7998-4528-7.ch009

couldn't help but laugh. It took me so off guard. Never have I seen so many weapons in a safety sweep. The mother was starting to get embarrassed toward the end of the session. However, as the therapist, I replaced the flat uncomfortable facial expressions that naturally come with invading someone's home, with a smile that came from a genuine place of amusement of just how many weapons were in the home. It's serious business and the mother gets that, locking up the weapons that are scattered in the home, but allowing myself to laugh and smile at the amusement of the situation lets the mother know I am human. The mother did not say anything at the time that would indicate appreciation: How could she, considering how she stressed probably was at the time? But I had confidence that using natural humor would pay off in the long run when it comes to building much needed rapport with a stressed-out mother.

A few sessions after this is when I met the dog. A little side note about dogs and family therapy: dogs don't tend to follow the usual rules of society when it comes to a guest or stranger entering your home. I sit at the dining room table, a typical workstation for therapy and self-reflection when it comes to in home therapy, and the mother is checking in with me after what was a worse than normal day for her and the family. This is when the dog declares that this period of emotional divulgence is a swell time to let his primal urges get the best of him. Or to put it in the words of the mother, "Oh no! Don't hump the therapist's leg!" After something like that, I feel as though humor is the only option and so I laughed. The mother was embarrassed for something her furry little friend did. There was very little she could have done to predict or prevent it from happening, but she still wanted to take ownership of it. This is actually a concept that makes us human but often causes guilt and shame. Just like how she takes complete ownership of her two boys acquiring assault charges when she is but one part in a massive system. Nevertheless, my laughter gave her permission to laugh instead of being embarrassed. Challenging a belief that she had to be in or was in control of everything (the boys, the enthusiastic dog, etc.) needed to be challenged.

As time went on, these moments built up. In the program I work it is normal to have 60 plus sessions with a family. Little moments of humor mending feelings of embarrassment add up until they start to paint a larger picture. In a session much later in treatment, the older brother starts to tell a story about a time during the week where he was attempting to help his younger brother with a homework assignment. The mother was there to help verify the story. As he went on, he explained that in the middle of trying to help his brother he had to pee, so he stepped outside and peed off the porch, onto the bushes. Mother steps in and laughed, allowing the older brother to simply be himself. Notice what was missing this time? The mother never apologized, showed disgust on her face, or stated she was embarrassed. The mother had shown with her actions that she was comfortable with her son's humanity in front of someone who ultimately was still somewhat of a stranger. This moment was like the therapist was not even present, showing a level of comfort that can be hard to find in therapy. A moment slipping away like this without emotional confrontation through embarrassment was difficult for her two months before. She embraced the unpredictability of human nature, specifically the human nature of her two boys whom she loves dearly. Humor came into sessions, welcome or not, and my choosing to welcome it rather than shun it has paid off, allowing me to use the moment as evidence to prove to the mother, that the barriers preventing her from connecting with her son in front of other people can be broken down over time and in a way that is slow, gradual, and not at all confrontational.

There are an ocean of stories that could be told just like this one. Where little moments of humor find their ways into counseling sessions. This family was able to use those moments to their advantage. Sure, I was there to help these kids get off of probation, avoid future fights, and treat the anxiety and emotional issues that caused them to resort to physical aggression as a coping mechanism. However, I was also there to help this family, which was shattered to pieces by bad choices, unforeseen stressors, and a flawed system, become a normal family again, a family that could dive into instances of humor and swallow them up with open arms. It is incredibly hard to be human again after your humanity is taken from you. However, humor in the counseling process can be that way to get that humanity back in a way that leaves the family feeling an unconditional positive regard, which is the essence of client centered therapy.

Chapter 10
Response: "Humor in Family Therapy"

Nicholas T. Iannarino
University of Michigan, Dearborn, USA

LITERATURE REVIEW

Surprise Liberation Theory

In her book on playful conversations between patients and providers across seven different healthcare settings, du Pre (1998) argued that humor can function as a signal that things are "not so bad" for those involved. She defined humor according to her surprise liberation theory (SLT): When something is interpreted as funny, it's because we've encountered a surprising deviation from our expectations, and because we've perceived that deviation as pleasurable and liberating. Du Pre also specified that we possess fluid upper and lower boundaries that define our willingness to see our expectations for different situations and phenomena subverted. If a surprise goes beyond those thresholds and violates an assumption that we cherish (e.g., our loved ones' safety) or are indifferent to (e.g., being asked for the time by a stranger on the bus), we would consider the surprise too threatening or too trivial to be considered humorous. However, especially when we're committed to an expectation that something is menacing or restricting, an unexpected event can provide us with a sense of profound relief (du Pre, 2018). But what would bring a doctor or a patient to include humor in a "serious" setting like a hospital room or medical office, and what effect could it have on the rest of their conversation?

Relational Perspective of Communication

Du Pre (1998) argued that medical routines, especially those that are tense and formal, can actually lend themselves *more* to the use of humor than other less threatening situations. Because even the smallest surprise in cold, distant, sterile, and regimented medical settings can seem unexpected and comical, both patients and healthcare providers can experience humor as a temporary reprieve from their anxiety, and

DOI: 10.4018/978-1-7998-4528-7.ch010

its use can help redirect their conversation going forward (Schöpf et al., 2016). This phenomenon can be explained by the relational perspective of communication (Bateson, 1972), which views communication as a transactional, collaborative process in which both sender and receiver influence and interpret the meaning of a message together.

For example, a message receiver can send feedback that helps determine the ways in which a sender's initial statement is ultimately interpreted. Du Pre (1998, pp. 95-96) described a humorous exchange that she observed in a breast care center before a patient received a mammogram, which takes x-ray images of a patient's breast tissue while two flat x-ray decks compress the patient's breast. As the technician explains to the patient that the machine has "automatic compression" that will prevent it from crushing her breast, the patient delivers an ambiguous statement ("I don't know that that's such a good idea!") that could be interpreted as "I'm actually nervous" or "I'm just joking around." When the technician chooses to laugh along with the patient rather than seriously explain why that wouldn't happen, she communicates to the patient that her fear was unreasonable, and the patient laughs off as a joke her initial statement.

When both the patient and the technician treat a potentially serious message as funny following the technician's feedback, we see that communication is a collaborative process in which meanings are mutually managed, and that humor can be a persuasive guide to interpretation. In fact, du Pre (1998) noted that following the introduction of humor in healthcare exchanges, patients and providers tend to appear more relaxed and casual with one another. The rest of their conversations are often filled with more eye contact, smiles, personal stories, and humor attempts than before. Thus, she argued that humor can help us change the "sense" of a distressful, threatening, embarrassing, impersonal, "uncommonly weird and emotionally charged" (p. 153) situation in a radically different way.

Normative Rhetorical Theory

Du Pre (1998) concluded her book by arguing that the patients and providers she observed seemed to prefer counterparts who were funny. She even proposed that humor could potentially enhance patients' and providers' satisfaction with one another. But what makes some humorous messages in medical encounters more "successful" than others? Normative rhetorical theory (NRT) focuses on *what* communicators say and *how* they say it within a particular context. It is a theoretical framework that explains why some messages are perceived as more "effective" than others (Goldsmith, 2019). NRT shares the assumption that communicators often pursue multiple goals in their conversations (Clark & Delia, 1979), and that sometimes these goals can threaten or interfere with one another to create complex *dilemmas* that require communication *strategies* to manage.

For example, physical therapists might have to communicate to patients that they need to "hurt" them with certain procedures to help them heal from an injury (i.e., achieving particular tasks; instrumental goals). However, having this conversation can unintentionally challenge the therapist's preferred identity as a "caring, helpful" provider and the patient's preferred identity as a "brave, cooperative" patient (i.e., managing identities; identity goals). Pursuing this task can also cause the patient's and therapist's preferred relationship as "close allies pursuing a common goal" (i.e., negotiating relationships; relational goals) to be marked with complaints and criticisms as one partner unilaterally inflicts pain upon the other. For these conversations to be "successful," the therapist and patient need to develop strategies to solve the dilemmas that occur as a result of their conflicting goals. While du Pre's (1998) book was written before the original NRT scholarship was published (Goldsmith, 2004), some of the examples of humor use that she observed across physical therapy units seem to function as helpful management strategies to the dilemmas explored above. For example, du Pre described how patients' winking exclamations that their therapy is "torture" and that their therapist is "the devil" allowed them to complain about their therapy in ways that helped them maintain their identity as a "brave, cooperative" patient. Therapists' ability to joke back while also picking up on the underlying "truth" of their patient's humorous statements enabled them to reduce the intensity of the therapy when appropriate. This allowed therapists to validate, rather than threaten, their own identity as a "caring, helpful provider," reinforce the patient's identity in return, and bolster their relationship as "close allies" while continuing to help the patient achieve the task of healing.

Communicating Dignity and Compassion Through Humor

By helping transform a stiff and unpleasant episode into something more relaxing, familiar, and playful, joking around can serve many broad functions in healthcare interactions. Two of these functions include (a) reducing threatening emotions to maintain one another's dignity, and (b) minimizing social distance by showing compassion (Francis et al., 1999). Both functions can lead to more open, collaborative communication between patients and providers (du Pre, 1998), which can improve patient satisfaction, adherence, and health outcomes (Ha & Longnecker, 2010).

First, patients and providers use humor to create a non-threatening environment that can help manage the awkwardness and discomfort of medical examinations and procedures. In other words, both patients and providers can work together to recharacterize a potentially serious situation as being unserious. For example, patients might use humor as a socially acceptable way to express fear or complain about a painful procedure, or to downplay the threats to their dignity during an examination that requires them to be nude. Providers "play along" to help protect the patient's individuality and preferred identity as a brave and dignified patient. Joking in return can also help providers perform painful or embarrassing procedures without threatening their identity as a "helpful" caregiver and becoming an enemy to the patient. Humor that communicates dignity functions as if to say, "This situation is normal. You're doing well, and it's not so bad anyway" (du Pre, 1998).

Second, patients and providers use humor to gain a sense of intimacy and familiarity with one another. Providers might start joking around to show compassion to patients who seem intimidated by the power differences and stiff formality that can sometimes be part of healthcare interactions. When their providers don't do this, patients might use humor to encourage their providers to work to identify with them, give them more personalized attention, and be less distant. Humor that communicates compassion functions as if to say, "I like you. Open up to me" (du Pre, 1998).

In sum, humor is defined by surprise liberation theory (SLT) as an unexpected and pleasurable liberation from our preconceived notions. According to a relational perspective of communication, humor use in healthcare settings is collaborative, and it can be a persuasive signal that things are actually not what they seem. Normative rhetorical theory (NRT) is a framework that can be used to explain why humor might be an effective way to manage the instrumental/task, identity, and relational goals that are common in healthcare interactions. Finally, humor is often used by patients and providers to maintain one another's dignity and show compassion.

APPLICATION TO THE CASE STUDY

What's So Funny About Nunchucks, Dog Humping, and Taking A Leak Anyway?

The narrator selected three examples from "an ocean of stories" to describe the ways in which small moments of "unforeseen humor" can make their way into family in-home counseling sessions. To understand how each of these instances of humor function within the narrative, and to help explain how they could have affected some of the outcomes described below, we can apply SLT and its components (i.e., encountering a surprising deviation that falls within one's fluid thresholds and experiencing a pleasurable liberation from one's expectations).

The narrator sets the scene by describing the family's difficult situation as being decidedly unfunny. I can see where the narrator is coming from: after all, I haven't seen many CBS sitcoms about single-parent households who, in the wake of the father's suicide 10 years earlier, have two kids who are each facing assault charges. The setting itself—with an uninvited stranger swooping in to observe the daily lives of a "troubled" family—also likely compounded the therapist's and mother's expectations that these meetings would be marked by stress and unpredictability, formality and detachment, power imbalances and unspoken judgments. The narrator says, ironically, that it's "hard to consider [in-home family therapy] therapeutic." However, we know from du Pre (1998) that—in much the same way a breast exam can be embarrassing, intimate, and frightening for those involved— difficult situations like these can sometimes prime interactants for the richest humor.

During one of his first sessions with the family, the therapist likens himself to a S.W.A.T. officer (and, by extension, the family to potentially-dangerous suspects with limited rights) as he scours their bedrooms in search of contraband. I can imagine that it's not a good feeling to believe you're a major source of stress and intimidation for others. I can also imagine that the emotional nakedness of revealing the most intimate details of your life with a decidedly non-intimate acquaintance wouldn't be pleasant either. Certainly these things were true for both the mother and the therapist as they began this meeting, if the therapist's natural tendency to employ a "flat uncomfortable facial expression" whenever he had to "[invade] someone's home" was any indication.

Imagine the profound relief, though, when the therapist did not encounter clients who viewed him as a threatening intruder there to judge, lecture, and correct their ways of life, or as a naïve sap who could be fooled with the "beautiful masks they have adorned" just for him. With their seemingly "authentic" inability to be intimidated or falsely charming, the siblings' prideful brandishing of exotic weapon after exotic weapon took the therapist "so off guard," not simply because it was rare for him to see nunchucks and throwing stars on his day job, but because he for once wasn't viewed as a villainous outsider. It also probably helped that he finally encountered a family who wasn't as concerned with making "themselves look 'right'" to him. It was a weight off his shoulders.

However, the mother was not ready to see humor in the situation. Perhaps the stimulus was not surprising to her (i.e., she knew that her sons possessed the weapons and would not be ashamed of them in front of the therapist). More likely, the mother's mounting shock as the therapist counted the 40-50 unlocked sharp objects possessed by the boys with a history of aggression transcended her upper threshold for humor because she felt such a great responsibility for the situation—even though the therapist's laugh challenged that expectation. It remains unclear whether the boys' actions that day were an intentional bid for humor, a way of soliciting feedback from or testing the waters with the therapist, or (as the therapist believes) an unintentional byproduct of their choice not to "stop being us just because you are here." But by matching his clients' authenticity and not stifling his natural tendency to laugh when his expectations were violated, the therapist interpreted the boys' reactions as humor all the same.

The second instance of humor, in which the family dog decides that the therapist's leg needed some TLC, violated "the usual rules of society when it comes to a guest or stranger entering your home." The emotional intensity of the conversation about the mother's "worse than normal day for her and the family" certainly helped prime the situation further and make the unexpected deviation more profoundly relieving. Again, the therapist believed his decision to embrace the humor of the situation further softened the mother's fluid thresholds. Yet, he felt the mother was still committed to her expectation that she "had to be or was in control of everything."

However, the mother not only laughed at, but participated in, the third described instance of humor, in which the boys recounted a story that the therapist likely found additionally liberating for its unabashed talk of open urination. It's clear that by this instance the mother had consciously switched her perspective from viewing the situation as threatening (which required displaying apologetic looks of disgust for the therapist to see) to viewing it as funny. The presence of *this* surprise could have increased the boys' liberation from their expectation that their mom was ashamed of them in front of strangers and supported the therapist's hope that he was no longer really a stranger to this family. In sum, across all three instances, humor dispelled the strict categorization the mother held about aloof authority figures and the therapist held about "inauthentic" clients who were threatened by him, which led to a pleasurable liberation from the confines of their expectations.

How Relational Communication Turned A Tense Situation into a Lighthearted One

Du Pre (1998) argued that medical communication can be inflexible when interactants mutually accept the expectation that patients are supposed to acquiesce to the providers' dominance, and that everyone involved agrees to follow the typical routines and agendas of these interactions. However, if the clients and therapists participating in these transactions realize that their own communication choices define the tensions present in their relationship in the first place, they also can understand that together they have the power to break free and change these dynamics. It's not clear whether the two boys *intended* to be funny to cope with the embarrassment of having a stranger enter their home to potentially judge them, or whether they did it to purposely "break the ice" and campaign for a less somber relational climate. But their brazen lack of shame and deference in proudly showcasing their weapons revealed to the therapist that they weren't playing by the traditional power structure rules that usually accompany this game. The boys' lightheartedness seemed to serve as a persuasive bid for the therapist to treat this problematic situation (after all, those were *a lot* of weapons) as less threatening and somber than it could've been.

In turn, the therapist actively chose to make sense of this situation by interpreting the boys' reactions as being genuinely, absurdly funny rather than threatening or scary. It's likely the therapist knew it was appropriate (and preferable) not to squelch his natural tendency to laugh in this instance because the boys had already shown that they were not wearing masks and were not on their best behavior, which gave the therapist permission to match their authenticity with his own. Thus, the therapist likely fed off the boys' communicative energy and converged (rather than diverged) with their naturalism.

Because humor is "an observable, rational means of organizing and interpreting a healthcare experience" (du Pre, 1998, p. 146), the therapist's *laughter* (and not his *own* attempt at humor) was enough to kickstart the mother's cumulative sense-making process. Maybe the therapist making a joke of his own would've been too much too soon and caused the mother to think the therapist was mocking the family or not taking his job seriously. At any rate, it's clear that the therapist's subtle acknowledgement of the boys' humanity was not only *not* offensive to the mother, but actually persuasive enough to begin having an effect on her. The more the kids and the therapist maintained a lighthearted atmosphere, the less the mother interpreted the interactions as threatening and institutional, which further marginalized her feelings of tension and embarrassment. In this case, humor's cumulative effect on the mother shows how transactional and collaborative communication can build a more relaxed and egalitarian relational climate.

How Humor Helped Manage Conflicting Goals and Communicated Compassion and Dignity

The narrator acknowledged that in-home therapy might not be the most therapeutic setting for achieving instrumental goals. While the therapist was faced with the task of helping these kids "get off of probation and avoid future fights," he and the family also had to find a way to manage the threats and barriers that accompanied the pursuit of this task. The example described in this case was rife with the potential for threatened identities. Depending on how messages were sent, an interloping and threatening (or gullible) therapist could have been positioned against a pair of unmannered delinquents and a hapless mother. Unproductive and unbalanced relationships could have also been formed from this experience. For example, a paternalistic therapist who "knows best" could have been matched with a passive family whom he believed needed to be taught how to behave in society. The mother also could have remained ashamed and controlling of her kids. And the troublemaking boys could have had to cope with their mother continuing to treat them differently in the judgmental therapist's presence. Yet, the narrator described a situation in which all four interactants used humor as a communication strategy to endorse one another's identities and build their relationships, enabling everyone to lower their guard to allow for the completion of the task (i.e., to discuss and treat the boys' anxiety and emotional issues).

First, by choosing to respond to the absurd number of exotic weapons, the random dog groping, and the story about open-air urination in a playful manner, the therapist communicated to the family that he didn't identify them as being monstrous or horrifying. Instead, the provider's ability to be flexible and to show genuine amusement in the face of unpredictability signals that he knows his clients are human rather than stock delinquents who he needs to "fix" before he can move on to another "messed up family." Perhaps most importantly, the therapist's laughter allows the stressed-out mother to maintain her valued identity as "loving caretaker" instead of feeling like she's a "negligent failure." By avoiding the "flat uncomfortable facial expressions" common in family home therapy sessions, the therapist side-steps the potential to seriously challenge or deny the preferred identities of the children and the mom. Additionally, the therapist's acknowledgement of the humorous situations allows him to manage his identity as a provider who tries not to inflict outside judgment and paternalistic control ("therapist knows best!") over what's best for the family.

Second, the therapist's laughter not only reduced tension, but it also began the process of changing the family's perception of their relationship with him. For starters, subtly acknowledging the absurd number and exotic breadth of unlocked weapons strategically aligned the therapist with the nervous mother in communicating that he understood the situation is serious, but that it's something they can address together (Schöpf et al., 2016). Laughter allowed the mother to recognize that the therapist was on the family's side, and unifying the communicators as cohorts (instead of adversaries) enabled them to recognize and pursue a common goal together (Meyer, 2000). While humor was used to build a mutual relationship and create a more relaxed atmosphere, it also helped prevent damage to the relationship by continually "mending feelings of embarrassment." Evolving from strangers to co-agents and avoiding threats to one another's identities helped the interactants reduce power imbalances and avoid creating animosity in the relationship, which "paint[ed] a larger picture" of trust and empathy over time. All of these factors were instrumental in facilitating the collaborative and serious talk necessary to complete the task while finding greater satisfaction in their relationships (Phillips et al., 2018).

Finally, the therapist's acknowledgement of humor was a message of compassion that helped the family re-discover its dignity and humanize what could have been an impersonal transaction. The narrator said, "It is incredibly hard to be human again after your humanity is taken from you." Affording a small laugh at several crucial moments in their relationship allowed the therapist to communicate an understanding that the family "may be overwhelmed by the situation in which they find themselves, and may need help coping with it" (du Pre, 1998, p. 140). The therapist's laughter compassionately let the mother off the hook, which allowed her to reduce her embarrassment, drop her need to control the situation, recognize that "she is but one part in a massive system," and fully embrace the opportunity that therapy afforded her to connect with her sons as humans. Additionally, the therapist's laughter was a sign of his own dignity as well. It communicated to the family that he was human too, and that he had the ability to laugh at their "rule-breaking" behavior. This helped the family feel increasingly comfortable and accepted in his presence, which lessened the threat of talking to him about serious matters. As a show of dignity and compassion, humor helped the therapist and the family more openly broach difficult topics and maintain solidarity in their therapeutic relationship, and it enabled the family to repair years of self- and other-inflicted degradation.

PRACTICAL APPLICATIONS

First, when participating in therapeutic or evaluative interactions—particularly if you're the one "invading" someone's home turf—don't be a black hole for humor. When something strikes you as funny, treat it as such! Across her years-long investigation into clinical humor, du Pre (1998) did not observe an interaction in which a patient or provider seemed upset or anxious by the introduction of humor. In all three instances of potentially unintentional humor described above, the therapist couldn't think of a more preferable response than to match his clients' authenticity and truthfully acknowledge that his expectations were subverted. After all, the practitioner is a person, and the family he was treating are people, and it's clear that the practitioner views the free expression of authentic reactions as a sign that a person is accepting of their own and others' humanity. Du Pre (1998) argued that it's easy for those familiar with a particular therapeutic setting to know when people are joking around. Even if the boys' initial lightheartedness was not an intentional bid for humor, the therapist likely interpreted from their smiles, posture, and the outlandishness of their comments related to the weapons that displaying his human reaction would be a risk that wouldn't be interpreted negatively (du Pre, 1998).

Conversely, in situations where patients attempt humor with a practitioner to build a relationship or to create a more relaxed environment, the patient could take the practitioner's refusal to laugh or to add a humorous comment as a sign that the provider is aloof, socially awkward, and doesn't care for the patient's attempt to be seen as a person (du Pre, 1998). Like the therapist in this case study, practitioners should work to increase their humor "strike zone" and minimize the SLT boundaries beyond which patients' attempts at humor would be considered bland or threatening. If providers are able to ward off their cynicism or resist offense, they would be better able to develop a healthier appreciation for their patients' diverse humor styles. After all, patients can't fully assert their autonomy and individuality unless healthcare providers are collaborative and embrace their attempts to do so in return, particularly by shedding their own traditionally stoic and stern demeanor. The unpredictable "bombs" detonated by the boys in this case study would certainly present a challenge for a less communicatively flexible therapist. At any rate, if humor really is "going to find its way to wiggle and worm its way in, whether it is welcome in or not," the benefits of humor in patient-provider communication (e.g., building rapport, minimizing embarrassment) suggest that it might as well be welcome. Different things may be funny to different people, but having an opportunity to explain one's laughter is still a chance to display one's humanity and build a more personal relationship.

Providers should also remember, however, that humor can be used by patients to soften, or to make more socially palatable, the disclosure of serious or emotional messages. While humor was likely acknowledged by the two boys and the therapist to open up discussion of the family's difficulties, research has shown that those in distress also use humor to mask (or subtly allude to) the chaos in their lives. Because humor is not always a sign that a message is meant to be interpreted less seriously, providers should be careful not to overlook the potentially important emotional meanings hiding beneath the surface of their patients' seeming humor attempts (Schöpf et al., 2016). While providers' responses to patients can also be humorous, they should not forget to address the issues at the root of their patients' bids for assistance.

When practitioners initiate humor with clients, they should remember that spontaneity is their friend. Conversely, relying on canned, contrived jokes that are less relevant to the client or situation at hand can elicit more groans than laughs. Imagine visiting a primary care clinic with a terrible stomach flu, only to hear the doctor immediately ask, "Did you know that diarrhea is hereditary? Yeah, it runs in your genes!" The most pleasant response the doctor could hope for would probably be a massive eye roll. Instead, providers can use SLT to avoid simply "telling a joke" and instead introduce humorous statements and actions that are spontaneous, situational, and more closely tailored to the client. Patients who are expecting to be seen by a traditionally stoic provider who adheres to a rigid medical routine might be particularly primed to experience profound relief when their provider initiates humor and avoids using the same greetings, asking the same questions, and making the same statements as always. For example, du Pre (1998) recommends that providers attempt to subvert patients' preconceived notions by telling funny stories about relevant life episodes, engaging in relevant playful banter or verbal play like humorous puns, using exaggerated playacting and feigned emotions, and improvising other absurdities and comical expressions. Even in interactions where the provider feels like "the public eye" and humor is otherwise absent, remaining flexible and looking for opportunities to interject situational humor that plays with expectations and addresses their various patients' specific situations can be extremely liberating.

Finally, practitioners should remember not to exceed patients' upper SLT thresholds or threaten their valued identities and relationships when using or acknowledging humor. This might require practitioners to adjust the tone and timing of their humor attempts to adapt for different patients, situations, and contexts. In the humorous interactions described in this case study, it's clear the therapist was laughing *with*, and not *at*, the family. Practitioners should similarly treat their clients with caution and respect, and avoid making comments or allowing laughter that could demean, mock, and degrade them. If patients show an unwillingness to use humor, providers should tread carefully. For example, if the mother had displayed negative body language when the therapist responded to the boys or the dog with laughter, he might acknowledge that the mother interpreted his reaction as threatening to her valued identities and relationships (even though it was not intended) and he should consider refraining from reacting similarly in the future. Humor should also not be used in situations where messages could be confusing or easily misinterpreted (e.g., in crisis situations, other instances of extreme emotion, and in intercultural transactions). But when push comes to shove, providers would do well to remember that humor should be used to protect and bolster valued identities and relationships, and it should never impede the instrumental goals of a medical interaction.

REFERENCES

Bateson, G. (1972). *Steps to an ecology of mind.* Ballantine.

Clark, R. A., & Delia, J. G. (1979). TOPOI and rhetorical competence. *The Quarterly Journal of Speech, 65*(2), 187–206. doi:10.1080/00335637909383470

du Pre, A. (1998). *Humor and the healing arts: A multimethod analysis of humor use in health care.* Lawrence Erlbaum Associates.

Francis, L., Monahan, K., & Berger, C. (1999). A laughing matter? The uses of humor in medical interactions. *Motivation and Emotion, 23*(2), 155–174. doi:10.1023/A:1021381129517

Goldsmith, D. J. (2004). *Communicating social support.* Cambridge University Press. doi:10.1017/CBO9780511606984

Goldsmith, D. J. (2019). Normative rhetorical theory. In S. Wilson & S. Smith (Eds.), *Reflections on interpersonal communication research* (pp. 211–230). Sage.

Ha, J. F., & Longnecker, N. (2010). Doctor-patient communication: A review. *The Ochsner Journal, 10*(1), 38–43. PMID:21603354

Meyer, J. C. (2000). Humor as a double-edged sword: Four functions of humor in communication. *Communication Theory, 10*(3), 310–331. doi:10.1111/j.1468-2885.2000.tb00194.x

Phillips, K. A., Ospina, N. S., Rodriguez-Gutierrez, R., Castaneda-Guarderas, A., Gionfriddo, M. R., Branda, M., & Montori, V. (2018). Humor during clinical practice: Analysis of recorded clinical encounters. *Journal of the American Board of Family Medicine, 31*(2), 270–278. doi:10.3122/jabfm.2018.02.170313 PMID:29535244

Schöpf, A. C., Martin, G. S., & Keating, M. A. (2016). Humor as a communication strategy in provider-patient communication in a chronic care setting. *Qualitative Health Research, 27*(3), 1–17. 10.1177%2F1049732315620773 PMID:26717942

Chapter 11
Outside the Inside Humor:
Mixed Messages for Medical Spouses

Susan M. Wieczorek
University of Pittsburgh at Johnstown, USA

During my 40 years of marriage to a family practice physician, friends and family frequently insisted that my position as a "doctor's wife" afforded me unique advantages. If one considers my ability to get a quicker appointment with a specialist friend or the opportunity to discuss my personal medical issues over an evening out with multiple physicians at a pharmaceutical dinner, perhaps this is true. For the most part, however, I found myself categorized in a way I did not see myself. Many assumed I was a nurse, worked in my husband's office, understood medical jargon, and knew the day-to-day jokes behind the scenes. Some of this is true: I manage his office, but from home; I overhear a lot of medical jargon, but never studied it; and I witnessed a few medical quips over drinks out, but not as many as I have when seeking my own personal medical care.

My first medical appointment as a married woman was with my husband's family practice residency director. In my brief visits he was polite, instructive, and quite serious. Soon, however, I began my health journey with my first obstetrics appointment. My pregnancy seemed to go as planned until my contractions started prematurely on a Saturday evening during grocery shopping at 5:00 pm and continued through morning. My husband, quite familiar with delivering babies, noted that I probably just had back pain since the cramping was not across my stomach like I learned in Lamaze classes. He was exhausted from a 48-hour stint on call and moonlighting in the Emergency Room. Groggily he gave me a long medical explanation about the position of the baby against my back and the likelihood of this all just being Braxton Hicks. He mumbled, "Take a few Tylenol and go back to bed." I decided to wait it out. By morning, despite my pains being consistently two minutes apart, we walked a few blocks to church to see if they would stop. When we returned, I was no better and insisted I needed an internal exam. He called his attending, my OB/GYN doctor, saying that he was bringing me in. As we drove to the hospital, the pains completely stopped making me question whether I really was in labor. This upset me, because I did not want to embarrass my husband in front of his teacher for not knowing this was just an early scare. Upon entering the hospital room, the doctor looked at me, smiled broadly,

DOI: 10.4018/978-1-7998-4528-7.ch011

and said, "She's not in labor! Look at that big smile of hers!" He started joking with my husband about how good I looked and teasing him that he should have just examined me and "saved himself the trip." Being my first baby and not knowing what to expect, I felt foolish. After the examination, however, I surprised everyone when he found I was eight centimeters dilated and approaching delivery. Although I felt somewhat validated, my husband and the doctor continued to banter back and forth about how they got fooled. I lie there, feeling dismissed and objectified.

Two babies later, we moved to a small rural community where my husband began working as a board-certified physician. Again pregnant, I selected another family doctor for my first prenatal visit. Before he even examined me, he chatted a bit asking how we liked the new area and remarking about how he must be careful about me since I am a doctor's wife. "I've been fooled a few times by them. If anything is going to go wrong, it will go wrong with the doctor's wife." He then alluded to my husband's partner's wife who had many unexpected things go wrong during her labor and delivery. I felt very uncomfortable with him discussing her private case and poking fun at doctor's wives in general. I vowed not to return for a second visit despite his being the only "baby doctor" in the small town. Fortunately, my husband took another job in a different area; so, I no longer felt obliged to see him again and to become further proof of his hypothesis.

Several years and moves later, we returned to our rural hometown and started a solo private practice. Happy to be back with my family and old friends, we enjoyed being a part of a community of physicians who seemed to be respectful towards us both. We had three more children, his business started taking off, we built a new home, and I regained my self-esteem teaching full time at the local university. All was well until I fell down a flight of stairs, breaking my ankle in three places and requiring a metal plate and five screws to stabilize my leg. Although I thought this was a permanent fix, additional complications arose, forcing me to seek a secondary opinion at the city university hospital two hours away. Not accustomed to a teaching facility, I was surprised when the doctor barged into my room with a group of five other medical students and residents. Without even introducing himself, he turned to them and said, "Now here is an interesting case...... However, I must warn you, that this patient is also a physician's wife, and for some reason they tend to face all sorts of unexpected complications. Beware of Murphy's Law when it comes to them!" He chuckled, turning my way as if he thought I would confirm his assertion. I looked back at the blank faces of his students who did not join in his amusement. I was mortified. Yet again, I felt like the brunt of a joke. Only this time, I facilitated "student learning."

It perplexed me as to why physicians openly and unapologetically teased me so much, as if my husband and I frequently laughed about this piece of common knowledge. In fact, I never once heard him speak of this. Perhaps they thought they could tease me because I was "one of them." I do not know why this happened so many times; but I do know it made me very uncomfortable every single time.

Finally, as I approached menopause, I began to have some rather serious gynecological issues requiring me to make numerous visits with yet another physician. At first, he seemed quite congenial, often talking about my husband being a "good guy" and asking about how he handled various patient issues concerning those who talked too much or who never paid their bills. I figured he was trying to make small talk by identifying with me; but over time I kept noticing the twinkle in his eye and wondered if his poking fun at my responses was more amusing to him than to me. I decided that perhaps I was overreacting. "Sometimes, when you are sick you can take things the wrong way," I told myself. Soon, my condition worsened, causing me to require a total hysterectomy. On surgery day, my husband got tied up at the hospital and was not able to be at my side throughout the procedure. Keeping a strong front,

I joked that he was always late, brushing off his absence as "typical." When I returned to the recovery room, my gynecologist greeted me with an enthusiastic smile and told me there were no complications.

"Except," he said, "you sure were mean when you got out of anesthesia!"

"Really? Why do you say that?" I asked.

"Oh, you were just terrible!" he said. "It was embarrassing. You were really cussing me out. I've never seen anything like it."

I took a long pause gazing into his eyes, trying to determine if he was joking with me or not. I argued that it was totally out of character for me to ever do such a thing. Grinning, he assured me that I really was "terrible." I yet again was mortified. Here was a physician who took me into the operating room without my husband at my side, removed my female organs while I was asleep, and then accused me of embarrassing him when I could remember nothing. Was he making light of my condition when I myself was already feeling alone and vulnerable? "Surely," I convinced myself, "he had to be joking!" His eye twinkled just as it had during my earlier office visits; however, this time, he accused me of something that I did outside of my memory that was apparently quite funny to him—but not to me.

To this day I will never know if my gynecologist was telling the truth. Maybe he was just teasing me like the others did about my status as a doctor's spouse. Maybe the intent was to help me feel included in the hidden world of medical humor. In each of these examples, I never once felt as if the physician was purposely trying to insult me. In every instance I reacted with a smile on my face as if I shared in the amusement, despite how uncomfortable and embarrassed I really was. All too often I felt as if I were being laughed *at* rather than laughed *with*. Are doctor's wives really a unique challenge or just an available object of inside jokes? Perhaps as I navigate the healthcare system in the future, I will be treated differently; or perhaps the pattern will continue. One thing for sure I remain perplexed by my experience and hope to find answers in the years to come.

Chapter 12
Response: "Outside the Inside Humor: Mixed Messages for Medical Spouses"

Eugenio Zaldivar
Santa Fe College, USA

INTRODUCTION

In this case, it is clear that the author feels that she has been treated badly by quite a few doctors throughout her life. At first read, the locus of her concern is perhaps a bit less clear. After all, many of her concerns seem to center around uses of humor in which she was not the butt of the joke. Indeed, she was included in the inner circle, treated as a confidant, by her doctors. From the perspective of someone accustomed to being in the inner circle, it may not be immediately obvious why the attempts at humor failed. After all, isn't humor meant to be a good way to help patients relax? Isn't it a good way to bond with patients and to make them more comfortable? As Berger (2004) notes "humor offers modes of intimate communication through which these objectives can be achieved. Physicians' use of quiet, respectful humor may provide patients with the "social license" to enter personal or sensitive content areas" (p. 827). If humor, or joking, is an effective tool in establishing channels of communication, then how or why did it go wrong here? The answer, in brief, is that not all humor is created equal.

Before going any further, we should acknowledge a few things. First, in this case the only form of humor that is on offer is joking, but humor is not limited to jokes. Usually, when we refer to humor broadly, as in the quotation above, the point can be taken to apply to jokes. However, if we refer specifically to jokes or joking the point may not apply to humor more broadly. This is so even if the jokes are meant to be humorous. Care should be taken lest we generalize in haste. Second, not all jokes are humorous, nor are all jokes intended to be humorous. Finally, much of what we will consider here—the purpose of joking, the orientation of care, the consideration of content—will be generally applicable to other forms of communication and, mutadis mutandis, should not be restricted to joking and humor.

DOI: 10.4018/978-1-7998-4528-7.ch012

Ethics

Medical practice, as any with any other human endeavor, has an obligation to minimize harm (Maccarone, 2010). To do this, medical professionals have not just a duty to do what is medically best for their patients, they must be also aware of their patients' needs and dispositions. The latter requirement is especially important, if medical professionals are to use humor effectively. Contemporary ethicists generally work with one of four ethical frameworks: utilitarianism, deontology, virtue ethics and ethics of care. In this case we will rely on deontology and ethics of care, so it would be useful to briefly consider them in some detail.

Deontology is perhaps the most compatible with important medical principles such as beneficence, non-maleficence and respect of patient autonomy. So, we can use it to form a strong theoretical backbone for our analysis of the case study. Following that we shall consider how Held's (2006) ethic of care can then help us to flesh out our understanding of the central issues (grounding the often obtusely abstract nature of deontology) to help us better understand how to evaluate and guide our actions in situations like the ones described in the essay. When combined these concepts will offer a grounded, guiding framework which can be fruitfully deployed to improve quality of care. In the final section we will turn to a critical examination of the humor in the example case and consider how to avoid similar errors in practice.

Deontic ethics considers the fulfillment of duties as that defining characteristic of ethical behaviors (Borchert, 1999). So, if an action, or more specifically the intention motivating the action, accords with our obligations toward others then it the action is good. In healthcare the outcomes are very often probabilistic. We simply cannot predict exactly how well a treatment plan will work. So, the intentions of the medical professional are often the only thing we can get a good account of. This, if nothing else, would be a good reason deploy deontic reasoning in cases involving doctor-patient interactions.

Care ethics are primarily concerned with practical issues of real-world relationships and the incorporation of non-rational dimensions of decision-making (Borchert, 1999). Because of its focus on individual circumstances and the actual effects of our decisions (instead of blind devotion to abstract principles) care ethics make a very good corrective to some of the short comings or traditional ethical frameworks.

Kant's (1996) ethical system is perhaps the most well known and most often deployed deontic system. The heart of his framework is the categorical imperative. This is a command that is meant to be the preeminent instruction in his framework. In his works it takes several forms, but in this analysis, we will focus on formulation that centers humans as ends: act so that "you use humanity, whether in your own person or in the person of any other, always at the same time as an end, never merely as a means" (1996, p. 38). In other words, briefly, it is our duty to promote the best interests of others. We must never see other persons as merely instruments for achieving our goals, instead everything we do ought to be in the service of helping others (and ourselves) achieve what is best for them. You might think of this as a very strong version of the virtue of beneficence. The intuitive appeal of this mindset is fairly clear; if, when we are dealing with others, we always act to promote their best interests we will almost certainly make their life better. Of course, we must be careful not to allow the categorical imperative to justify extreme forms of paternalism. It is rarely, if ever, in a person's best interests to have their autonomy significantly curtailed.

Held (2006) argued for an ethical framework she labels the ethics of care which eschews strict adherence to abstract moral principles in favor of incorporating emotions into our decision-making. This means that emotions like disgust, rather than being shunned in favor of abstract calculations, are a regarded as a useful part of moral decision-making. Held (2006) also argues for the notion that the particular relationships between individuals are morally relevant. "The central focus of the ethics of care is on the compelling moral salience of attending to and meeting the needs of the particular others for whom we take responsibility" (2006, p. 10). This is to say that we ought not to simply pretend that caring for one's mother is morally identical to caring for a stranger. That the patient is your mother and that you love her are both salient parts of moral decision making. This is a stark departure from traditional western moral tradition, but it is a beneficial departure. It encourages us to not just place patients at the center of our thinking [as Kant (1996) does], but to take into account the fullness of the patient's circumstances. Care ethics reminds us that all patients are individuals who have specific circumstances and who demand bespoke treatment plans. For example, two patients with the same illness but different home environments—two patients with very different relationships to particular others—might respond very differently to the prospect of a treatment plan like chemotherapy that often leaves them needing assistance.

The argument here is that combining Kant (1996) and Held (2006) give us the best chance to achieve beneficial, patient-centered outcomes. Via Kant's (1996) deontology we arrive at a thorough, rational argument for placing the patient's interests at the center of our decision making especially in the context of medical treatments wherein outcomes are often uncertain. Via Held's (2006) ethic of care we come to understand the importance of relating with patients as particular individuals, not merely as abstract entities. So, while the strict demands of the categorical imperative to respect individuals above all else helps us to avoid many of the pitfalls of the modern healthcare, the contextually away perspective of care ethics allows us to form singular, caring bonds that improve the doctor-patient relationship and help ensure better health outcomes.

So, then, while we are duty-bound to do what is best for each patient, doing that requires getting to know them in their individual contexts. Had Wieczorek's doctors operated with these guiding principles in mind, it is likely that she would have better experiences and offered much more positive responses.

Humor

A little reflection shows us that jokes can be used for any number of purposes besides amusing an audience. They can be intended to belittle, to show off, and to relieve tension, etc. (Richards, 2013). So, what are the jokes in this case intended to do? I believe the intent of the jokes was to create, or acknowledge, an intimacy between the doctors and their patient and I will argue for this in the next section. Before that, however, let us take a look at some important concepts that will help us to see how joking could be used to do this.

Jokes, regardless of the intent of the joker, only work if they are offered within a common context (Cohen, 1999). Thus, shared jokes are a reliable sign of a bond between the joker and their audience (Richards, 2013). To put it another way, joking simply fails if the audience and the joker do not share a common understanding of the concepts deployed in the joke; the audience simply will not get it. A mutual understanding of the relevant concepts is a necessary condition for successful joking.

Elsewhere Cohen (1978, p. 28) describes the process of sharing jokes in this way:

Three aspects are involved: (1) the speaker issues a kind of concealed invitation; (2) the hearer expends a special effort to accept the invitation; and (3) this transaction constitutes the acknowledgment of a community...The property in common with metaphor...is the capacity to form or acknowledge a...community and thereby to establish an intimacy between the teller and the hearer.

In other words, the joker invites their audience to form a community with them, a community formed around the humorous appreciation of the topic of the joke. As Gordon (2014) describes Cohens' view "jokes create intimacy between two people by highlighting the beliefs and feelings they share in common as well as by providing proof that what one person finds funny is a genuine human absurdity that the other recognizes too" (p. 7). This is a different point than the one just above. Gordon's point here is that act of telling a joke can be used to establish a closer relationship. It is an invitation to strengthen an existing bond or establish a new bond that signifies agreement and allegiance, not just understanding.

Beyond the goals and conditions of joking, we should consider some elements in the ethics of joking. When thinking about what sorts of jokes we ought, or ought not, to tell, we sometimes come across notions of *punching up* and *punching down* (Gimbel, 2018). Punching up, is the act of using humor to make fun of groups that are in positions of power with respect to the joke teller. For example, an hourly employee of a large corporation punches up when they make jokes at the expense of the executives. Punching down is making fun of someone who is in some way socially inferior to you. A member of an ethnic majority making fun of an oppressed ethnic minority is punching down. In this case the doctors might be taken to be punching down, but it's a mistake to think so. Punching down (or up) is an act of laughing at a group that neither the joke teller nor the audience—at least not usually—are a part of.

Finally, we should consider the phenomenon of gallows humor, joking about terrible things. This is a well-known and long-standing way to relieve stress and to help deal with circumstances that are sometimes too hard to look at soberly (Richards, 2013; Watson, 2011). As Watson (2011) points out "Joking and laughing together can establish or affirm intimacy. But when joking reveals that we do *not* see the world similarly, it can harm relationships" (p. 38-39). Gallows humor can serve the role of kinship formation highlighted by Gordon. Gallows humor is most successful when there is already a bond or community in place, when you are amongst medical residents, for example. Here the humor serves to strengthen the bond. However, when the joker misjudges the situation and deploys gallows humor in a group without a preexisting bond, the joke may be mistaken as an attempt to punch down.

Both the notions of punching up or down and gallows humor rely on the notion of an in-group and an out-group. For our purposes we can define an in-group is a group of people similar enough in status and mindset to see themselves as one group. An out-group, then, is any person or group of people that is outside the boundaries of the in-group. When we punch up or down, we punch at people outside of our group. When we share gallows humor, we share it with persons in our group. Attention to these elements of joking will help us to understand the case at hand.

Analysis of The Case

We should start by acknowledging that, generally speaking, when working within a medical context and we ought to consider what is best for doctors, caregivers, patients and the broader community. However not all of these stakeholders will be weighted equally in each case. For example, if we were looking at a problem in the context of a drug testing trial, the effect on doctors would likely weigh much less heavily than the concern for the subjects and the general community. In this case, we will mostly consider what is best for patients as that is the theme of the case and the focus of our ethical framework. We'll start by briefly shining a light on some lesser problems and then taking a look at the main concern.

There are two types of transgressions by the doctors against Wieczorek that we ought to acknowledge even though they aren't specifically related to humor. To begin with, we can note the doctors' disturbing inclination to talk about Wieczorek as if she were not present. We see this in her story of her first delivery—where the attending physician ignores her to banter with her husband—and we see it again at the teaching hospital—where she is treated as a case instead of a person. It should be clear that this is problematic. While doctors may sometimes have reason to consult with other doctors in front of their patient, it should never be done in a way that makes the patient feel as if their agency doesn't matter. The consultation shouldn't make the patients feel as if the doctors don't see them as important participants in their own care. We also see a doctor very likely violating a patient's privacy, not to mention HIPAA, by discussing an acquaintance's medical history with Wieczorek. I hope the problematic nature of these transgressions is fairly obvious and will not dwell on them any further. We can take them as examples of how easily things can go awry when a doctor attempts to create an informal atmosphere. It is also worth noting that the physicians are very unlikely to have been crossing these lines on purpose or with malice. They simply didn't see that what they were doing is wrong. That said, if these transgressions are not the main cause of concern, what is?

To start to build a picture of what went wrong, we ought to note that the jokes told by the doctors to Wieczorek are not particularly funny. This is a subtle but important key to what is going on in the case. The jokes are worn out clichés clearly repeated often among doctors within their peer group. Indeed, in this context the purpose of the jokes was clearly not to be funny or amusing. This might suggest, as Wieczorek concludes, that the doctors were making fun of her in some way. However, it seems unlikely that this was their goal. What, then, were the doctors trying to do? Why did it fail (presuming that their intention as not to insult and alienate)? Let's examine the latter question first.

The main problem is likely a case of using in-group humor based on mistaking the nature of the relationship that Wieczorek has with medical professionals. In each of the attempts at humor the doctor seems to have taken Wieczorek to be a part of the medical community in a broad sense. They saw her as one of their own. This means that they assumed that she shared their sensibilities, perspectives, and default attitudes.

I think this really is the heart of the matter. The physicians simply misunderstood the nature of the relationship. So, what's the case for this analysis? We can see Wieczorek, herself, relate how her friends and family "frequently insisted that my position as a 'doctor's wife' afforded me unique advantages," and that many simply assumed that she either was a medical professional herself, as a nurse, or that she was intimately familiar with the workings of medical offices, as an administrator. Any of these descriptors can be reasonably taken to denote someone who is intimately familiar with doctors and medical settings. Someone who is part of the medical community and who might appreciate the gallows humor of that community. However, Wieczorek, clearly did not take herself to be in that club. Note her observation that she "found myself categorized in a way I did not see myself." It is not surprising, therefore, given the break between how people identified her and how she identified herself, that misunderstandings and concomitant problems would arise.

Consider, briefly, how you might react if a person assumed that you were an auto-mechanic and started making jokes about *gear heads.* At best you would be baffled. If you were consistently mistaken for a mechanic, and that was used as an excuse for making jokes about your greasy hair or poor driving skills, you might very well respond, as Wieczorek does, with consternation and offense—clearly, I have no idea what sort of self-deprecating humor mechanics employ. Indeed, it is clear that she absolutely did not approve of the attempts at humor. As she notes "it made me uncomfortable every single time." The first instance of mistaken comradery occurred in the office of the doctor during her fourth pregnancy; the doctor who declared that he "had been fooled a few times" by doctors' wives. Here was a doctor who is clearly at ease with their patient. He certainly would not have offered that line of humor if he hadn't been.

But the comments were so off-putting that Wieczorek never returned to his office. The doctor's plan, to lean on their presumed bond in order to make her more comfortable, clearly backfired. The doctor at the teaching hospitable who joked with his students about doctors' wives and their unexpected complications made the same mistake. As Wieczorek put it "I was mortified. Yet again I felt like the brunt of a joke."

Finally, in the most egregious example, Wieczorek's gynecologist ribbed her during her visits and especially after her surgery. As she relates "he assured me that I was 'terrible.'" Presumably, this attempt to tease her, in a lighthearted way, was meant to offer her a moment of levity at what was surely a stressful moment. Perhaps he meant to demonstrate that he could joke with her because the surgery had gone well, and she was past any moment of great concern. He might even have been trying to reassure her that *he was not offended* by her vulgarity, because, after all, they understood each other. And yet his efforts had the opposite effect. Wieczorek notes that the jokes were "apparently quite funny to him—but not to me."

The diagnosis of what went wrong in these examples is clear: they thought Wieczorek was a member of their in-group, but she did not share that perspective. Thus, jokes that rely on the in-group bond were received in a very different light. Wieczorek seems to think that the doctors are punching down by making jokes at the expense of women who may have very limited options for defending themselves. Was she right?

To answer that question, we should note a further, important element: jokes are communicative acts. As we have noted Wieczorek's doctors were attempting to signal to her that she and they were part of a group and that she should feel at ease. More importantly, the messages were part of their medical practice and thus, as any part of their practice, were governed by moral standards (Maccarone, 2010). Which is to say, in the context of a medical practice, jokes must be evaluated for the harm they may cause. More importantly, we cannot try to deflect blame for any harm caused by offensive or derogatory jokes as inconsequential simply because they are jokes. But then, how should we evaluate her doctor's actions? Should we condemn them for causing harm or should we praise them for trying to put her at ease?

Intent matters in terms of whether a person can be morally condemned for telling a joke (Gimbel, 2018). If I intend to harm a group or to cause offense, then I ought to be condemned for my intention, if nothing else. However, if my intent is to promote your best interests, then you ought not to condemn me, even if my actions have negative consequences. To see this distinction an example would be helpful. Imagine that you are exquisitely dressed in preparation for a formal event and then imagine that I douse you with a full blast from a fire extinguisher. Should you be mad at me? Well, if my intention is to ruin your outfit and your evening, then, yes, you should condemn me. I have failed to act in your best interests. However, if I honestly believed that you were on fire, and my intention was to save your life, you ought not to blame me. I was acting in your best interests, as I understood them. It is the same with jokes. If I tell a joke in violation of my duty to do right by you, I am blameworthy. If I tell a joke that harms you, but my sincere intention was to benefit you, then I am not blameworthy. Of course, this is true only if I can plausibly claim to not know that my joke might be offensive. If I knowingly incorporate a racial slur into a joke, it is hard for me to claim that I have that groups best interests in mind when I tell the joke. In the case at hand, it seems plausible to me that the doctors did not realize that their jokes might upset Wieczorek. They believed they were serving her interests, and their obligations to support her interests, by creating a more welcoming space for her.

But while intent is important with respect to blame, it is not the salient element with respect to the question of offense. Offense is a response to an action or expression, and like any consequence it is determined, at least in part, by factors beyond the control of the agent. I may intend to state something clearly, but despite that intent, the person I'm speaking with may still be confused. It's the same with joking, I may intend to put a person at ease by telling them a joke, but I might simply fail and cause offense instead. That I didn't intend to confuse or to offend does not mean that I didn't confuse or offend. So, that the doctors did not intend to offend does not mean that they did not offend.

It may be tempting to simply argue that Wieczorek is too sensitive, that she's overreacting. I would urge against this conclusion; looking to her as the cause of the misunderstanding misses the point. Alternatively, you might think the takeaway is that she should have spoken up to let the doctors know that she didn't appreciate their humor (I. Lutticken, personal communication, December 10, 2020), but, again, this is taking your eye off the ball. With respect to the latter concern, specifically, it is wrong to place the burden of speaking-up on patients. It is not enough to be passively receptive to feedback. Even if we ignore the strong history of paternalism in the field, doctors today are often given significant deference. We contradict them at our own peril. More importantly, Wieczoreck was often exposed to these jokes in moments of crisis or significant stress. It is unrealistic to expect a person stressed form legitimate medical concerns to have the wherewithal to speak out against perceived slights or rude comments. And, more importantly, focusing on whether a patient should have been offended or should have spoken up in their own defense obscures the real problem.

Recall from our discussion of ethics that medical professionals have an obligation to place the patient's needs at the center of their practice. It simply does not matter that a patient is sensitive or unwilling to express discomfort, even if it is true that patients should advocate for themselves, you must treat the patient that you have in your office, not the patient that you would like to have. If a patient has trouble reading, you would not proceed to give them nothing but written instructions. If a patient is sensitive, you must respect their sensibilities. Thus, there is no refuge for the doctors in the fact that they were joking.

We certainly can accept that they were joking. We can accept that they did not intend to harm. Indeed, it seems clear that, contrary to Wieczorek's implication, the doctors were not inviting her to join them in laughing at doctor's wives, they were inviting her to laugh with them about the travails of being a part of the medical community. They were not trying to insult doctor's wives, at all. The doctors were, instead, attempting to share a moment, to demonstrate a kinship, centered on the, to them absurd and amusing, observation that doctors' wives have unusually difficult medical histories. That Wieczorek did not see herself as one of them was the main stumbling block. She did not accept their invitation to form a community. So, the jokes caused offense instead of leading to greater intimacy.

Seeking to deepen the bonds of trust and community between a patient and their doctor is a laudable goal. One which is likely to improve outcomes for patients. So, we should not criticize the doctors for their intent. But, good intentions aside, what they actually did was harm the relationship. This led Wieczorek to avoid further contact with her doctor in at least one case. This leaves us with two questions: should they have tried to deepen the bond through humor at all, and what could they have done better?

Takeaways For The Healthcare Professional

By telling such jokes the doctors were, very likely, attempting to deal with stressful situations in a way that was meant to be helpful. They assumed that Wieczorek shared their perspectives as a member of the medical community. This assumption, warranted or not, led them to communicate with her in a way that was meant to signal solidarity and foster intimacy, but which would be inappropriate with someone who was not a medical professional. The mistake they made is, at bottom, that they did not pay enough attention to their patient.

Medical professionals must actively assess their patient's comfort. In general, it is wrong to place additional burdens—the expectation that they will correct your inappropriate behavior—on patients that are already stressed and even frightened by their medical concerns. As a medical professional your goal is what is best for the patient *as they are* not as you would like them to be. If this means modulating how you communicate, then that is simply what you must do.

This is the culmination of our earlier discussion of ethical frameworks. It is wrong to burden your patient because doing so is not in their best interests. You do not fulfill your duty to do what is best for them by putting them in a position to correct you. You do not fulfill your duty to do what is best for them by failing to treat them as particular individuals with distinct concerns. An ethic of care acknowledges that respecting their emotions, insecurities, concerns, etc. is a vital part of treating them and treating them well. Whether or not a patient's fear is well-founded it is still a very real fear to them. Failing to acknowledge that and to treat it with sensitivity is failing to fulfill your duty to them.

In a similar vein, in any setting in which there is a power imbalance it is the responsibility of the person in the superior position to establish feedback loops so that the persons in the inferior position have a chance to be heard. The current fashion for customer satisfaction surveys is an example of this. It is sometimes difficult to have a sense of what a good communication process looks like, but we can say something that should be helpful. The best advice is likely this: make room for your patient to be heard. When you ask them questions, be silent and patient. Do not be in a rush to ask the next question. Do not expect them to communicate efficiently and concisely. They do not have your training. Do not try to rob them of their individuality. Surveys that reduce individual experiences to scores are likely to do nothing so much as get in the way of meaningful communication. Be respectful of their perspective and respond to them, not just their illness. These general comments aside, what more can we say about the use of humor, specifically?

Given what we noted earlier about the effective use of humor as a tool for relieving tension, we should be loath to give it up. As Cohen (2009) and many others point out humor, and joking, can be a powerful tool for establishing intimacy and relieving stress. The solution then is reasonably straightforward.

In the main, when using humor as part of a patient-centered approach medical professionals must establish a good understanding of who their patients are before using humor that is specific to the patient. What does this look like in practice?

First, we must be honest about what a joke or humorous aside can accomplish. The deeper, more effective bond that you seek to establish with your patients cannot be established in a twenty-minute visit. It may take years. It will be formed by demonstrated concern for their well-being, and by consistently and continuously placing their needs at the center of your practice. The goal of using humor during a consultation is, at most, to set them at ease in the moment. It is not a substitute for excellent care.

Second, don't make the mistake of thinking that you can rely on your intuition to accurately assess who will or won't be offended by just reading the room. Our intuitions in these matters are highly likely to be self-serving and chock full of implicit bias. More importantly, patient responses are not reliable guides to whether or not they have taken offense. Again, consider how often Wieczorek kept silent or even nodded along because she was shocked by the doctor's rudeness. It is likely that if we were to poll her caregivers each of them would report that she was amused or put at ease by their wit, but, of course, they were wrong.

Third, avoid making any jokes about your patients, their conditions, or contexts unless or until you have gotten to know them. The odds of inadvertently casting a pall over your relationship is simply too high. You may believe that you have a great sense of what is or is not offensive, but this assumes that there is an objective standard for offense, there is not. Instead of setting yourself as the arbiter of taste, it is probably best to follow your patients' lead. If they make jokes about their illness or some other personal topic, it is a good sign that you can take similar liberties. Of course, you are under no compulsion to make these sorts of jokes and even if a patient makes them first, you might still cause offense by taking things too far or simply misreading their mood. There is no harm in playing it safe.

It is tempting to say that you should also avoid having canned jokes that you repeat over and over, but, honestly, we are not professional comedians. Coming up with humorous, off the cuff observations for each patient is too high a bar. Feel free to have a few good jokes at the ready and deploy them as needed. Just try not to let them get too stale.

You can, safely, make jokes at your own expense. As Mordechai (2014) notes, "In sharing some private details about ourselves, including ones that are not particularly flattering, we allow ourselves to be vulnerable in the face of our significant others and thus open ourselves to cultivating intimacy" (p. 10). Self-deprecating humor has a humanizing effect which may help your patients see you as less intimidating, less an authority figure, and thus make them more likely to be honest and forthcoming with you. Though, a word of caution, it is likely not a good idea to make jokes about how bad you are at being a doctor.

Finally, I'll offer a word on behalf of the down-trodden, cornball humor of *dad-jokes*. There is an admirable humanity to telling a joke that is obviously bad and inviting someone to laugh with you at how bad it is. If a patient rolls their eyes at a terrible pun, roll your eyes with them. Acknowledging that your joke was indeed terrible is just another a way to form a bond. Which is, after all, what the doctors in our sample case were trying to do all along.

REFERENCES

Berger, J., Coulehan, J., & Belling, C. (2004). Humor in the physician-patient encounter. *Archives of Internal Medicine*, *164*(8), 825–830. doi:10.1001/archinte.164.8.825 PMID:15111367

Borchert, D. M. (1999). *Philosophy and ethics*. Macmillan Library Reference.

Cohen, T. (1978). Metaphor and the cultivation of intimacy. *Critical Inquiry*, *5*(1), 3–12. doi:10.1086/447969

Cohen, T. (1999). *Jokes: Philosophical thoughts on joking matters*. University of Chicago Press. doi:10.7208/chicago/9780226112329.001.0001

Gimbel, S. (2018). *Isn't that clever*. Routledge.

Held, V. (2006). *The ethics of care: Personal, political, and global*. Oxford University Press.

Kant, I. (1996). *Groundwork of the metaphysics of morals* (M. Gregor, Trans.). Cambridge at the University Press.

Maccarone, E. M. (2010). Ethical responsibilities to subjects and documentary filmmaking. *Journal of Mass Media Ethics*, *25*(3), 192–206. doi:10.1080/08900523.2010.497025

Mordechai, G. (2014). Friendship, intimacy and humor. *Educational Philosophy and Theory*, *46*(2), 162–174. doi:10.1080/00131857.2012.721732

Richards, R. (2013). *A philosopher looks at the sense of humor*. Healing Time Books.

Watson, K. (2011). Gallows humor in medicine. *The Hastings Center Report*, *41*(5), 37–45. doi:10.1002/j.1552-146X.2011.tb00139.x PMID:21980898

Chapter 13
Party in the Front

Kaylie George
Independent Researcher, USA

As an LPN, I completed one year of classroom and clinical training, with classes including Anatomy and Physiology, Pharmacology, and Fundamentals of Nursing as well as many other classes and over 1000 clinical hours in the course of one short year. The initial four months were all lessons, and after successfully completing those courses, we started new classes two days a week, with 3 days of clinical at one of the hospitals in our area. Nursing management clinical was the first opportunity I had as a nursing student to provide nursing care for a full load of five to six patients. This was done under the supervision of a preceptor, which is a nurse that works at the hospital. I was assigned to work in the Neuro Progressive Care Unit (NPCU). The NPCU housed primarily stroke victims, with an occasional head trauma or someone recently out of neurosurgery.

It was during this nursing management clinic in the NPCU that an instance of humor occurred that stands out strongly in my memories against other patient interactions. In this case, my patient was a woman around 70 years old, who had fallen and hit her head, causing a rather large subdural hematoma. A subdural hematoma is a condition that may occur after head trauma in which blood pools between the brain's middle and outer covering. This can be very dangerous because it can compress and damage brain tissue. This one was a massive 74 millimeters, which is nearly three inches! Luckily, this patient had no significant brain damage. By the time I began assisting with her care, the patient had had the back of her head shaved and needed quite a few staples inserted.

The first morning I met this patient was a few days after her accident. She was talking about her hair, which was around shoulder length, and how she was sad that it had to be shaved. In an attempt to make a joke I said, "It's pretty cool though, almost like a reverse mullet!" I immediately realized that may have not been the best thing to say and was mortified waiting to see her response. We locked eyes for what seemed like an eternity while she thought about how to interpret what I had said. Luckily, she had a good sense of humor, laughed, and said, "You're right!" Relieved, I breathed a sigh of relief.

Later that day, I heard her telling a family member about her reverse mullet. They both laughed about it, so it was clear the patient was in a much better humor about her hair. It was a small joke, but it worked as an inoculation for her sadness, taking her mindset from being sad about her poor haircut, to

DOI: 10.4018/978-1-7998-4528-7.ch013

allowing her to make jokes about the new trends she might be setting. My small joke empowered her to find the light side of her situation.

As a nursing student, I was always so focused on not messing up by a breach in professionalism that I rarely used humor. This experience taught me how humor can positively affect these relationships though, and I try to strategically use humor working with patients now. Yet, the concern still exists that using a joke threatens the nurse-patient relationship if not interpreted in the way it was intended. Now, I take a little more time to learn about the patient before making jokes, especially ones focused on their appearance, so I can carefully calculate whether humor is appropriate for them.

Chapter 14

Response: Building Resilience Through Humor – Positive Impact on Stress Coping and Health: "Party in the Front"

Florian Fischer
https://orcid.org/0000-0002-4388-1245
Institute of Public Health, Charité - Universitätsmedizin, Berlin, Germany & Institute of Gerontological Health Services and Nursing Research, Ravensburg-Weingarten University of Applied Sciences, Germany

HUMOR IN THE CONTEXT OF SALUTOGENESIS, COPING, AND RESILIENCE

Humor can be used when individuals are under stress or perceive discomfort in others. In the midst of these moments, people rely on laughter and humor when attempting to remedy, cope with and buffer a wide range of awkward, sensitive, embarrassing, fearful, anxious, atypical, strange or abnormal situations (Beach et al., 2005; Beach & Dixson, 2001; Beach & Prickett, 2017). Therefore, humor may act as a powerful adaptive coping mechanism when confronted with adversity and is found to be positively correlated with resilience (Abel, 2002; Abrams et al., 2016; Fine, 1991; Romundstad et al., 2016).

The way one deals with stressful situations is highly important for well-being. The concept of salutogenesis, first introduced by Antonovsky (1979; 1987), contains a theoretical foundation for factors promoting health and well-being. This is in contrast to the perspective of pathogenesis, which emphasizes those factors causing a disease. Furthermore, it abandons the dichotomous view on health vs. illness by describing and explaining the relationship between health and illness as continuous – indicating that health is not a fixed state but a process. The salutogenic model is concerned with the relationship between health, stress and coping (Antonovsky, 1979).

According to this model, the appraisal of individual life situations plays a major role in the subjective feeling of health. Antonovsky (1996) used a river as a metaphor of life and called it the "River of Health"

DOI: 10.4018/978-1-7998-4528-7.ch014

(p. 14). Rather than preventing us from swimming or rescuing from a dangerous river, the salutogenic intention is to improve our individual skills to make swimming safer. From this perspective, health is a dynamic, ever-present relation between the swimmer and the river (Eriksson & Lindström, 2011). The river metaphor includes the following stages moving up the river: (1) cure or treatment of diseases, (2) health protection/disease prevention, (3) and finally health promotion. All of these three stages – which are kinds of approaches in public health – ultimately strive to improve health, but out of different perspectives. This is the classic image of the River of Health, where the *downriver bias* is focusing on processes where the risk exposure already may have caused a damage (Eriksson & Lindström, 2008).

However, the River of Health has been developed further to a "Health in the River of Life" by Eriksson and Lindström (2008, p. 194): At birth, we drop into the river and float with the stream and over life learn how to swim. Some are born at *ease* where the river flows gently and where they have time to learn how to swim. Other children are born close to the waterfall, at *dis-ease*, where they have to struggle to survive. Where we end up in the river is based on the orientation and learning through life experiences. This, in turn, is closely related to the concept of resilience, which is the ability to exercise constructive life skills to meet the challenges of life (Zautra et al., 2010). Resilience might be seen as a personality characteristic, as a positive, distinct feature of an individual that prevents negative effects of stress (Konaszewski et al., 2019). An additional theoretical foundation is the sense of coherence, which is defined as the capability to perceive that one can manage in any situation independent of whatever is happening in life. Sense of coherence is not constructed around a fixed set of coping strategies, but is flexible (Antonovsky, 1993). The understanding of a problem, a way out and the answer to the question whether life makes sense to an individual define how he or she can handle a situation and how ill he or she feels (Antonovsky 1979). The key components for the sense of coherence are comprehensibility, manageability and meaningfulness: People have to understand their lives and they have to be understood by others, perceive that they are able to manage the situation and perceive it is meaningful enough to find motivation to continue (Antonovsky, 1979; 1987).

Humor, as such, can lead to resilience, which is understood as the ability of humans to spring back from stressors in the environment. By not taking oneself too seriously, one is able to let go of excessively perfectionistic expectations, while remaining motivated to achieve realistic goals. For that reason, humor can enable us to encounter stress and to return to previous levels of functioning (Lefcourt & Thomas, 1998). Four styles of humor have been identified: affiliative, self-enhancing, aggressive and self-defeating. Adaptive humor, which is associated with the benefits that result in better health, can be affiliative. In this case, amusement is used to enhance interpersonal bonds by decreasing tension. Self-enhancing humor is when amusement is derived from pointing out the incongruities in life. Maladaptive humor, which has negative effects on mental health, can be aggressive (criticizing others) or self-defeating (making fun of oneself; Martin et al., 2003). Affiliative humor, for example, is vital to sustaining a sense of resilience and buffering the effects of stress (Cheung & Yue, 2012),

Having a good sense of humor is thought to be a healthy and desirable personality trait, as it refers to the readiness to respond positively to serious, uncomfortable and stressful situations and may, therefore, be used as a coping strategy (Forabosco, 1998). This goes along with another explanation of humor with health-related outcomes which is derived from positive psychology, wherein humor is viewed as a personal quality promoting resilience and well-being by means of cognitive reappraisal of stressful events (Kuiper, 2012).

Humor has a broad range of effects on perceptions, attitudes, judgments and emotions, which may mediate directly or indirectly to be beneficial for the physical and psychological state of health. The anticipation of indirect effects fits within the framework of the buffering hypothesis, which asserts that social support helps to protect against distress by providing the perceived resources needed to manage stressful situations (Cohen & Wills, 1985). The general use of humor buffers against the negative effects of rumination and depression (Olson et al., 2005). Research suggests that some of the psychological challenges during recovery from illness are inherently social. Perceived social support, for example, particularly the presence of close companions and friends, has measurable effects on depression following myocardial infarctions (Lett et al., 2009). The beneficial functions of humor in this context are the connectedness with others and a sense of hope, joy and relaxation (Claxton-Oldfield & Bhatt, 2017). As humor helps to build relationships and promotes perceptions of social support, humor enactment could support coping with stress (Lockwood & Yoshimura, 2014). Humorous interactions between patients and service providers can also support the therapeutic relationship (Haydon et al., 2015; Haydon & van der Riet, 2014) and positively influence patients' experiences (Haydon et al., 2015; McCreaddie & Payne, 2014; Tanay et al., 2013). However, humor in healthcare interactions still is a relatively understudied area (McCreaddie & Payne, 2014).

CONNECTIONS BETWEEN ACADEMIC CONTENT AND THE CASE

The functions of humor are closely related to several theoretical foundations highlighted above. It is obvious that the patient with the subdural hematoma was worried about the shaving of her head. The nursing student used a simple comparison which led to the patient changing her perspective on the issue. This comparison making use of the incongruity of humor led to a cognitive shift in the patient. She was no longer worried about the situation. Instead, the use of humor – like other positive emotions – broadened the focus of attention. This fostered exploration, creativity, and flexibility in thinking, which is illustrated by the example that the patient has been able to make jokes about the new trends she might be setting.

Therefore, humor can actively lead people to confront, proactively reframe, and at times transform stressful situations, because humor provides a distance to the problem and may lead to a changing perspective. However, one needs to keep in mind the distinction between adaptive and maladaptive humor (Martin & Ford, 2018) – as mentioned before in the four styles of humor. Based on previous research, we can understand humor as a stable personality tendency referring to a sensation (amusement), to a behavior (laughter or smiling), to its use as a way of coping (humor as a coping mechanism), to an ability (production and creation of stimuli) and, finally, to an aesthetic sense (sense of humor, appreciation of humor; Hehl & Ruch, 1985).

Sense of humor involves a series of cognitive and emotional appraisals, behaviors, attitudes, and values. Moreover, it influences the relations we establish with others and our communication and persuasion (Martin & Ford, 2018). There is a line of research aimed at analyzing the affective and cognitive dimensions in relation to the sense of humor (Ruch & Köhler, 2007). It is important to understand the personality of a person to apply humor in a way that is understandable and beneficial. In this regard, positive psychology is a scientific approach within psychology that focuses on research on what is best in people. Within this framework, humor is understood as a character strength (Santos et al., 2013). Referring to the case of the patient with the subdural hematoma, the type of humor used by the nursing student worked well, although he was not familiar with the patient's personality and sense of humor. The nurse has been worried about the situation. Although people with illnesses or disabilities may find relief due to humor in making light of their often life-threatening situations, humor and joking are sometimes still seen as socially unacceptable (Demjén et al., 2016). Nurse's perceptions regarding the use of humor indicate that humor is seen as something very personal. Whereas one person might laugh about a joke or funny statement, the same verbatim may cause discomfort in others (Haydon & van der Riet, 2014). Therefore, the use of humor must be appropriate to each individual within his or her situation. This requires a thorough training to allow for an appropriate use for each situation (Pinna et al., 2018). The case described above emphasizes the problem that the nurse did not know the patient at all. Due to the missing information about patient's characteristics – related to his or her personality, psycho-social situation, and cognitive appraisals (e.g., leading to fear) – the humorous statement, which might be seen as kind of an "intervention," is not necessarily – or even unlikely – based on the needs of the patient. This illustrated that humor is not per se effective and does not per se lead to the intended effects, although the case is a positive example, where the humor worked well. Humor and empathy are closely related, as a previous study has also shown that a sense of humor and empathic concerns are associated for people with emotional intelligence who use these two personality characteristics to interact effectively with other persons (Hampes, 2001).

There is a connection between positive psychology and the concept of salutogenesis, because both concepts reconsider the resources of healthy functioning (Joseph & Sagy, 2017). Therefore, in this specific case the impact of humor is also related to coping and resilience: As already described in the precedent subchapter on the functions of humor, humor enables people to cope better with stress. This relationship has been established in a study by Abel (2002), who described that study participants with a high sense of humor appraised relatively lower amounts of stress and anxiety. This refers back to the relevance of sense of humor – and further personality characteristics – for coping with adversities. However, the impact of humor on positive stress coping is also strongly linked with the concept of resilience. Resilience is typically defined as the capacity to recover from difficult life events. It is the ability to withstand adversity and bounce back and grow despite life's downturns. People who are resilient tend to be flexible and creative. The case shows that the patient accepts what cannot be changed and how to positively reframe the adversity. This in turn regulates her emotion. The creativity enables to explore a totally different viewpoint and the flexibility embraces a positive but realistic assessment of the challenging situation. Furthermore, due to the flexibility, resilient people can shift from one coping strategy (e.g., problem-focused vs. emotion-focused) to another – depending upon the circumstances. An important component of cognitive flexibility is accepting the reality of each situation. In addition, resilient people are able to cognitively reappraise a situation. A positive reappraisal requires a person to find alternative positive meanings for negative or stressful events, situations, and/or beliefs.

For these reasons, the theoretical and practical foundation of resilience is highly important for salutogenesis, because it focusses on (resistance) resources (Idan et al., 2017), which are needed to swim in the River of Health, as outlined by Antonovsky (1996) in his salutogenetic model. Overall, there are seven pillars of resilience, which exist side by side, are mutually dependent and complement each other:

- Realistic optimism
- Acceptance
- Solution orientation
- Self-regulation
- Assuming responsibility
- Network orientation
- Future planning

The seven pillars of resilience are all directly related to the basic attitude of humor and can be exemplified based on the case of the patient with the subdural hematoma.

Realistic optimism, as the first pillar, consciously deals with what has been experienced. Optimistic people accept the circumstances, but do not give up hope for a positive turn of events. Humor not only promotes optimism, humor even means being optimistic. With humor the circumstances can be positively reassessed. A humorous attitude helps to increase the tolerance, as it is visible that the patient no longer worries about the haircut, but emphasizes the new trend she might be setting.

To consciously deal with adversities, it is necessary to accept what is happening. Humor is a basic attitude that helps us to accept ourselves and surrounding – irrespective of adversities. Therefore, humor is also related with empathy and a benevolent attitude. Acceptance, however, does not mean to accept something defenselessly, but to open up to reality. Nevertheless, the inner distance, which humor helps us to maintain, enables us to look at the situation from an outside perspective and thus to reflect despite our own involvement. In the case the acceptance of the situation becomes clear due to the agreement of the patient ("You're right!") towards the reassessed view on the haircut.

Solution orientation is a further pillar of resilience. It is future-oriented and directs attention to possible solutions. To this end, it is particularly important to formulate goals. In this regard, humor helps to question entrenched structures and thought patterns. Furthermore, it encourages initiative and creativity in discovering and testing new solution models. Again, within the reported case, this can be seen in the goal to act as a trend-setter.

Self-regulation is another issue of resilience. Only those who see themselves as actors are capable of action. Leaving the role of victim is therefore indispensable for overcoming difficulties and strengthening resilience. Humor can help us to reassess the situation. The example illustrates that the patient is no longer a victim, but faces the adversity with autonomy.

The fifth pillar is responsibility. Assuming responsibility means becoming aware of one's own actions within a specific situation and bearing the consequences. This is easier with humor, because it helps us to become more relaxed. Humor enables us to break through the boundaries that restrict thinking, feeling and acting. Viewing the shaved hair as a reverse mullet would have been no option for the patient before the humorous interaction. Therefore, humor opens the opportunity to assume responsibility for the situation and the consequences.

Social networks, whether family, friends, or even professional helpers, are among the social resources. Humor as a social competence is particularly suitable for building and maintaining relationships with other people. Humor has a loosening and sympathetic effect, while a sincere laugh limits conflicts and calms down. This kind of network orientation is obvious in the case, because the patient benefits from the positive attitude of the nursing student and shares this experience afterwards with her family.

Looking to the future includes active future planning. Humor helps to be more flexible in dealing with the demands of life and to free ourselves from rigid coping strategies. The empowerment experienced by the patient is a demonstrative example of the power humor has. All of the pillars of resilience described above complement each other and allow, in combination with humor, for developing and implementing new solution strategies.

TAKE AWAY

The case encompasses several take-away-messages. First of all, humor does not ignore difficulties, but it makes them tolerable. Humor has the strength to weaken negative emotions – and it may even turn a negative emotion into a positive one. The humorous situation does not solve the incriminatory situation by curing the subdural hematoma. But it allows for redirecting the perspective on this situation and may, therefore, lead to kind of a solution of the problem that has created negative emotions. This allows the patient to control the challenges she is faced with. Laughter liberates, leads to an inner distance and a higher tolerance for adversities and thus helps in coping with difficult and crisis-ridden life events.

The second message is that laughter is contagious. Sharing a laugh with family members or friends creates joy and affection for each other. The case describes this aspect due to the fact that the patient shared the funny moment with her family. Thereby, it creates a connection to others and helps to remain focused and alert. It is important to understand that just because you find something to laugh about during tough times does not mean you are not serious about the respective issue.

Thirdly, and very important, humor plays an important role in improving psychological balance and strengthening resilience. For example, the power of laughter is particularly obvious in a stressful situation such as treatment in a hospital. As described above, laughter dissolves negative emotions (e.g., fear), keeps problems in perspective, puts the people involved in a positive frame of mind, and enables them to better deal with the situation. As it has been shown in several studies, resilient people even manage to experience positive emotions in the middle of stressful and challenging situations. Therefore, humor is a coping strategy and protects from the damaging impact of stress.

Fourthly, the case is an example of positive humor and its effects. Studies have shown that the tendency to use negative humor is associated with lower interpersonal competence, self-esteem, and psychological well-being, as well as higher levels of depression and anxiety. The positive kind of humor, which allows individuals to find pleasant aspects or unexpected benefits in difficult and stressful situations prevents negative emotions from taking over.

In summary, the case is an excellent example of how humor might empower resilience, and, therefore, act a coping mechanism. The humorous "intervention" has just been part of a conversation which has not been prepared. Therefore, it belongs to the conversational humor, which is a spontaneous reaction within a trivial situation, although this specific situation is linked to many uncertainties and sorrows from the patient. However, the use of humor in such a situation helps to overcome fears and rotating thoughts focusing on the burdening condition of dealing with the consequences of the patient's subdural hematoma, which impacts her outer appearance. The major advantage of conversational humor – compared to performance humor – is its availability in everyday situations in terms of humorous personal anecdotes, irony, and other funny comments that tend to occur spontaneously in all sorts of social interactions. In the case described above, the nursing student serves as the person who relieves the tension. And this funny situation also leads to the fact that the patient talks with her family members about this moment. The ease of handling this situation also facilitates further social support from the family members, because group stability is strengthened.

Coping does not necessarily mean to be able to fix all situations: Problem-focused coping is not always possible. However, the case is an example of emotion-focused coping. It concentrates on changing one's mood or frame of mind. This has been achieved by creating a cognitive-affective shift by the use of humor. Reframing the perspective leads to an emotional shift, and, following from this, to a more positive direction for dealing with stressful situations. Therefore, humor is the ability to look at unpleasant things and everyday difficulties in a calm and cheerful way. We cannot avoid feelings of disillusionment or sadness depending on the situation, but we are free to let go of such feelings and look optimistically and hopefully into the future. By accepting and/or rephrasing difficulties, we can create an appreciative atmosphere in order to face the challenges more calmly but also more courageously.

REFERENCES

Abel, M. H. (2002). Humor, stress, and coping strategies. *Humor: International Journal of Humor Research, 15*(4). 365-381. doi:10.1515/humr.15.4.365

Abrams, T. E., Ogletree, R. J., Ratnapradipa, D., & Neumeister, M. W. (2016). Adult survivors' lived experience of burns and post-burn health: A qualitative analysis. *Burns, 42*(1), 152–162. doi:10.1016/j.burns.2015.09.011 PMID:26527372

Antonovsky, A. (1979). *Health, stress, and coping*. Jossey-Bass.

Antonovsky, A. (1987). *Unraveling the mystery of health – How people manage stress and stay well.* Jossey-Bass.

Antonovsky, A. (1993). Complexity, conflict, chaos, coherence, coercion and civility. *Social Science & Medicine, 37*(8), 969–981. doi:10.1016/0277-9536(93)90427-6 PMID:8235741

Antonovsky, A. (1996). The salutogenic model as a theory to guide health promotion. *Health Promotion International, 11*(1), 11–18. doi:10.1093/heapro/11.1.11

Beach, W. A., & Dixson, C. N. (2001). Revealing moments: Formulating understandings of adverse experiences in a health appraisal interview. *Social Science & Medicine, 52*(1), 25–44. doi:10.1016/S0277-9536(00)00118-0 PMID:11144915

Beach, W. A., Easter, D. W., Good, J. S., & Pigeron, E. (2005). Disclosing and responding to cancer "fears" during oncology interviews. *Social Science & Medicine, 60*(4), 893–910. doi:10.1016/j.socscimed.2004.06.031 PMID:15571904

Beach, W. A., & Prickett, E. (2017). Laughter, humor, and cancer: Delicate moments and poignant interactional circumstances. *Health Communication, 32*(7), 791–802. doi:10.1080/10410236.2016.1172291 PMID:27420294

Cheung, C.-K., & Yue, X. D. (2012). Sojourn students' humor styles as buffers to achieve resilience. *International Journal of Intercultural Relations, 36*(3), 353–364. doi:10.1016/j.ijintrel.2011.10.001

Claxton-Oldfield, S., & Bhatt, A. (2017). Is there a place for humor in hospice palliative care? Volunteers say "yes"! *The American Journal of Hospice & Palliative Care, 34*(5), 417–422. doi:10.1177/1049909116632214 PMID:26917788

Cohen, S., & Wills, T. A. (1985). Stress, social support, and the buffering hypothesis. *Psychological Bulletin, 98*(2), 310–357. doi:10.1037/0033-2909.98.2.310 PMID:3901065

Demjén, Z. (2016). Laughing at cancer: Humour, empowerment, solidarity and coping online. *Journal of Pragmatics*, *101*, 18–30. doi:10.1016/j.pragma.2016.05.010

Eriksson, M., & Lindström, B. (2008). A salutogenic interpretation of the Ottawa Charter. *Health Promotion International*, *23*(2), 190–199. doi:10.1093/heapro/dan014 PMID:18356285

Eriksson, M., & Lindström, B. (2011). Life is more than survival: Exploring links between Antonovsky's salutogenic theory and the concept of resilience. In K. M. Gow & M. J. Celinski (Eds.), *Wayfinding through life's challenges: Coping and survival* (pp. 31–46). Nova Publishers.

Fine, S. B. (1991). Resilience and human adaptability: Who rises above adversity? *The American Journal of Occupational Therapy*, *45*(6), 493–503. doi:10.5014/ajot.45.6.493 PMID:2063939

Forabosco, G. (1998). The ill side of humor: Pathological conditions and sense of humor. In W. Ruch (Ed.), *Humor research. The sense of humor. Explorations of a personality characteristic* (pp. 271–292). De Gruyter Mouton. doi:10.1515/9783110804607.271

Hampes, W. P. (2001). Relation between humor and empathic concern. *Psychological Reports*, *88*(1), 241–244. doi:10.2466/pr0.2001.88.1.241 PMID:11293036

Haydon, G., van der Reit, P., & Browne, G. (2015). A narrative inquiry: Humour and gender differences in the therapeutic relationship between nurses and their patients. *Contemporary Nurse*, *50*(2-3), 214–226. doi:10.1080/10376178.2015.1021436 PMID:26073613

Haydon, G., & van der Riet, P. (2014). A narrative inquiry: How do nurses respond to patients' use of humour? *Contemporary Nurse*, *46*(2), 197–205. doi:10.5172/conu.2014.46.2.197 PMID:24787253

Hehl, F.-J., & Ruch, W. (1985). The location of sense of humor within comprehensive personality spaces: An exploratory study. *Personality and Individual Differences*, *6*(6), 703–715. doi:10.1016/0191-8869(85)90081-9

Idan, O., Eriksson, M., & Al-Yagon, M. (2017). The salutogenic model: The role of generalized resistance resources. In M. B. Mittelmark, S. Sagy, M. Eriksson, G. F. Bauer, J. M. Pelikan, B. Lindström, & G. A. Espnes (Eds.), *The handbook of sautogenesis* (pp. 57–69). Springer. doi:10.1007/978-3-319-04600-6_7

Joseph, S., & Sagy, S. (2017). Positive psychology in the context of salutogenesis. In M. B. Mittelmark, S. Sagy, M. Eriksson, G. F. Bauer, J. M. Pelikan, B. Lindström, & G. A. Espnes (Eds.), *The handbook of sautogenesis* (pp. 83–88). Springer. doi:10.1007/978-3-319-04600-6_10

Konaszewski, K., Kolemba, M., & Niesiobędzka, M. (2019). Resilience, sense of coherence and self-efficacy as predictors of stress coping style among university students. *Current Psychology*, 1–11. doi:10.100712144-019-00363-1

Kuiper, N. A. (2012). Humor and resiliency: Towards a process model of coping and growth. *Europe's Journal of Psychology*, *8*(3), 475–491. doi:10.5964/ejop.v8i3.464

Lefcourt, H. M., & Thomas, S. (1998). Humor and stress revisited. In W. Ruch (Ed.), *The sense of humor: Explorations of a personality characteristic* (pp. 179–202). De Gruyter Mouton. doi:10.1515/9783110804607.179

Lett, H. S., Blumenthal, J. A., Babyak, M. A., Catellier, D. J., Carney, R. M., Berkman, L. F., Burg, J. A., Mitchell, P., Jaffe, A. S., & Schneiderman, N. (2009). Dimensions of social support and depression in patients at increased psychosocial risk recovering from myocardial infarction. *International Journal of Behavioral Medicine*, *16*(3), 248–258. doi:10.100712529-009-9040-x PMID:19288205

Lockwood, N. L., & Yoshimura, S. M. (2014). The heart of the matter: The effects of humor on well-being during recovery from cardiovascular disease. *Health Communication*, *29*(4), 410–420. doi:10.1080/10410236.2012.762748 PMID:23829386

Martin, R. A., & Ford, T. (2018). The psychology of humor: An integrative approach (2nd ed.). Elsevier Science & Technology.

Martin, R. A., Puhlik-Doris, P., Larsen, G., Gray, J., & Weir, K. (2003). Individual differences in uses of humor and their relation to psychological well-being: Development of the Humor Styles Questionnaire. *Journal of Research in Personality*, *37*(1), 48–75. doi:10.1016/S0092-6566(02)00534-2

McCreaddie, M., & Payne, S. (2014). Humour in health-care interactions: A risk worth taking. *Health Expectations*, *17*(3), 332–344. doi:10.1111/j.1369-7625.2011.00758.x PMID:22212380

Olson, M. L., Hugelshofer, D. S., Kwon, P., & Reff, R. C. (2005). Rumination and dysphoria: The buffering role of adaptive forms of humor. *Personality and Individual Differences*, *39*(8), 1419–1428. doi:10.1016/j.paid.2005.05.006

Pinna, M. Á. C., Mahtani-Chugani, V., Sánchez Correas, M. Á., & Sanz Rubiales, A. (2018). The use of humor in palliative care: A systematic literature review. *The American Journal of Hospice & Palliative Care*, *35*(10), 1342–1354. doi:10.1177/1049909118764414 PMID:29587520

Romundstad, S., Svebak, S., Holen, A., & Holmen, J. (2016). A 15-year follow-up study of sense of hand causes of mortality: The Nord-Trondelag Health Study. *Psychosomatic Medicine*, *78*(3), 345–353. doi:10.1097/PSY.0000000000000275 PMID:26569539

Ruch, W., & Köhler, G. (2007). A temperamental approach to humour. In W. Ruch (Ed.), *The sense of humor: Explorations of a personality characteristic* (pp. 203–228). De Gruyter Mouton. doi:10.1515/9783110804607-011

Santos, V., Paes, F., Pereira, V., Arias-Carrion, O., Silva, A. C., Carta, M. G., Nardi, A. E., & Machado, S. (2013). The role of positive emotion and contributions of positive psychology in depression treatment: Systematic review. *Clinical Practice and Epidemiology in Mental Health*, *9*(1), 221–237. doi:10.2174/1745017901309010221 PMID:24358052

Tanay, M. A. L., Roberts, J., & Ream, E. (2013). Humour in adult cancer care: A concept analysis. *Journal of Advanced Nursing*, *69*(9), 2131–2140. doi:10.1111/jan.12059 PMID:23215893

Zautra, A. J., Hall, J. S., & Murray, K. E. (2010). Resilience: A new definition of health for people and communities. In J. R. Reich, A. J. Zautra, & J. S. Hall (Eds.), *Handbook of adult resilience* (pp. 3–30). Guilford Press.

Chapter 15
RIP 2855

Elena Gabor
Bradley University, USA

Octavian Gabor
Methodist College, USA

My 46-year-old husband, a philosophy professor, vegetarian, non-smoker, daily gym goer, soccer player of average weight with genetically inherited high cholesterol, underwent double coronary bypass surgery in June 2020. After conducting an angiogram, the cardiologist wrote bafflingly in his file: "Octavian is the image of health. However, …" His LAD (left arterial descending artery), also called the "widow-maker," was completely blocked, and his RCA (right coronary artery) was partially obstructed. The blockage contained calcifications, so placing a stent would have brought the risk of "heart attack, stroke or death." The only reason he had not dropped dead in March when the LAD became completely occluded, was that, over time, his heart had developed its own bypasses, or secondary vascularization, thus compensating for the diminished blood flow through the arteries. All that athletic activity paid off. As soon as COVID-19 rules allowed elective procedures, we scheduled a coronary artery bypass graft (CABG) with a left internal mammary artery (LIMA) graft for the LAD bypass and a saphenous vein graft (SVG) for the RCA bypass. He spent five days in the hospital and by the end, the nurses made sure he could walk, shower, and go up the stairs on his own. The story below is in his words:

'6:00 am. I'm at the hospital. In two hours, I go into the surgery room for open heart surgery. I receive the hospital armband. I look at it, and I see the number: RIP 2855. I am doomed. Have 2854 people died before me? Am I going to "Rest in Peace" as well? Of course, the armband was not the sign of my demise, but just an identification tool. It reminded me of the ambulance I once saw with the word "END" on its license plate. Within the gloomy pandemic context, with nothing to do, the "Rest in Peace" armband provided the occasion for humor and human connection with the nurses in the Cardiac ICU. Everyone

DOI: 10.4018/978-1-7998-4528-7.ch015

is tired in the cardio-vascular ICU units. The patients don't sleep much after surgery, and the nurses' shifts can be eventful. In my five hospital days, I began to know the nurses and their daily demeanors.

One day, a technician nurse came to see me for a daily activity: an oxygen mask on my face through which I was supposed to breath for five minutes. I noticed she was sad, although very professional, when she came to put the mask on, so I thought I would make her laugh. After five minutes, while she may have helped other patients with their oxygen, she came back into the room to take off the oxygen mask. I took a very serious demeanor as well, and, with my voice still weak after the ventilator had scratched my vocal chords, I said, "May I show you something?" "Of course," she replied, coming toward me. "Look, this is the armband they gave me: Rest in Peace 2855." And I started to laugh despite the pain, clutching the pillow to my sternum-long scar that my wife had nicknamed "the zipper." Her face lit up, she covered her mouth with her hand, surprised, and started laughing as well. She said, "My, my, I've never seen that!" And we continued laughing together, while I was guarding my chest from opening up again. "I'll have to check all the other numbers, now!" she said, laughing. "Why would they give you such a number?"

Making her smile made me feel like I was not just a passive recipient of her care, but a giver of care as well. There is one more aspect of it. She was a woman, I was a man. She was black, I was white. All of them reasons to create distance between us. The RIP armband brought us at the same level. There was no more nurse-patient, woman-man, or black person-white person difference. It was just two human beings enjoying a moment of communion.

The story repeated a couple of times with different nurses over the next few days in ICU, and it always ended in laughter. But this particular nurse was the most memorable. Perhaps, it was so because she was not particularly happy. Our interaction was short, just a few minutes, since she was there just for the brief breathing exercise. To some extent, it was the occasion for each of us to bring something good in the life of the other, and the Rest in Peace armband did that for both of us. For some reason, I believe I will remain in her life, and she will remember the encounter even if she doesn't know my name and I don't know her name (well, she knows my "name": RIP2855). I also believe that this memory will bring a smile on her face whenever she will think of it. It certainly gives me reasons to smile. And even if I do not know her name, I remember her face, especially the light that was absent when she came in the room, and the light that was present when she left.

If we think about this moment as creating memory, we may wonder whether such moments of humor have ripples beyond the moments themselves. Of course, if we consider that moment only, we can say that it produced for both patient and nurse a certain relaxation, a break away from problems, even if only for a few moments. But since the moment was memorable—and the light on my nurse's face and the change in demeanor gave me all the reasons to believe that it was so—it may also be that "funny" moments have a much larger influence, even beyond themselves. The memory of the shared laughter in the Cardiac ICU unit may have had a curative aspect: it made both of us forget the pain of the moment; it brought back a "lightness" of human interaction, and it thus gave me the possibility to bring goodness to myself and those around me once again.'

Fortunately, Octavian's young age and the good work of his medical team have allowed him to recover quickly. The armband with the "RIP" initials is stored in our "bypass file," and the "image of health" expression is now a cautionary joke in our family.

Chapter 16
Response:
'RIP 2855'

Galen Foresman
North Carolina A&T State University, USA

LOVE, JOKES, AND COMPASSIONATE CARE

Telling jokes is a mixed bag at times. Sometimes telling jokes can be meant in a friendly fashion and other times, jokes can be meant to ridicule or make fun. For this paper we will focus on joke telling as an expression of a type of love philosophers have called "*agape*" (Helm, 2017, para 3). When we "get" a joke, we share a connection with the joke teller that can make us feel included and valued. Originating from an ancient Greek concept of love, *agape* has come to mean a love stemming from a genuine regard for all people (Helm, 2017, para 5). As an overarching love for humanity, *agape* also makes us feel included and valued. When we tell someone a joke, we express *agape* through tacit assumptions we make about our audience. For example, we typically assume they will think our joke is humorous, which depends on a great many other assumptions about a person, like whether or not they will get the joke at all. As a joke is told, these assumptions are revealed and by the conclusion a shared understanding manifests, hopefully acknowledged through mutual laughter and enjoyment.

The Gabors' account illustrates how even basic attempts at humor in a healthcare environment can be compassionate acts. There are, of course, pitfalls to joke telling, and while Octavian Gabor's account of the case appears to avoid them, a slight reinterpreting of the scenario will show how things could have gone wrong. While Octavian's account is unique in that he, the patient, expresses compassion through a joke to his nurse technician, the role could easily have been reversed. In which case, offending a patient is always a potential risk in joke telling, but that risk is manageable when you know your audience (Creative Commons, 2016, para 9-10). Often, offence results when a joke's humor hinges upon incorrect assumptions about the identity or character of an audience, not malign intent by the joke teller (Creative Commons, 2016, para 15). Ostensibly, a joke is told to make you feel good. An offensive joke may mischaracterize the audience, but it is still an attempt to share and connect with them. The nature of this connection may be friendly, as in the case of agapic love jokes, or it may be a joke meant to ridicule

DOI: 10.4018/978-1-7998-4528-7.ch016

or demean. While it may seem counterintuitive, telling an offensive joke is perfectly compatible with being compassionate and respectful. Of course there are plenty of jokes where the humor is quite the opposite of respectful.

An Analogue of A Joke

A*gape* and joke telling work together, but to understand this, it will first help to understand how *agapeic* love is unlike other loves. Previously, a*gape* was described as the love we have for others simply because they are human like us. Unlike romantic love, *eros*, or the love we have for our friends, *philia*, the object of our *agapeic* affection is worthy of love because it belongs to a category of things we respect and value (Helm, 2017, para 5). We love our friends, in part, because we like them, and so there are identifiable features of our friends that we point to as reasons for liking them. Strangers aren't our friends, because we don't yet know anything specific about them worth our liking. *Agape* is a love that we can have for strangers, because strangers share an important feature common to everyone we love, including ourselves. They are human.

Being human may seem like an unusual reason for loving someone, but it is this love that drives our compassion for the less fortunate and those in need. When we help strangers, we often do so because we would want the same help if the situation were reversed. In other words, we are intimately familiar with our own intrinsic worth, the depth and breadth of joy and suffering we can experience. *Agape* is a recognition that all humans share in those capacities. Popularized primarily through Christianity, *agape* is understood as bestowal of value (Helm, 2017, para 5), which means it is a type of love that creates value in its object. Our care and concern for ourselves, our families, and our friends is responsive to features we find valuable in each of them, but by virtue of being human, we extend and bestow value to all of humanity.

A joke expresses *agape* in two ways. The first is simply by virtue of the joke teller's intention in telling the joke. For our purposes, it will suffice to define jokes broadly as, "something, such as a funny story or trick, that is said or done in order to make people laugh" (Cambridge University Press, n.d., para 1). Therefore, someone telling a joke intends, in part, to make their audience laugh. Intentionally creating joy in others simply to brighten their day or improve their mood is an expression of *agape* that C. S. Lewis (1895 – 1963) called, "charity" or "gift-love" (Lewis, 1960, p. 82). The audience may not show their gratitude to the joke teller as they would when receiving a gift with a verbal, "thank-you," but their amusement confirms their appreciation all the same.

The second and commonly overlooked way a joke expresses *agape* is by virtue of the audience's experience of getting and enjoying the joke. While a joke that goes over well with an audience provides shared enjoyment, it also creates connection through commonalities shared by the audience and anticipated by the joke teller. The audience derives pleasure in finding a joke humorous, and the joke teller enjoys successfully bringing this about in the audience (Cambridge University Press, n.d.). Although the experience is different for the joke teller and the audience, it is all derived from the joke teller's ability to accurately predict what the audience will find humorous. Building on Lewis' (1960) analogy, a joke is like a gift in this way. There is joy in both giving a gift and in receiving a gift. There is greater joy when you accurately predict what someone will like, but even if you fail at giving a good gift, we tell ourselves, "it's the thought that counts."

Despite its overuse, this platitude is correct for both gift giving and joke telling. The thought behind a gift and a joke is all important. Gifting my wife a vacuum for Mother's Day is a bad idea. In fact, there is no good occasion to gift my wife a vacuum. If I know her, then I should know to celebrate her with a fun experience, like a trip to the beach. Similarly, I should also know when she will not find a joke humorous. This is how a good joke can be intimate. It reflects the joke teller's understanding of their audience. You can joke more with friends because you know and understand them better. An audience experiences *agape* through a joke because the joke reflects the joke teller's assumptions and understanding of the audience. From the audience's perspective, getting a joke feels like the joke teller really gets your sense of humor and who you are as a person. And so, it is true, "the thought does count," but it is the thought that connects that matters.

Importantly, connecting through joke telling is reciprocal. The audience has a part to play, and so, telling a joke to make someone feel better depends on their willingness to participate. Engaging the joke takes mental effort. An audience must follow along to find the humor in a joke's "punchline," which is particularly difficult when the audience doesn't know a joke is being told. For example, to successfully deploy sarcasm in a conversation, your audience needs to understand that an assertion you are making is inconsistent with what you actually believe or endorse (Literary Devices, 2020, para 1). Oscar Wilde (1854 – 1900) is often quoted as having said, "Sarcasm is the lowest form of *wit* but the highest form of intelligence," and while I never understood what he meant, it struck me as *apropos* here (Literary Devices, 2020, para 4). It illustrates that the less a person knows you, the more difficult it is to know when you are being sarcastic. If you want to be sarcastic with people you don't know, you need to use more inflection in your voice to indicate the facetious nature of your remarks. I was, for example, being sarcastic and ironic when I wrote, "…and while I never understood what he meant, it struck me as *apropos* here." Although, it is next to impossible to tell unless you know me well or I ham-handedly point it out in subsequent text.

Another popular form of humor that depends on the audience's mental acuity is deadpan humor. Deadpan humor occurs when we deliberately make humorous remarks in a sterile, emotionless manner (Cambridge University Press, para 1). If the audience believes the joke teller is speaking earnestly, they will miss the joke. The audience must actively suspend their disbelief to understand that the seriousness of the spoken word is funny precisely because the content is amusing or absurd. A faculty member may successfully engage in deadpan humor among colleagues and yet, as often happens, have no such endorsement among their students. For example, strapping twenty babies to a car to create a "baby-bumper" is a horrific idea to consider. Yet, it makes a humorous example. The absurd and horrific nature of the example makes it humorous to some people, precisely because we are not taking it seriously. The audience must be engaged and connect with the joke teller as well. They must play their part to share in the humorous experience.

Arguably, the reciprocal nature of telling jokes bolsters the connection created between a joke teller and their audience. While the joke teller makes the effort to connect and understand the audience in order to create for them a humorous joke, the audience affirms that connection by understanding the joke. Subtly and repeatedly over time this creates rapport and intimacy between the audience and the comedian. On stage, a great comedian will tell jokes for hundreds of strangers, and those that reciprocate are bound to like the comedian as though they were a close friend they have yet to meet.

Case: RIP 2855, Live, Love, Joke

Positive human connection is an obvious upshot of having humor in our lives, so functionally, humor can be used as a tool to make people closer and their lives better. In framing her husband's narrative,

Response

Dr. Elena Gabor highlights the irony of a husband who is the picture of health, maintains a healthy lifestyle, but who would otherwise be dead if not for double coronary bypass surgery. According to Elena, the expression "image of health" has become something of a "cautionary joke." A humorous anecdote warning against a cavalier assessment of one's health based on one's lifestyle. Arriving at a hospital emergency room only to learn an unanticipated heart surgery is in the immediate future, the Gabors' experience would have been frightening for anyone. On a daily basis, many healthcare workers experience the events in our lives that we are never fully prepared to confront, so the Gabors' experience was not unique. It was, nevertheless, shocking for them.

Elena's cautionary joke probably originated as something of an inside joke initially shared among family and close friends. Including it in this book, framing Octavian's personal experience, the joke will resonate with others who have experienced something similar, and it may serve a small comfort to someone who finds themselves similarly positioned. Sharing the joke to a broad audience of readers, shares and connects the Gabor's experience with anyone willing to relate and engage. A shared experience neatly packaged in a joke goes a long way to initiating a space for connection and comfort.

Octavian Gabor's effort to share something humorous with his nurse was an expression of *agape*. Octavian's armband was not particularly remarkable on its own. As he points out, there very well may have been 2854 others before him who bore the mark of RIP. However, they may not have been in the hospital for life threatening reasons. Others may have seen it, noticed the RIP, and dismissed the coincidence as unworthy of additional intellectual attention. Each of us finds humor in different things, which makes our senses of humor unique expressions of our character. Furthermore, it is revealing that Octavian shares his experience, along with the humorous other questions that initially sprung to his mind. In a hospital, it is not unusual to experience some anxiety over any potential indicator that the end may be near, and he had plenty of time to ruminate over what the armband may have foretold. In the moment, in the hospital, just prior to surgery, thoughts we would otherwise dismiss as irrational tend to take on an outsized role in our thinking. It is, nevertheless, funny that we had them. Sharing those thoughts with others, especially when they are ridiculous, is a form of self-effacing humor that is humble, relatable, and connects people. Perhaps even more so when you are a professor of philosophy, since the job is anything but relatable.

In the spirit of *agape* and self-improvement, it is worth revisiting Octavian's interaction with the technician nurse. He says, "There is one more aspect of it. She was a woman, I was a man. She was black, I was white. All of them reasons to create distance between us," which seems like a joke because there are clearly two aspects and possibly a third in the nurse-patient dynamic. But seriously, this is a situation where it's reasonable to be concerned about using humor in healthcare or the workplace more broadly. Power dynamics can transform a person with a terrible sense of humor into the most hilarious person in the room. Race, sex, gender, religion, ethnicity, occupation, etc. can play a massive role in how a person responds to your use of humor, and there are at least three of these aspects present in the situation. The technician nurse may placate those patients who tell her yet another RIP armband joke, feeling unable to respond the way she actually feels for fear of reprisal.

I think it would be unfair to assume that any aspect other than shared humanity played a role in Octavian's scenario with the technician, but it is certainly important to be mindful of these dynamics when we use humor. Our efforts at *agape* through humor—especially repeated efforts—can cause discomfort and even suffering if we aren't actually connecting with the audience. As we have seen, successfully using jokes to express *agape* begins and ends with knowing your audience, which includes the social context within which the joke is uttered. If we aren't being sensitive to that, then we are failing to connect with very important aspects of our audience's identity. Beyond knowing your audience and a sensitivity to the social context within which the joke is told, the last crucial recommendation for using humor or jokes in healthcare is practice. The best jokes seem natural because they are practiced. Practicing a joke or two gives you an opportunity to test it. It can help you get a sense of the type of person who finds it humorous and the circumstances that are best suited for its use. And whether your audience knows it or not, the time you invest in perfecting your jokes is ultimately time you've invested in making others happy.

Octavian made an effort to connect and lift the spirits of the person who was there to ensure his health and safety. Regardless of whether he was funny, his act was an expression of *agape*. Nevertheless, the joke played an important role. In his retelling of events, Octavian says, "Rest in Peace 2855," when he shows the armband to the nurse, which is important, because there is very little context for the technician to indicate Octavian is trying to bring some levity to her life. Beyond that, the technician must make sense of the joke for herself, like solving a puzzle. We already know Octavian is expressing *agape* simply because he is trying to make the technician feel better, but the joke does this by revealing shared assumptions and possibly hidden similarities. Clearly, RIP is an unfortunate reminder of death for someone who just underwent heart surgery. When the technician gets the joke, she shares Octavian's thoughts and humorous experience. What is more, Octavian anticipated the technician's response, because he made accurate assumptions about the way she was like him, sensitive to the irony of the circumstances. Ultimately, the nurse technician experienced someone successfully relating to her, because Octavian accurately predicted she would find the armband humorous.

Telling a joke respects an audience's competence to get it on their own, which is why people are bothered when you try to explain a joke to them. In getting the joke, the audience confirms the comedian's assumptions. But, more importantly for an expression of *agape*, it demonstrates to the audience that the comedian believed they were capable of getting the joke and that the joke was gifted to them for their enjoyment. When you tell a joke, you are trusting the audience will figure it out on their own. When you get a joke, you confirm that the trust was well placed. Octavian shows *agape* for the technician through the joke. In the act of telling the joke, he expresses trust and respect and demonstrates how they share a similar sense of humor.

PUNCHLINE DEAD AHEAD

Jokes can go wrong and often do. But good or bad, telling a joke like Octavian's still demonstrates a level of trust and respect for his nurse, which is to say nothing of the very real intention he had to try to cheer her up. Even if he had not noticed she was sad, he would have still expressed *agape* through the joke. Whoever tells a joke may have nothing but selfish motives for doing so, but ultimately, the comedian's motives make little difference. Their ability to connect with the audience through humor is what matters, even if that connection is disingenuous. The audience's experience only depends on whether they get the joke and find it funny. The only time the audience has reason to question the comedian's motives for telling a joke is when the joke offends them. Then they may want to know if the offence was intentional.

So, what exactly is the risk of telling a joke in a healthcare environment? In some cases derogatory humor or humor that ridicules a patient or target an individual can create problems. Such humor can distance a health care worker from the patient and thus decrease the (Aultman, 2009; Morreall, 2009). These findings comport well with other research on the use of divisive or derogatory humor (Meyer, 2000). It can also create room for an impression among patients and health care providers that those environments where derogatory humor is used are less welcoming places (Wear et al., 2008). On the other hand, you might make someone laugh, which will not only bring a smile to their face but also express respect and connection with them (Anderson, 2015). Of course, you may also offend them or make them feel as though you are being flippant in a situation they find very serious. This result is bad for the audience, and some audience members will no doubt work to make the result bad for the joke teller. However, an accurate analysis of jokes and the way they express *agapeic* love, illustrates why this should not be the case. Again, every joke starts with some intention on behalf of the comedian to make the audience laugh, along with some assessment of the character and capacities of the audience.

A joke offends when there is a misalignment of the comedian's assumptions about the audience and what is actually true of the audience. Offence occurs when the audience thinks to themselves, "why would you think that I would find that funny?" People take the joke personally, because it trivialized or demeaned something they hold dear. This sends an openly hostile message: "What I think you care about is dumb." In a case of an offensive joke that was unintentional, the joke teller has misunderstood the audience, and the audience is upset about being mischaracterized. Misunderstandings of the audience also occur when we use a form of humor the audience feels is "beneath" them, like sarcasm, dick jokes, or slap-stick.

In many circumstances, the act of telling a joke is an attempt at connection. As we've seen, the problem arises when we make incorrect assumptions about the person's sensibilities. Throughout this essay, telling a joke is described as an interplay between the comedian and the audience, and one of the first assumptions an audience member must understand to get a joke, is that a joke is being told. Once that happens, the audience should also understand that it is implied by the very act of telling a joke that the joke teller is trying to make them laugh. In other words, the joke—offensive or not—is presumed by the audience to be for their benefit. The fact that it offends them bears not on the fact that it was intended for their benefit.

When we stifle our joke telling because we are concerned that people will be offended, we are assuming that an audience's offence at a joke indicates we have wronged them somehow. Based on the preceding analysis quite the contrary is true. The fact that we were telling them a joke is evidence that we were trying to connect and bring them some happiness. That we misjudged the person's sensibilities simply means we didn't know them well enough, not that we intended to offend or are generally offensive. You can, of course, keep to jokes that require very few assumptions about your audience, but that also reduces the number of personal connections you can make with them. It also tends to produce awkward or just plain bad jokes. To connect and to show compassion, sometimes you must risk making assumptions about your audience. At minimum, if the assumptions are based on a shared humanity, the only people who will be offended are those who quite literally don't get the joke.

It may seem like the safest bet is to refrain from humor in a healthcare environment. No jokes mean no chance of offending someone with your jokes. Simple though the math may be, the reasoning behind it is akin to never undergoing treatment so you will never experience any side effects. The reasoning is also based on a false assumption. It assumes avoiding offense from not telling jokes is a better way to treat people than telling jokes that could potentially offend them. In truth, whether you risk telling the joke or refrain from telling the joke, you are making assumptions about your audience. In refraining from telling a joke, you are assuming your audience isn't capable of getting it or incapable of recognizing your well-meaning intentions if you accidentally offend them. In telling the joke, you assume your audience can get the joke or will at least understand you meant well even if the joke offends. The former understanding of the patient or colleague is patronizing and paternalistic, while the latter is trusting, respectful, and expresses *agape*. Spoiler: I prefer the latter from my healthcare providers.

So taking this all together, what can healthcare practitioners take away from this case? Overall, there are three important messages to remember:

1. Be bold enough to attempt humor as part of your patient care. One of the important aspects of *agape* and humor is that they are parts of how we reach out and connect with folks.
2. Expect that not every joke you attempt with your patients will land, and recognize that when humor fails, it's because you have misread something about your patient and need to clarify that you were attempting humor. This also opens up more avenues of communication. Even a failed joke can lead to a closer connection when you try to find out why the person didn't like it.
3. Likewise, recognize that when patients attempt to use humor with you, regardless of whether you find the humor to be funny, that they are attempting to connect, which is as much self-care as care for you.

The base of all of these is *agape,* which is a fundamental component of care.

REFERENCES

Anderson, G. (2015). Humor in treatment is no joke. *ASHA Leader, 20*(7). Advance online publication. doi:10.1044/leader.HYTT.20072015.np

Aultman, J. M. (2009). When humor in the hospital is no laughing matter. *The Journal of Clinical Ethics, 20*(3), 227–234. PMID:19845193

Cabridge University Press. (n.d.). Joke. In *Cambridge English dictionary*. https://dictionary.cambridge.org/us/dictionary/english/joke

Cambridge University Press. (n.d.). Deadpan. In *Cambridge English dictionary*. https://dictionary.cambridge.org/us/dictionary/english/deadpan

Creative Commons. (2016, November 8). *5.1 why conduct an audience analysis*. https://open.lib.umn.edu/publicspeaking/chapter/5-1-why-conduct-an-audience-analysis/

HelmB. (2017, August 11). *Love*. https://plato.stanford.edu/entries/love/

Lewis, C. S. (2017). *The four loves*. HarperOne.

Literary Devices Editors. (2020, November 12). *Sarcasm - definition and examples of sarcasm*. https://literarydevices.net/sarcasm/

Meyer, J. (2000). Humor as a double-edged sword: Four functions of humor in communication. *Communication Theory, 10*(3), 310–331. doi:10.1111/j.1468-2885.2000.tb00194.x

Response

Morreall, J. (2009). *Comic relief.* Wiley Blackwell. doi:10.1002/9781444307795

Wear, D., Aultman, J., Zarconi, J., & Varley, J. (2008). Derogatory and cynical humour directed towards patients: Views of residents and attending doctors. *Medical Education*, *43*(1), 34–41. doi:10.1111/j.1365-2923.2008.03171.x PMID:19148979

Chapter 17
"Your Doctor is Right": Using Humor to Manage Uncertainty With Unknown Illnesses

R. Tyler Spradley
https://orcid.org/0000-0002-4026-9755
Stephen F. Austin State University, USA

My story begins a little more than a dozen years ago when a bone scan performed to discover underlying causes of pain resulted in images of extreme bone loss throughout my body. As a result, I was diagnosed with *osteoporosis in a young male*, which is rare and not a primary disease. Much to my concern, the diagnosis led me to transformations from patient to guinea pig, moving from doctor to doctor and expert to expert. The anxiety of referral after referral is not an inviting emotion. All I wanted was a clear cause and path to recovery. Afterall, is not the purpose of medicine to heal? I wanted to be on with my life and back out on the streets running and biking and in the pool swimming. Pain and fragile bones are not conducive to outdoor living nor performing triathlons. I have work to do as a professor. I could not help but feel an emptiness, "What was wrong with me?"

Only time and the presence of other aliments would connect my chronic kidney stone production to the bone loss. Essentially, the rapid overturning of bone production results in the formation of hypercalciuria, elevated calcium in the kidneys and chronic kidney disease. With renal stones forming as a result of the hypercalciuria, the health of my kidneys became an alarming concern. Yet, leaving no stone unturned, osteoporosis and chronic kidney disease were just the beginning. In the years to follow, a team of doctors would perform whole genomic sequencing to try to find an underlying genetic abnormality for the state of my health along with a bone biopsy extracted from my spine. The tests resulted in a variety of markers that could point to similar conditions, but no genetic markers really stood out as the root cause. You have a real hell of a war when you add lifelong battles with allergies and eosinophilic asthma and a dose of fibromyalgia to explain the multiple points of pain, brain fog, and depression. Top doctors at major research hospitals still believe all of these aliments to be secondary to a unifying primary issue,

DOI: 10.4018/978-1-7998-4528-7.ch017

which is most likely a rare disease with no name. What about this health war of mine could possibly be humorous?

In the absence of meaningful prognoses, pain became the enemy and these secondary issues became the daily battles that would come to define my health and my feelings of hopelessness. At times I would cry in despair, and other times I would just laugh at the unbearable nature of the situation. The absence of a technical primary diagnosis is not a peaceful or funny health situation. Nevertheless, in all the struggles, there have been three humorous phrases that have brought laughter and clarity in clinical encounters.

First, Dr. Anderson, head of internal medicine at a world-renowned research hospital is the lead investigator and specializes in bone health under the banner of endocrinology. His expertise has provided a baseline for fighting my unknown illness by addressing bone loss and low growth hormone levels. At one visit, Dr. Anderson began discussing results from various tests. His conclusion could be summarized in his quick-witted retort, "You are disappearing before my eyes." We chuckled as he proceeded to share the results that over a span of a couple of years my bone density decreased at uncanny rates. The thought of becoming boneless was not a pleasant thought and elicited a slightly cartoonish image of me. The humorous phrase brought with it a clearer understanding of the gravity of my condition and began to provide a sense of reality to all the questions that go with undiagnosed primary health conditions. For those who lack experience in the war with the unknown, having moments where observable data is presented to prove you are not imagining all the pain are often as meaningful as a clear disease name. For a brief moment, the fact that I was disappearing before the eyes of experts comforted me because I had a nameable disease, even if it was secondary.

Second, when new secondary symptoms arose that resulted in diplopia, I was referred to a neuro-ophthalmologist Dr. Houston at another prominent research hospital. After introductions and discussion of test results, he turned to my wife and asked for her diagnosis. Seemingly befuddled, my wife quipped back, "I just think his body does not like him." As if an epiphany occurred, Dr. Houston simply exclaimed, "Your doctor is right!" It was clear he was referring to my wife, who is a Ph.D., not an M.D. With the humorous method, Dr. Houston simply affirmed that, as my wife said, "My body does not like my body." Whether the daily pain, the migraines, the fragility of body, or, in this case, diplopia, I can testify there is most certainly a problem. Now, the problem was not the seemingly endless list of secondary diseases; instead, the problem all along has been me. That's right, my disease is myself. Unfortunately, that is not a confidence booster or vote for the sanest in the room. If anything, I felt like a bifurcated body and soul - a product of dissection. My body hates me. Give a chuckle, but I am in a war here. Of course, with all the adjectives asides, my immune system thinks healthy parts of my body are invaders.

Lastly, another visit with Dr. Houston provided the final humorous comment that has uniquely framed my war with myself, "One day, we will find out what causes Spradley syndrome." The final humorous comment, and most recent, occurred during the COVID-19 pandemic as we met through telemedicine on a phone call. Across the airwaves, Dr. Houston reached out and touched us by making us all laugh. The laughs constituted a material reality: knowing the primary cause of these continuing health battles is not at an end. As with the pandemic, the unknown is the known. Yet, a few laughs have provided more clarity in contemplating and conversing about the war in my body that has me pinned down to a bed many days in recent months. Whether in jest or in making sense, Dr. Anderson and Dr. Houston offered knowing in the form of laughter and sober reality. Along the way, I have a list of phrases and cracks to assist me in answering the casual questions, "What is wrong with you'"

Chapter 18

Response: "'Your Doctor is Right': Using Humor to Manage Uncertainty With Unknown Illness"

Elizabeth L. Spradley
Stephen F. Austin State University, USA

LITERATURE REVIEW

Having read "Your Doctor is Right!" written by R. Tyler Spradley, this case response is distinctively composed by one who had a front row seat for all three instances of physician humor. I am, if you did not already surmise, the spouse, and as both spouse and health communication scholar, I have a unique vantage point to weigh in on both the patient-provider humor and the relevant literature. To contextualize,

My version of "Your doctor is right!" begins slightly over twenty years ago when my husband and I became engaged. I was riding with his mother to deliver a wedding cake to a wedding venue and sneak a peek at what could be our wedding venue at the end of the year. She was telling me a story about him as we drove. Then, she paused, and quite seriously she said, "You should know. Strange things happen to his health." I laughed it off as I was marrying a very healthy young man who had recently been an active triathlete.

Fast forward twenty years, scores of doctors practicing in the best research hospitals, and countless diagnostic testing and imaging, I have a bit more inkling what she meant. However, her humor is not the humor to be analyzed.

Patient-provider humor literature indicates that patients and providers initiate humor in their clinical interactions most often pertaining to the patient's health condition (Phillips et al., 2018). This speaks to the content of healthcare humor; however, the literature to be reviewed speaks more to the function of healthcare humor. Humor can function to break the ice, provide cathartic release, identify/relate with

DOI: 10.4018/978-1-7998-4528-7.ch018

one another, engage in face saving correction, and draw attention to or introduce a difficult message (Phillips et al., 2018; Schöpf et al., 2017). While the outcomes of humor run the gamut between positive and negative, healthcare humor scholarship demonstrates that humor is both frequent and useful for providers and patients alike. This section further examines the functionality of humor with regard to managing emotions, uncertainty, and relationships. This case analysis centers on patient-provider humor and three case-specific intersecting topics: dark humor, uncertainty management, and narrative medicine. As healthcare providers aim to use humor artfully and skillfully, this case study analysis illustrates how humor may enhance the communicative management of emotions, uncertainty, and relationships.

Using Dark Humor to Manage Emotions

Emotion management poses a communicative challenge for healthcare interactions, especially given the gravity of circumstances that oft surround them. Francis (1994) work posited the value of humor as an interpersonal approach to manage emotions. From this perspective, Francis (1994) argued that humor demonstrated expert cultural performance, strengthened or restored norms, generated positive emotions, and provided a way to exclude some persons, events, or things. Francis et al. (1999) extended this work focusing their data collection on a hospital setting to study the effectiveness of humor at eliciting an emotional shift. The authors emphasize that healthcare interactions including conversations about severe, life-threatening, disabling, and chronic conditions generate intense negative emotions for which humor may be an effective emotion-focused communication strategy. Thus far, much of the research reviewed has foregrounded positive outcomes associated with therapeutic humor, but what about dark humor and its ability to manage emotion?

Dark humor in healthcare settings is typically associated with morbid health statuses and consequences, and for this case, dark humor excludes the taboo (c.f., Tomlinson, 2015). Scholarship in this area tends to feature provider-provider instances or patient-initiated instances of dark humor rather than patient-provider instances of dark humor. In Cain's (2012) analysis of hospice providers, participant observation of backstage behaviors – those behaviors performed out of view from the public including patients and their loved ones – featured dark humor. Hospice providers joked about death, even their own deaths, laughing about cremation preferences. These backstage uses of dark humor were primarily used in provider-provider communication. In Dean and Gregory's (2005) study of humor in palliative care, they noted several different types of humor including dark humor. Their observations of dark humor occurred when patients introduced humor referencing their terminal status. For example, Dean and Gregory (2005) include a patient's use of dark humor in their article, "Someone said to me, 'You need to get a life.' I said, 'In my condition, that's a great idea! Do you know where I could get one? Could you loan me yours?'" (p. 294). In comparison to therapeutic humor, the work on dark humor is scant in healthcare scholarship, and especially, with regard to patient-provider communication and provider-initiated dark humor. Yet, as Cain (2012) and Dean and Gregory (2005) indicate, dark humor plays a functional role in emotion management, therefore implying its plausible functions for managing emotions in patient-provider communication.

Using Humor to Manage Uncertainty

When problems are knowable and controllable, coping energy is most effectively directed at the solution, but when problems are unknown, uncertain, or uncontrollable, coping may focus on stress relief as a means to manage uncertainty (Brinkmann, 2019; Francis et al., 1999). Uncertainty is a term used by a number of scholars varying in its implications. In Berger and Calabrese' (1975) work with uncertainty reduction theory, uncertainty is conceptualized as a cognitive state resulting from the lack of information to assess an individual's behavior in social situations. This iteration of uncertainty neglects emotional dimensions in favor of cognitive dimensions. Then, in the work of Babrow (2001) and colleagues with problematic integration theory, uncertainty is treated as a broader and more complex construct, extending its applications beyond interpersonal relational contexts to include an assessment of an outcome, event, or attribute (Bradac, 2001). Whereas, uncertainty reduction theory's use of the term insinuates a parallel between uncertainty and ambiguity. This theory asserts that uncertainty is assessed as a "bad" state, subsequently, motivating individuals to reduce it (Bradac, 2001). In these different uses of the construct, the underlying assumptions related to uncertainty are that it is perceived negatively and should be reduced through some cognitive or social activity. However, critics have inquired, "Is uncertainty reduction always the best communication goal?"

To unpack what is meant by uncertainty in healthcare interactions, attention turns to Babrow's (2001) extensive scholarship on uncertainty and the problematic integration theory, which has been primarily applied in healthcare contexts and to patient-provider communication. Uncertainty typifies illness as Babrow et al. (2000) point out,

Illness raises questions about how the body will feel and perform; about how relationships with others will change; and most generally, about who we are in the world, what we are doing, and where our life is going (p. 42).

Given uncertainty's persistent presence in healthcare contexts, Babrow et al. (1998) offer a typology of uncertainty as insight into its complexity and functionality in patient-provider communication. They identify five types of uncertainty: 1) illness-related complexities, 2) quality of illness information including sufficiency, reliability, and validity, 3) decision-making capacity or judgment to affect outcomes termed probabilistic formulations, 4) integration or structuring of information, and 5) subjectivity of certainty. The complexity and pervasiveness of uncertainty makes it germane to patient-provider interactions; yet, humor remains an underexplored means by which patients and providers can manage their uncertainties.

Using Humor to Relate In Narrative Medicine

Patient and relationship-centered approaches to patient-provider communication have advanced a more participative and interactive perspective on the more traditionally power-imbalanced, didactic relationship. One such approach within this body of literature is narrative medicine. Pioneered by the scholarship and practice of Charon (2001), narrative medicine is no longer a fringe approach to patient-provider communication. Instead, narrative medicine certificates, workshops, and classes are integrated into medical education. As such, narrative medicine asserts that healthcare communication is inherently storied, and healthcare providers may use narrative skills (otherwise referred to as competencies) to elicit and respond to patient stories (Charon, 2001).

Humor healthcare scholarship is negligible within the body of narrative medicine literature, unless you include fiction, nonfiction, or field note pieces in medical humanities journals or a special section of the *Journal of the American Medical Association*. In these personal stories of health, the author may introduce humor into the storyline, maybe to reflect the actual dialogue or situation deemed humorous or maybe as a writing technique to appeal to readers. While humor is novel rather than the norm in narrative medicine literature, there is a body of literature on humor in patient-centeredness that is applicable. Patient-centered studies that focus on humor demonstrate that humor can reduce social distance and increase perceived immediacy between patients and providers (Coser, 1959; Scholl, 2007), enhance patient's active participation in clinical encounters (Davidhizar & Shearer, 1996), and facilitate greater patient satisfaction with their healthcare experiences (Sala et al., 2002) resulting in positive affect between patient and provider (Scholl, 2007). Therefore, it stands to reason that the role of humor in these patient-centered studies may also apply to narrative medicine. Humor may play a role in narrative competencies as providers listen to the ways patients use humor in their illness stories and respond with situationally appropriate humor that enhances feelings of affiliation between the patient and provider.

The Communicative Accomplishment of Managing Emotions, Uncertainty, And Relationships

Just as the patient-provider relationship is constructed through their communication with one another, patient-provider humor patterns are constructed through their communication. Patients and their healthcare providers verbally and nonverbally exchange messages that comprise their relational histories, and, in their message exchanges, patients and providers inject humorous messages into their interactions. As Scholl (2002) indicates, the communication exchanges that comprise the patient-provider relational context impact the use and perception of humor. When a patient or provider communicates using humor for the first time, a precedence occurs. If positively perceived by the other person in the communication exchange, then it is likely that reciprocity will occur. Reciprocity is a communicative response. When a communicator uses a message type or strategy such as humor, reciprocity occurs when the receiver responds, not necessarily immediately, with a similar message type or strategy. While Burgoon and colleagues (1993) have developed more operationalized and nuanced ways of measuring and applying the term reciprocity, it is generally understood that reciprocity in interpersonal interactions could elicit either negative or positive communication responses, thus cautioning patients and providers in considering how humor is perceived and reciprocated by one another.

Additionally, as patients and providers reciprocate humorous messages their communication patterns resemble what Giles (2016) refers to as convergence in his theory Communication Accommodation Theory. Applying Giles work to patient-provider communication, Haidet (2007) discusses how providers may converge with patients' communication messages and strategies for delivering those messages, which could be matching humor with humor. However, providers may diverge with their patients' communication messages and strategies to change the content, tone, or direction of a conversation whilst still communicating within a set of messages that compliments the patient-provider relationship and communicative history. Haidet points out how divergence may occur as providers choose to diverge from the topic at hand to explore an observation such as shortness of breath. In the context of humor, the first person to use humor is diverging from previous patterns and may find that the other reciprocates to converge communication patterns through humor, or the divergence may not be reciprocated.

In sum, humor's vital function in managing emotions through dark humor, managing uncertainties, and relating through narrative medicine are scant threads in the patient-provider literature and are dependent on the communication that constructs the patient-provider relationship. In the case study presented, the patient-provider humor in question demonstrates that these scant threads may be instrumental in understanding certain healthcare relational dynamics and positive coping.

CASE ANALYSIS

Shifting the focus back to the case, the following section examines Dr. Anderson's dark humor and Dr. Houston's affirming humor more closely.

Dr. Anderson's Dark Humor: "You Are Disappearing Before My Eyes."

When faced with delivering the bad news that bone density was rapidly depleting rather than improving, Dr. Anderson used dark humor, bordering on the ridiculous, through his quick-witted comment, "You are disappearing before my eyes." While some patients and providers may have shied away from riskier dark humor as it is more associated with backstage provider-provider communication (Cain, 2012; Tomlinson, 2015), Dr. Anderson's comment rolled off his tongue with ease and resulted in amusement just as quickly as the utterance was out of his mouth. Osteoporosis was not life-threatening, as many dark humor references make jest of, but it was life-altering. The noted bone loss generates increased risk of fracture, longer healing times, greater risk of complications (including death) from fracture, and other related problems including bone pain (Ebeling, 2008). Dark humor was assessed as productive along two different functions: clarifying and comforting. First, the case study notes this reaction to the dark humor, "The humorous phrase brought with it a clearer understanding of the gravity of my condition and began to provide a sense of reality to all the questions that go with undiagnosed primary health conditions."

In addition to clarity, the dark humor elicited a strange, possibly antithetical for some, outcome – comfort. Throughout the case, we learn more and more about the mysterious nature of the patient's health condition. When reflecting on Dr. Anderson's dark humor, R. Tyler Spradley comments, "For a brief moment, the fact that I was disappearing before the eyes of experts comforted me because I had a nameable disease, even if it was secondary." Osteoporosis was an identifiable disease. It had a name – a label. It had diagnostic testing that could confirm its physiological presence in his body. In other words, osteoporosis was more concrete and, even if for a moment, gave the patient a sense of legitimacy for what he was feeling and his extent of testing. Juxtaposing the osteoporosis to the unknown primary disease causing it, the patient takes comfort in what is knowable. He may not be able to tell people what is causing the osteoporosis, but when people ask what is wrong, he can tell them he has osteoporosis.

Dr. Houston's Affirming Humor: "Your Doctor is Right" and "One Day We Will Find Out What Causes Spradley Syndrome."

When faced with no determinate causal relationships for test results and the symptoms, Dr. Houston, on two different occasions, used humor to acknowledge uncertainty and affirm probabilistic associations (Babrow, 2001) that the patient and his spouse asserted to manage uncertainty. "One day we will find out what causes Spradley syndrome," is reminiscent of the uncertainty related to illness information – the lack of an inclusive, unifying diagnosis – and probabilistic formulations – the diagnosis exists but has not been formalized through evidence-based medicine. Still, humor is not functioning in either case to reduce uncertainty per say. Instead, humor is functioning to acknowledge it, which in and of itself, is a communicative approach to managing uncertainty. Oft when we think of uncertainty management, we think of uncertainty reduction. In the field of communication, theories, like uncertainty reduction theory and uncertainty management theory referenced above in the literature, reinforce the association between the perceptual existence of uncertainty and the behavioral response of reduction (Bradac, 2001). The underlying assumption is that uncertainty tends to produce negative emotions and outcomes, and thus, individuals seek to reduce uncertainty. Uncertainty reduction is accomplished through a variety of indirect and direct information seeking behaviors. Instead, this case demonstrates the value of uncertainty. Humor transforms the way uncertainty is perceived. Through humor, uncertainty is not reduced, but it is acknowledged. There is a cathartic release when the doctor acknowledged the war with the unknown.

In this case, rather than offer either absolutes or conjectures about a unifying diagnosis that would have reduced uncertainty, the physician elected to use humor to acknowledge the uncertain underlying causes of the patient's symptoms. In doing so, the interaction shifted from information seeking-providing to legitimacy seeking-granting. To clarify, consider the situation once more. It is a telemedicine visit evaluating extant diagnostic testing, symptoms, and other physicians' notes on the patient. The physician asks a series of questions, and the patient provides a series of answers. Repeat. Overall all, the interactional exchange features information seeking, gathering, and providing that should reduce both the provider's uncertainty about the patient's condition and the patient's uncertainty about diagnosis, symptoms, and treatment. But, this case features a different kind of interaction. The patient chooses to feature how Dr. Houston humorizes uncertainty and how the humor pointed to what everyone already knew – there was no definitive or diagnostically evident unifying explanation for the diplopia or other symptoms. Yet, that did not negate the patient's experience or suffering. Dr. Houston drew on humor as a means to acknowledge the patient's experience, lighten the frustration of the moment, and point to a probabilistic, even if unverifiable, future diagnosis.

An initial reaction may assume that the humor exacerbates uncertainty, negatively impacts patient-physician confidence, and diminishes the patient's coping. That is not accurate in this instance and likely not so for others experiencing similar humor. What made the humor "work" or "function" constructively is hinted at in several different ways in the case. First, this is not the first instance of humor for this patient-provider relationship. The relational history and patterns of communication suggest that humor will be received positively by the patient. Second, the humor's direction and content do not denigrate or evaluate the patient; instead, the humor is directed at the illness rather than the person with its content creating a probabilistic evaluation. Finally, the humor addresses patient uncertainty through acknowledgement. Given these factors, humor provided a constructive communicative strategy for the physician.

Dr. Houston's use of humor was described in another instance as well. Now, reconsider how the patient cognitively and emotionally appraises the "Your doctor is right" humor.

Now, the problem was not the seemingly endless list of secondary diseases; instead, the problem all along has been me. That's right, my disease is myself. Unfortunately, that is not a confidence booster or vote for the sanest in the room. If anything, I felt like a bifurcated body and soul - a product of dissection. My body hates me. Give a chuckle, but I am in a war here. Of course, with all the adjectives asides, my immune system thinks healthy parts of my body are invaders.

The patient's reaction to "Your doctor is right," is reflective. The patient ponders what it means to have a body that attacks itself – that is to have an unnamed auto-immune disease wreaking havoc across the body with the latest victim being muscles around the eyes resulting in diplopia. "Your doctor is right," invited reflection cathartically expresses the emotional and cognitive appraisal of embodied illness.

Additionally, this use of humor by Dr. Houston extended patient-provider communication to the patient's guest as a communicative act of inclusion. The guest became an active participant in healthcare communication and was affirmed as a positive, welcomed presence with valuable contributions to the clinical visit. Humor was a light-hearted way to include the guest without either over-emphasizing the guest's role or contribution or overshadowing the patient-provider's relational development and informational exchange. In considering Dr. Anderson's and Houston's humor, the constructive and functional role of humor was foregrounded in patient-provider and patient-guest-provider communication to fulfill emotional affirmation, uncertainty acknowledgment, and relational development.

LESSONS LEARNED FOR HEALTHCARE

Translating case-based evidence from analysis to practice, there are three applied recommendations to consider and implement: 1) relationally contextualized humor use, 2) acknowledgement or affirmation of uncertainty, and 3) narrative medicine competence.

Recommendation 1: Relationally Contextualized Humor Use

Patient-provider humor is widely cited for its role in managing healthcare relationships (Schöpf et al., 2017), and it is through relational contextualization that providers, and really patients and their guests too, should consider how the humor may be interpreted as it is received. As Dean and Gregory (2005) note in their study with palliative care humor, "Receptivity to humor clearly depend[s] on the individual and on the circumstances" (p. 296). Therefore, the first recommendation is to relationally contextualize humor use to enhance the probability of its receptivity. Francis, Monahan, and Berger (1999) suggest that humor choices account for a wide array of factors including: actors (e.g., statuses, relationship), content, culture, emotional outcomes, exclusions, norms, setting, and timing. In other words, given these factors, do you think that the use of humor will have the desired outcome? If you take a walk on humor's dark side, will the patient and the patient's guests find value in the humor?

Implementation of Recommendation 1: Look For Relational Patterns To Cue Humor

To put the first recommendation into practice, healthcare providers should consider the relational context with the patient and their guests, which may be years of regular appointments or the immediate interaction as it unfolds. In Scholl's (2002) words, "without adequate familiarity with the patient, it is difficult to know what a patient perceives as funny versus offensive" (p. 171). A wide range of strategies have been suggested to help with determining when and what type of humor to use in healthcare (c.f., Dean & Gregory, 2005). With that said, one of the most important considerations in implementation is to monitor the communication patterns of patients to determine if humor is among their communication strategies and when, where, why, and with whom are they using humor. Two terms come to mind stemming from the communicative accomplishment of managing emotions, uncertainty, and relationships section above: 1) reciprocity, which is matching messages as they are exchanged (Burgoon et al., 1993) and 2) convergence, which is adopting similar communication patterns in interaction episodes (Giles, 2016). Using reciprocity and convergence in healthcare interactions, providers have the relational context to help cue humor use. Furthermore, this is a good indicator of the appropriateness of dark humor in patient-provider communication as providers can use patient's interaction patterns with dark humor to cue the appropriateness of their own use.

Recommendation 2: Acknowledgement or Affirmation of Uncertainty

Considering uncertainty's complexity and pervasiveness in healthcare communication, it seems counterintuitive to avoid acknowledging or affirming uncertainty. Rather than ignoring, avoiding, or denying uncertainty, uncertainty-related humor is a path toward acknowledgement and affirmation. In the same way that Dr. Houston acknowledged the patient's uncertainty and legitimized the patient's suffering through humor, practitioners may similarly use humor. This example leads to the question, "How can humor be used in conjunction with other communication to acknowledge or affirm patients' uncertainty?"

Implementation of Recommendation 2: Address Uncertainty Directly, Through Humor

To this end, Berger et al.(2004) remind healthcare providers to use humor within a broader repertoire of communication strategies with patients. To implement humor with patients to address uncertainty, consider how humor may accompany other communication strategies like patient education or therapeutic communication. If accompanying a diversified set of patient communication strategies, humor is contextualized through them rather than isolated from them. Next, to implement humor with patients to address uncertainty, providers should consider their own vulnerability and power being willing to admit their limitations – limitations of themselves and medicine. Afterall, limited knowledge, practice, and technology further complicates uncertainty. Finally, to implement humor with patients to address uncertainty, there is value in understanding what type(s) of uncertainty the patient and their loved ones are trying to manage. Recall that Babrow et al.(1998) identified five uncertainty types reviewed in the literature section. Rather than assuming uncertainty type, consider asking patients a series of questions such as, "What do you wish you could know about ___________?" or "If you knew _________ this about the future, how would that effect your decision making?" In other words, ask probing questions to learn more about the uncertainty that is affecting the patient. This type of information may elicit different timing, types, and outcomes related to humor.

Recommendation 3: Narrative Medicine

As reviewed earlier, narrative medicine is a storied approach to understanding how health accounts are expressed and interpreted, especially in patient-provider interactions, and to accomplish its aims, narrative medicine practitioners apply a set of competencies intended to enrich their patient-provider relationships (Charon, 2005). Narrative medicine education and workshops hone in on three communication competencies: attentiveness, representation, and affiliation (Charon, 2001; 2005). First, attentiveness elicits patient storytelling through an invitation for patients to express who they are and their experiences, and attentiveness also involves active, empathic listening as providers consider storied accounts (Spradley, 2020). Second, representation occurs as providers, typically after the interaction that elicited storytelling, write about patients creating a narrative notation rather than or in addition to a traditional notation (Charon, 2005). Eventually, providers share narrative notations with patients as an open-ended communicative act that recognizes patients' voices, acknowledges their experiences, and welcomes continued storytelling. Third, affiliation describes the relational connection forged through vulnerable disclosure and collaborative storytelling catalyzing future narrative patient-provider communication (Charon, 2005). It is no stretch of the imagination to conceive of patients' storied accounts as plausibly infused with humor. Whether a quick witted pun, sarcasm, or dark humor, storied accounts are likely to be laced with the same type of humor documented in patient communication. Questions emerge, what do providers do with humor? How is humor elicited in the attention competency? How is humor represented in the narrative notation? What role does humor play in affiliation?

Implementation of Recommendation 3: Apply Humor Within Narrative Medicine Competencies

When healthcare providers heed the call to develop narrative medicine competencies, they usher in patient-provider relational transformations. Competencies are skills needed to appropriately and effectively perform an activity, and in this case, attention, representation, and affiliation competencies have been identified as narrative medicine competencies. In more intimate and trusting relational contexts, the communicative history and patterns enable practitioners to discern when, where, and how to use humor in conjunction with these competencies. In the attention competency, practitioners may use humor to break the ice to help patients feel at ease with sharing their illness stories. In the representation competency, providers may use light-hearted self-deprecating humor as they are forgiving with their own writing about patients or as they ask patients for feedback on their written accounts of the shared illness stories. In the affiliation competency, humor may emerge as a sign of relational satisfaction, strength, and trust. Or, it may be that humor takes a backseat to other communicative skills needed to achieve attention, representation, and affiliation because the relational history and patterns do not provide the contextual impetus for it. It is likely that the uniqueness of illness accounts and patient communication patterns will be diverse and complex eliciting a repertoire of equally diverse and complex skills, of which humor may be quite constructive.

CONCLUSION

In closing, humor's functionality in healthcare interactions has become a given, but that does not mean its execution *in situ* is without concern. To use humor artfully and skillfully, providers should consider how humor may enhance their communicative management of emotions, uncertainty, and relationships. The positive example of patient-provider humor offered by R. Tyler Spradley's case demonstrates that when a provider considers the relational context, acknowledges or affirms uncertainty, practices narrative medicine competence, and fulfills narrative desire, the humor may function more productively for the patient. The outcome of humor is not a smile, smirk, chuckle, or belly laugh, the outcome of humor is its communicative implications for the patient-provider relationship and its functionality for patients and their loved ones to better manage uncertainty and intense emotions that characterizes their lives.

Reflecting on this case in terms of one present in the interaction, in some regards, "Your doctor is right," felt affirming to me. Dr. Houston took the "I told you so" face-threatening statement that I dare not verbalize, and he made it funny. Not only that, Dr. Houston sought my opinion as the patient's guest, which affirmed my experiential knowledge and its value in the medial encounter. Humor drew me into the patient-provider communication, thus, transforming it from dyadic to group communication. Simultaneously, the humor affirmed the patient's concerns regarding his immune system's attacks on his organs. Despite Berger et al.'s (2004) warning to healthcare providers rethinking humor in the presence of a third person, Dr. Houston's humor was received with appreciation by both patient and guest. Not only that, Dr. Houston's humor disaffirmed the medical narrative that leads to definitive answers, which helped in the ongoing work of uncertainty and emotion management. We were not much more informed about my husband's condition than when we started the patient visit. Nevertheless, Dr. Houston affirmed, albeit in a humorous way, that medical knowledge takes many different forms and that my role in my husband's health is consequential even if it evades labeling.

REFERENCES

Babrow, A. S. (2001). Uncertainty, value, communication and problematic integration. *Journal of Communication, 51*(3), 553–573. doi:10.1111/j.1460-2466.2001.tb02896.x

Babrow, A. S., Hines, S. C., & Kasch, C. R. (2000). Managing uncertainty in illness explanation: An application of problematic integration theory. In B. B. Whaley (Ed.), *Explaining illness: Research, theory, and strategies* (pp. 41–67). Lawrence Erlbaum.

Babrow, A. S., Kasch, C. R., & Ford, L. A. (1998). The many meanings of uncertainty in illness: Toward a systematic accounting. *Health Communication, 10*(1), 1–23. doi:10.120715327027hc1001_1 PMID:16370987

Berger, C. R., & Calabrese, R. J. (1975). Some explorations in initial interaction and beyond: Toward a developmental theory of interpersonal communication. *Human Communication Research, 1*(2), 99–112. doi:10.1111/j.1468-2958.1975.tb00258.x

Berger, J. T., Coulehan, J., & Belling, C. (2004). Humor in the physician-patient encounter. *Archives of Internal Medicine, 164*(8), 825–830. doi:10.1001/archinte.164.8.825 PMID:15111367

Bradac, J. J. (2001). Theory comparison: Uncertainty reduction, problematic integration, uncertainty management, and other curious constructs. *Journal of Communication, 51*(3), 456–476. doi:10.1111/j.1460-2466.2001.tb02891.x

Brinkmann, J. T. (2019). Humor in clinical encounters: It's not about being funny. *The O&P Edge.* Retrieved from https://opedge.com/Articles/ViewArticle/2019-07-01/humor-in-clinical-encountersits-not-about-being-funny

Burgoon, J. K., Dillman, L., & Stem, L. A. (1993). Adaption in dyadic interaction: Defining and operationalizing patterns of reciprocity and compensation. *Communication Theory, 3*(4), 295–316. doi:10.1111/j.1468-2885.1993.tb00076.x

Cain, C. L. (2012). Integrating dark humor and compassion: Identities and presentations of self in the front and back regions of hospice. *Journal of Contemporary Ethnography, 41*(6), 668–694. doi:10.1177/0891241612458122

Charon, R. (2001). Narrative medicine: A model for empathy, reflection, profession, and trust. *Journal of the American Medical Association, 286*(15), 1897-1902. doi:10.1001/jama.286.15.1897

Charon, R. (2005). Narrative medicine: Attention, representation, and affiliation. *Narrative, 13*(3), 261–270. doi:10.1353/nar.2005.0017

Coser, R. L. (1959). Some social functions of laughter: A study of humor in a hospital setting. *Human Relations*, *12*(2), 171–182. doi:10.1177/001872675901200205

Davidhizar, R., & Shearer, R. (1996). Using humor to cope with stress in home care. *Home Healthcare Nurse*, *14*(10), 825–830. doi:10.1097/00004045-199610000-00012 PMID:9052068

Dean, R. A. K., & Gregory, D. M. (2005). More than trivial: Strategies for using humor in palliative care. *Cancer Nursing*, *28*(4), 292–300. doi:10.1097/00002820-200507000-00009 PMID:16046892

Ebeling, P. R. (2008). Osteoporsis in men. *The New England Journal of Medicine*, *358*(14), 1474–1482. doi:10.1056/NEJMcp0707217 PMID:18385499

Francis, L. E. (1994). Laughter, the best medication: Humor as emotion management in interaction. *Symbolic Interaction*, *17*(2), 147–163. doi:10.1525i.1994.17.2.147

Francis, L. E., Monahan, K., & Berger, C. (1999). A laughing matter? The use of humor in medical interactions. *Motivation and Emotion*, *23*(2), 155–174. doi:10.1023/A:1021381129517

Giles, H. (2016). Communication accommodation theory. In K. B. Jensen, E. W. Rothenbuhrler, J. D. Pooley, & R. T. Craig (Eds.), *The international encyclopedia of communication theory and philosophy* (pp. 1–7). Wiley Blackwell. doi:10.1002/9781118766804.wbiect056

Haidet, P. (2007). Jazz and the 'art' of medicine: Improvisation in the medical encounter. *Annals of Family Medicine*, *5*(2), 164–169. doi:10.1370/afm.624 PMID:17389542

Phillips, K. A., Ospina, N. S., Rodriguez-Gutierrez, R., Cansaneda-Guarderas, A., Gionfriddo, M. R., Branda, M., & Montori, V. (2018). Humor during clinical practice: Analysis of recorded clinical encounters. *Journal of the American Board of Family Medicine*, *31*(2), 270–278. doi:10.3122/jabfm.2018.02.170313 PMID:29535244

Sala, R., Krupet, E., & Roter, D. (2002). Satisfaction and the use of humor by physicians and patients. *Psychology & Health*, *17*(3), 269–280. doi:10.1080/08870440290029520

Scholl, J. C. (2007). The use of humor to promote patient-centered care. *Journal of Applied Communication Research*, *35*(2), 156–176. doi:10.1080/00909880701262658

Schöpf, A. C., Martin, G. S., & Keating, M. A. (2017). Humor as a communication strategy in provider-patient communication in a chronic care setting. *Qualitative Health Research*, *27*(3), 374–390. doi:10.1177/1049732315620773 PMID:26717942

Spradley, E. L. (2020). Storying clinical interactions: Narrative medicine as an artistic intervention in medical training and education. In K. Afary & A. M. Fritz (Eds.), *More than words: Communication research on expressive arts and narrative as forms of healing* (pp. 241–262). Lexington Books.

Tomlinson, T. (2015 Sept. 29). Humor in medicine: Nasty, dark, and shades of gray. *Michigan State University's Bioethics in the News*. Retrieved from https://msubioethics.com/2015/09/29/humor-in-medicine/

Chapter 19
Just Kidding!

Christine North
Ohio Northern University, USA

Laura and I were in the pre-op bay. I was already in my gown and waiting for the nurse to come and start the IV. I had been given a marker and told to indicate which on which knee Dr. Brown was to perform surgery and which knee was *not* the correct knee. Laura, my medical student friend, wanted to be an orthopedist and had shadowed Dr. Brown in the clinic several times. Dr. Brown had performed both my right and left lateral release procedures[1], but when I needed to have a more involved modified Maquet[2] procedure which would take much longer and require an overnight stay in the hospital, Laura and I discussed her being in the operating theater to observe. I knew Dr. Brown well; he had done two knee surgeries for me before, and I trusted him. But this procedure was no outpatient surgery, and I was nervous. Laura had been cleared to come and observe, and I was thrilled my friend would be by my side the whole time.

Dr. Brown had been a Navy surgeon and had served on a floating hospital before coming to our community. As I began to mark my knees, Laura and I began laughing in that giddy kind of laughing people do in the face of a LOT of nerves, trying to hold back the flood gates of emotion that are just pushing to rush forth. All the way down my right leg we left Dr. Brown messages: GO NAVY! THIS ONE! BEAT ARMY! Arrows indicating the location pointing to my knee. On the left leg, we continued in a similar manner: DON'T EVEN THINK ABOUT IT! STAY AWAY! THIS SIDE CLOSED! And a giant circle with a slash through it right on the knee. We laughed and laughed. And time wore on. Anesthesia came in and asked their questions, then started the IV. Things were getting real now.

The nurse returned with the compression hose. Man, do I hate those things! Time to turn over the markers. On went the hose, and then the intermittent pneumatic compression (IPC) devices that work like blood pressure cuffs on your legs, squeezing and releasing, to prevent blood clots during and after surgery. By this time, I wasn't any longer laughing. Now, I just wanted everything to be over. My mind was racing with anxiety. We were in a waiting game now. Laura sat in the pleather chair next to me, and we were talking about her med school classes and her list of things she had to do before her upcoming exam week. Thinking about Laura and what was going on with her took my mind off of me—well, at least it distracted me a bit.

DOI: 10.4018/978-1-7998-4528-7.ch019

Finally, Dr. Brown popped his head around the curtain. He apologized that the surgery before mine ran long, but said that he was ready. With his familiar warm smile, he asked if I was. I told him I was as ready as I was going to be, and he wiggled my big toe and said he would see us back there.

My stomach was in knots, my palms were sweating, and the flood gates let loose. A torrent of tears flowed everywhere. I was utterly terrified. Laura grabbed my hand and told me that she would be with me the whole time—that everything would be okay. I blubbered, "I know," and kept crying. Then some angel came in and said, "We're going to give you a little *versed* [ver-séd] in your IV. That should take the edge off." Laura told me, laughing, "*versed* will make everything better! I will see you when you come out." I was still crying as they put the *versed* into the IV, but the next thing I really remember was being moved from the gurney to my hospital bed in my room—I didn't even really remember waking up in recovery.

As the nurses and Laura all took a corner of the sheet from the gurney to slide me over to my hospital bed, my right leg was in a large, hinged leg brace from ankle to hip and locked in the straight position. My left leg was also wrapped from toe to hip. Still somewhat out of it from anesthesia, I could not quite process everything. Once settled into my bed, I looked down at my legs. Slightly concerned with my left leg, I noticed a large piece of white tape that ran down the front of my ace-bandaged leg. Nicely printed on the tape was a message from Dr. Brown: "Just Kidding."

I started laughing so hard at that message and his sense of humor. Laura told me that the nurses were concerned about his wrapping my leg. "You can't do that! Did you see her? She was crying when she came in here. She isn't going to think that's funny!" But I thought it was hysterical. That extra gesture on Dr. Brown's part was an incredibly personal and playful gesture very much in line with the kind of relationship that had developed with him as his patient over the past year and a half and two prior surgeries. He loved to tease and give me grief. He was so easy to be around. He was a physician who always asked how school was going or how my job was. He knew my major and where I worked. He took an interest in his patients. I knew that I mattered to my doctor.

The Saturday morning after my surgery, Dr. Brown made a special point to stop by my room before he had to jump on a charter plane to go the University of Nebraska Cornhuskers game. He was the team orthopedist. He popped in early to see how I was doing because I had been so uptight. I thanked him for taking the time and being concerned enough to stop by, and I thanked him for the humor. I wished him a safe flight and told him I would watch the game.

I don't know, all these years later, if he realizes the impact he made, but he had a significant influence on this Health Communication and Public Health professional. Thanks, Dr. Brown, for just kidding with me!

ENDNOTES

1 "The patella (kneecap) is balanced in the front of the knee on the femur (thigh bone). In order to keep the patella centered in the middle of the knee, there are tissues on the inside and outside of the patella which are supposed to pull the patella equally each way. These tissues are call the medial (inside) and the lateral (outside) retinaculum. It is a surgical release of the outside or lateral retinaculum." [Washington University Orthopedics (2017). Lateral retinacular release. Retrieved from https://www.ortho.wustl.edu/content/Patient-Care/3184/Services/Pediatric-and-Adolescent-Orthopedic-Surgery/Overview/Knee-Education-Overview/Lateral-Retinacular-Release.aspx]

2 The Maquet procedure involves cutting the tibia tubercle (part of the tibia bone) while keeping the patellar tendon attachment intact. The tubercle is raised by wedging the loosened piece of bone with a bone block to help realign the knee toward the inner part of the leg to stop dilocations and create better knee alignment. [Flannagan, D. (n.d.). Distal realignment procedures: Maquet procedure. Retrieved from https://www.ohiokneesurgery.com/patellofemoral-procedures-davidc-flanigan-md.html#:~:text=Maquet%20procedure%20%E2%80%93%20In%20this%20procedure,inner%20aspect%20of%20the%20knee)]

Chapter 20
Response: "Just Kidding!"

Elizabeth Kaye Victor
William Paterson University, USA

LITERATURE REVIEW

There is a burgeoning literature on the positive function of humor on one's health, the appropriate use of humor in clinical encounters, and a growing debate over whether the use of humor by clinicians undermines standards of professionalism. Before diving into the debates about whether cracking a joke with a patient is (un)professional, we first have to briefly review the primary theories of humor and varieties of styles or forms can take more generally.

Different Styles or Forms of Humor

The form of humor is characterized by the way the joke is deployed (what is the tone of voice used, who is the audience, who/at what does the content aim). Humor in general is thought to be neutral and can be either positive or negative in form and style. The style of humor overlaps with and is informed by the form of the humor. As Vallade et al. (2013) explain, there are four different styles of humor intersecting on two spectrums of self/other directed and positive/negative content. This gives rise to four different styles of humor: (1) self-enhancing humor is positively directed at the self/in-group; (2) other-enhancing humor is positively directed at the other/out-group; (3) aggressive humor is negatively directed at the other/out-group; and (4) self-deprecating humor that is negatively directed at the self/in-group (Vallade et al., 2013). For example, if I am a doctor and make fun of myself during a patient consultation, I am using self-deprecating humor. However, this self-deprecation can be about my lack of knowledge about baseball or a neutral topic. Thus, even as the style is negative, since I am making fun of myself, it need not be sarcastic, cynical, or black humor.

As explained by Aultman (2009), the most common forms of negative humor include black, cynical, derogatory, gallows humor, and satire. Black humor is "characterized by grim, distorted or grotesque satire" (Aultman, 2009, p. 228). Cynical humor plays on the idea that human beings are inherently self-interested and ought to be distrusted. Derogatory humor aims at "detracting from the character or standing

DOI: 10.4018/978-1-7998-4528-7.ch020

of something" and often is used to express a low opinion of someone or something (Aultman, 2009, p. 228). Gallows humor makes light of horrific life circumstances or life-threatening situations. Finally, satire employs irony or sarcasm to "expose and discredit vice or folly" (Aultman, 2009, p. 228). These different forms of humor are all negative and are most often aggressive in style, making the patient the butt of the joke. But, *why* do we find such a wide variety of things funny?

Primary Theories of Humor: Superiority, Incongruity, and Relief

Superiority theory posits that humor is used to establish dominance or to draw a line between the in-group and others (Morreall, 2020). This form of humor, when deployed within organizations such as a hospital, can be used to enforce an existing hierarchy. As Aultman points out, "[t]hose who are at the top of this hierarchy, that is, attending physicians, implicitly control how and when [humor] is used and who should use it in the presence of the healthcare team" (2009, p. 229). When a joke is made at a patient's expense, or an attending physician makes a joke at the expense of a resident, these are instances where superiority theory might explain why the joke was successful. Thus, instances of derogatory humor, black humor, and aggressive styles of humor can be explained by the superiority theory of humor.

Incongruity theory is possibly the most obvious explanation of humor or why we find certain jokes funny (Morreall, 2020). Incongruity theory holds that humor is the product of the felt incongruity between what we expect to be the case and what actually takes place in a joke (Morreall, 2020). Sobel (2016), for example, relays an anecdote about a time when she and a group of fellow residents shared stories of the funniest page they had received while on call. Some of the contenders included, "Doctor, your patient is covered in ants" and "Doctor, your patient is on fire" (Sobel, 2006, p. 1114). In both instances, part of what made the pages so funny to the residents is the deadpan delivery of the call service or nurse relaying the information. Another aspect that invoked humor in both instances is the unexpected content—how is the patient covered in ants or on fire *in the hospital* (when, ostensibly, the patients were not in that condition upon arriving)? What these examples illustrate is that the incongruity can be placed at the level of the joke's content (what the joke is about), the delivery of the joke (tone of voice), or at the linguistic level (stating something as present tense instead of past tense; Watson (2011). Incongruity theory, then, explains why we find some instances of gallows humor, cynical humor, and aggressive styles of humor funny.

Relief theory holds that we laugh as a way to release tension, anxiety, or excess energy that is pent up in ourselves (Freud, 1990; Smuts, 2009; Spencer, 1911). One example of gallows humor is offered by Watson (2011) as she recounts one particularly difficult night where a group of residents order a pizza at 3 a.m. after a long shift—they are called back before their dinner arrives only to realize, to their horror, that they are working to save the life of the delivery boy who was shot while en route to deliver their dinner. Despite heroic interventions, they could not save the patient. As they sat in silence, one resident asked, "What happened to the pizza?"—another resident found the pizza, face up, outside the ER, brought it in and another resident asked "How much you think we ought to tip him?" The residents laughed and ate the pizza (2011, p. 37). Examples of gallows humor between physicians, out of view of the patients (i.e., backstage), is often explained as a way for physicians to blow off steam and release the tension that comes from caring for patients, losing patients to death or surgical complications, or releasing frustration that comes from caring for patients that seem to be unwilling to care for themselves. Watson offers just such an explanation as part of her analysis: "[w]hen a compassionate professional gets overwhelmed, gallows humor may be a psychic survival instinct…When a terrible joke is the only bridge between horror and necessity, gallows humor can be a show of respect for the work that lies ahead" (2011, p. 44). Relief theory explains why high-stress professionals, such as clinicians that face existentially intense situations, turn to humor as a release valve. This theory also allows for clinicians to express and feel complex moral emotions (Tomlinson, 2012), and can be a powerful tool for moving conversations forward or moving past trauma (Kaebnick, 2011).

These theories guide us to better understand what humor *is*, but none of these theories offer a framework for evaluating whether it is *moral* to use humor in the hospital. That is to say, these theories give us a framework for *describing* different forms of humor and competing explanations for *why* we find different jokes funny, but none of the theories tell us *if we should* tell a specific joke or use a specific kind of humor. There is some evidence that humor and joking "moderate the negative effects of stress and provide some benefit through enhanced interpersonal skills or social support" (McCreaddie, 2008, p.1), and can soften isolation and build connections between clinical staff and patients (Penson et al., 2005). Nurses are well placed to use humor given their increased interactions with patients, and yet, they have reported not wanting to take the risk of a patient feeling rejected for not getting a joke (Anonymous, 2008). The primary arguments against joking or using humor in clinical settings have focused on (1) the dehumanizing effect it can have on patients or act as a barrier to clinical sympathy (Aultman, 2009; Hardy, 2020), (2) that humor or specific forms of humor can cause moral injury or harm to colleagues, clinical staff, and medical students/residents (Piemonte, 2015), and (3) the erosion of professional standards or the claim that humor in the clinic or hospital can undermine professional relationships (Berk, 2009; Parsons et al., 2001; Sokol, 2012).

ANALYSIS: WHAT HARM COULD A JOKE CAUSE?

There are several instances of humor in the case above. First, the patient initiates humorous banter with Dr. Brown based on their friendly team rivalry (Go Army! Beat Navy!). Second, the patient herself employs this humor, along with over-the-top messages to alleviate her tension about the surgery. Her messages seek to ensure Dr. Brown knows which leg not to operate on, but, as explained, clearly acts as a form of relief. Finally, we have Dr. Brown who wraps both of the patient's legs and puts the long piece of tape over the leg he didn't operate on with the wording "Just Kidding!", which is clearly meant to convey to the patient that he is joking back. In this context, both the incongruity theory and relief theory of humor are in play. The patient acts out of the need to alleviate stress, and her stress is reportedly reduced when she engages in humorous acts directed toward Dr. Brown. In this way, she can be said to be employing self-enhancing humor (Vallade et al., 2013). When Dr. Brown enacts his joke, the patient awakens to see that both legs are wrapped—an incongruous context, that in combination with the taped message of "Just Kidding!" (another incongruous element), delivers the punchline and the patient laughs.

It is clear from the reporting of the case that there are no instances of derogatory humor or self-deprecating humor. The jokes, though, arise out of a fear that the doctor might operate on the wrong leg. Dr. Brown, in feeding into that fear, seems to dally in a bit of gallows humor. Even as there are no medical students mentioned, we could ask whether Dr. Brown is setting the right tone here—is he being professional? Does the staff agree with his use of humor? Is he undermining is doctor-colleague relationships with this joke?

Aultman (2009) looks at studies that focus on the uses of derogatory or cynical humor by different healthcare professionals in hospital settings. She argues that while humor itself may offer therapeutic effects for both clinicians and patients, gallows humor that is derogatory or cynical humor is unethical, nontherapeutic, and should be avoided. Such forms of humor, Aultman (2009) argues, communicate immoral attitudes that dehumanize and can negatively affect clinical relationships and hospital culture. Similarly, Hardy (2020) argues that unreflective use of aggressive humor "can lead to a pattern of disrespect, and by extension a lower level of care" (p. 188). In addition to reduced clinical sympathy, some uses of humor has been reported to increase distress in medical students, who report that those "…who engage in both derogatory and gallows humor, it seems, contribute to the process of deidealization and perpetuate the discrepancy between students' expectations of what it means to be a doctor and what they witness firsthand" (Piemonte, 2015, p. 380).

In regard to this case, on the one hand, it does not stand up to the objectivity test. The objectivity test asks us to consider the joke from anyone's point of view. In other words, if taken out of context, would this joke still be funny? From an objective observer's point of view, Dr. Brown could be said to be acting in a manner that is unsympathetic. If he does this regularly and in an unreflective manner, this could be an instance of displaying an immoral attitude toward a patient (not taking their fears seriously; using humor to poke fun at a serious issue). If he were a clinical educator, this could feed the kind of moral distress about which Piemonte (2015) is concerned. On the other hand, this is an established relationship and Dr. Brown clearly knows *this* patient. It is the personal relationship that has already been established through years of clinical care that suggests the doctor is acting *from sympathy* when he jokes in this manner. Thus, Hardy (2020) would likely say that this act of humor was reflective and unproblematic—we are not in danger of dehumanizing the patient. That said, this does not appear to be obvious from his colleagues' perspective. In the case details, the nurses urge Dr. Brown not to wrap the patient's other leg, stressing that the patient was visibly upset and stressed. This should signal to us that the nurses might think that Dr. Brown's actions are less than professional, and he is not taking his patient's concerns seriously, which may undermine the doctor-colleague relationship.

While many codes of ethics mention treating others, including colleagues, with respect, humor is not specifically mentioned as something to avoid. Beyond the patient-provider relationship, the use of humor in the hospital can undermine other working relationships. As Sokol (2012) notes, "[in] modern medical ethics the ethics of the doctor-colleague relationship is overlooked" (p. 1). As Sokol (2012) pithily puts it, "[o]ne doctor's 'banter' is another's offensive remark. A risqué joke might amuse most of the people but deeply offend one person" (p.1). Similarly, medical students have reported alarm and concern that humor and jokes about patients on the part of attending physicians (Parsons et al., 2001). Finally, Berk (2009) notes that negative humor is often justified as a coping mechanism when dealing with difficult or demanding patients, but "…derogatory and cynical humour as displayed by medical personnel are forms of verbal abuse, disrespect and the dehumanization of their patients and themselves… [Such humour] erodes any sense of professionalism and civility in the workplace" (p. 7). What this study indicates is that clinicians are *socialized* into the use of problematic use of humor, and this may lead to its unreflective use. In this case, the use of humor is a call back to an earlier discussion with the patient, but if another healthcare staffer overheard Dr. Brown this could contribute to deidealization identified in the studies above. As a result, we can ask whether Dr. Brown's use of humor is an instance of gallows humor, especially from an outsider's point of view? Is he being uncivil?

While the case makes clear that the patient did not view the joke as derogatory or ridiculing her as an individual, the case itself does not provide enough details to make a definitive judgment about the relationship between Dr. Brown and nursing staff. Still, we do know that humor can reduce tension in clinical situations (Anderson, 2015; McCreaddie, 2008; Penson et al., 2005). We also know that studies have reported that nurses are more conservative than their clinical counterparts to use humor out of fear of alienating patients (Anonymous, 2008; McCreaddie, 2008). This implies that this could just be an instance where a doctor is comfortable with humor and the nurses are more reluctant—both doing so out of a desire to act in the best interest of the patient. However, another point worth attending to is whether Dr. Brown's dismissal of the nurses' concerns is a pattern. If Dr. Brown regularly ignores or dismisses the nurses' concerns, this could erode collegial bonds and make the nurses less likely to speak up in the future. This is a risk that Dr. Brown should take seriously—patient care is improved by having all healthcare provider voices heard and promoting a respectful work environment. What, then, can we discern from this case? How do we balance the demands of collegiality with good patient care? There are clear recommendations we can draw from this case that many clinicians and health care providers can instantiate as best practices.

RECOMMENDATIONS

In this case, Dr. Brown has an established relationship with the patient, and they have established a history of lighthearted banter. However, this kind of dynamic is not a universal one. Clinicians cannot take for granted that they will have such common ground with all patients, or that all patients will want to joke about something as serious as mistakenly operating on the wrong limb. Furthermore, the relationship between Dr. Brown and the nurses could be strained if the nurses regularly suggest that the doctor's joke might not be funny, and he ignores them. In light of these features, I offer the following recommendations:

Recommendation 1: Nurses & Staff Need To Be Listened To and Respected

Any one instance of Dr. Brown dismissing the nurses he works with when they suggest he has taken a joke too far will not necessarily erode collegiality. However, if this is a pattern of behavior, Dr. Brown may be unconsciously undermining the expertise and experiences of the people he works with, and that is a problem. Keeping the lines of communication open between nurses and clinicians is imperative for patient care, and if Dr. Brown's funny bone is getting in the way of that, what can be done? How do we balance the need for open communication and professionalism with a doctor being funny?

Acting on Recommendation 1: Debrief Clinical Encounters Regularly

Concerning the case above, the nurses might have felt the humor was unprofessional. Furthermore, the nurses may have felt that Dr. Brown didn't value their opinion and was not taking the patient's fears seriously. Having an opportunity to explore the use of humor in clinical encounters more generally, and specific cases of humor usage within a hospital or clinic could be part of the continuing education and ethical reflection opportunities already at hand. For example, a clinic or hospital could make a point of focusing on humor in the workplace or patient encounters as the focus of a medical debriefing session or workshop series. Debriefings are common in hospitals and clinics after mass casualty events or a particularly significant clinical event has taken place. Some hospitals hold debriefings regularly, but this is less common. Debriefings are a space that can further medical knowledge, reexamine what happened in a particular case, and share different insights and emotions surrounding a specific event—it is not a space to call people out or review errors, but to objectively assess an event. Debriefings can take the form of a meeting, can be scheduled as part of a luncheon, or can be incorporated into other regular events offered by a clinic or hospital. Incorporating debriefings as part of a hospital or clinic's culture can help provide an outlet for staff to bring up issues and be heard. This can help maintain collegiality in the workplace, help Dr. Brown find a way to be funny within the bounds of workplace civility, and safeguard against issues that may erode professional standards.

Recommendation 2: Use Humor To Enhance Patient Autonomy and Trust

In this instance, rapport between Dr. Brown and the patient was set early on—the patient reports that they had an established and on-going relationship over a number of years. Dr. Brown knew what this patient was like and what kind of humor he could use with her. He did not go into the surgery trying something new, and this was not his first or even second clinical encounter with this patient. Three elements of the clinician-patient relationship that made Dr. Brown's use of humor successful in this case, then, are: (1) the patient was clearly supported and allowed to write messages on her own leg, (2) the use of humor clearly allowed the patient some much needed relief of the tension she felt prior to surgery, and (3) Dr. Brown followed the patient's lead and signaled very clearly that the bandage on the "wrong" leg was a joke.

Acting on Recommendation 2: Let the Patient Set the Tone and Type of Humor

When attempting to establish a new patient relationship, clinicians would do well to follow Dr. Brown's lead and get to know whether a patient responds well to humor more generally (Penson et al., 2005). Test the waters before launching a full-scale attack of the funny. Use humor to help establish a good rapport with patients and deepen the trust essential to any clinician-patient relationship.

What makes humor successful in this case is that it enhanced patient autonomy—the little jabs against the navy were a way to draw on the trust the patient already had and was based on her relationship with Dr. Brown. Dr. Brown, in turn, recognized the patient's fear for what it was, and further helped relieve that tension by making his joke—and, more importantly, making it known with the use of tape down an entire leg that he was "just kidding!" Clinicians would do well to treat patients as the active inquirers and agents in the clinical encounter that they are. If humor will not further support and enable patient autonomy and agency, better to check it at the door.

Recommendation 3: Humor Is Good, But Gallows Humor May Harm

To an outside observer that did not have access to the specific clinician-patient relationship in play, Dr. Brown's joke may have been perceived as a form of gallows humor. In this case, joking about operating on the wrong leg, especially given the pronounced fear the patient had of the doctor operating on the wrong leg, could arguably be a form of gallows humor. As discussed earlier, any use of gallows humor runs the risk of causing moral injury to fellow clinicians or patients. Furthermore, if this becomes a habit, it may prevent the clinician from cultivating and maintaining clinical sympathy. Dr. Brown was able to pull off this joke not because the joke was objectively funny, but because the patient and Dr. Brown had a pre-existing relationship that included friendly jabs and jests over an extended period of time.

Acting on Recommendation 3: Pay Attention To What is Joked About

Hardy (2020) offers the advice of paying attention to the intention and target of the humor. The goal is to ensure that the humor used in the clinic is other-enhancing, at best, or at the very least, does not risk undermining professional standards or patient care. As Hardy (2020, p. 189) notes,

[i]f the humor is intended to make fun of patients, then it would make sense for patients to be offended. However, if the jokes are meant to enhance patients or to merely make fun of symptoms and situations, then there can still be genuine sympathy towards patients.

In the case above, even if the joke played by Dr. Brown was an instance of gallows humor, it is not prima facie cynical, derogatory, or aggressive. It came from an established relationship built on trust and demonstrated sympathy for the patient at the same time that it lightened the mood. Drawing from insights offered by Anderson, the joke succeeded in part because it served as a social reinforcement and tapped into a familiar theme for this doctor-patient relationship (Anderson, 2015). In all of these ways, the joking in this case illustrates why the humor was well received by the patient and provides us with clues to help others navigate the difficult terrain that makes laughter the best medicine.

REFERENCES

Anderson, G. (2015, July). Humor in treatment is no joke. *ASHA Leader*, *20*(7), 42–43. doi:10.1044/leader.HYTT.20072015.np

Anonymous. (2008, June 11). Joking with patients seen as risky. *Nursing Standard*, *22*(40), 7. doi:10.7748/ns.22.40.7.s6

Aultman, J. M. (2009). When humor in the hospital is no laughing matter. *The Journal of Clinical Ethics*, *20*(3), 227–234. PMID:19845193

Berk, R. (2009). Derogathory and cynical humor in clinical teaching and the workplace: The need for professionalism. *Medical Education, 43*(1), 7-9. .1365-2923.2008.03239.x doi:10.1111/j

Freud, S. (1990). *Jokes and their relations to the unconscious* (J. Strachey, Trans.). W.W. Norton & Company.

Hardy, C. (2020). Humor and sympathy in medical practice. *Medicine, Health Care and Philosophy, 23*(2), 179-190. doi:10.100711019-019-09928-0

Kaebnick, G. E. (2011, September-October). From the editor: Laughter in the best medicine. *The Hastings Center Report, 41*(5), 2. Retrieved from https://www.jstor.org/stable/41241295

McCreaddie, M. (2008, April 23-29). You must be joking. *Nursing Standard*, *22*(33), 22–23. doi:10.7748/ns.22.33.22.s26 PMID:18540555

Morreall, J. (2020). Philosophy of humor. In E. N. Zalta (Ed.), *The Stanford encyclopedia of philosophy (online)*. The Metaphysics Research Lab.

Parsons, N. G., Kinsman, S. B., Bosk, C. L., Sankar, P., & Ubel, P. A. (2001). Between two worlds: Medical student perceptions of humor and slang in the hospital setting. *Journal of General Internal Medicine, 16*(8), 544–549. doi:10.1046/j.1525-1497.2001.016008544.x PMID:11556931

Penson, R. T., Partridge, R. A., Rudd, P., Seiden, M. V., Nelson, J. E., Chabner, B. A., & Lynch, T. J. Jr. (2005). Laughter: The best medicine? *The Oncologists, 10*(8), 651–660. doi:10.1634/theoncologist.10-8-651 PMID:16177290

Piemonte, N. M. (2015). Last laughs: Gallows humor and medical education. *The Journal of Medical Humanities, 36*(4), 375–390. doi:10.100710912-015-9338-4 PMID:26062447

Smuts, A. (2009). Do moral flaws enhance amusement? *American Philosophical Quarterly, 46*(2), 151–162.

Sobel, R. K. (2006). Does laughter make good medicine? *The New England Journal of Medicine, 354*(11), 1114–1115. doi:10.1056/NEJMp058089 PMID:16540611

Sokol, D. K. (2012). No laughing matter. *British Journal of Medicine, 344*(e2119), 1–2. doi:10.1136/bmj.e2119 PMID:22438391

Spencer, H. (1911). On the physiology of laughter. Essays on education, etc. *Dent, Contemporary Dentistry.*

Tomlinson, T. (2012, May-June). Uncomfortable humor. *The Hastings Center Report, 42*(3), 9. https://www.jstor.org/stable/23883181 PMID:22670292

Vallade, J. I., Booth-Butterfield, M., & Vela, L. E. (2013). Taking back power: Using superiority theory to predict humor use following relational transgression. *Western Journal of Communication, 77*(2), 231–248. doi:10.1080/10570314.2012.669018

Watson, K. (2011, September-October). Gallows humor in medicine. *The Hastings Center Report, 41*(5), 37–45. doi:10.1002/j.1552-146X.2011.tb00139.x PubMed

Chapter 21
India Is in Asia?

Monalisa M. Tailor
Norton Healthcare, USA

My hospital serves numerous patients from poor, underserved areas in Kentucky who come into "the city" to visit a doctor. The majority of my patients have a high school education or less. Many of these patients have never left the state of Kentucky, much less the U.S. Their world is local, and few have need to think much about the larger world.

Because so many of my patients have such small worlds, there are many things that come up in conversation that feel as though they should be common knowledge to the well educated medical staff at the hospital, but truly are not. When patients reveal a lack of knowledge, it is easy for them to become embarrassed. It is the job of the healthcare personnel with them to prevent them from feeling embarrassed, because if they do feel embarrassed, that may limit what additional information they share. Open communication between patients and their healthcare providers is essential for effective patient care.

An example of one such precarious revelation of ignorance happened when a patient was surprised to learn that I, his new Indian doctor, was from Asia. This particular patient, who I shall call *James*, came to visit me as a new patient. When I walked into the examination room and introduced myself, the immediate reaction was surprise, "You were not the doctor I was expecting!" He assured me that all was well though, and that we could proceed with the exam. He further explained that he had asked the front desk what I looked like and thought he understood them to say that I "looked Asian," which is why he was surprised to see me.

It was then that I realized that this patient had no idea that India was in Asia. I smiled kindly and replied, "Yes, sir my family is from India, so yes, therefore we are Asian." The patient looked confused and asked, "India is in Asia? I didn't learn geography good." So, I advised him in a non-judgmental tone that the Middle East, most of Russia, and India were all part of Asia and we would regroup for another geography lesson at his next visit. Reframing the next appointment as a geography lesson brought humor into the situation, diffusing any tension he might feel. Using the right tone to make the patient feel like he was not being disrespected allowed me to gently note the geographical mistake, acknowledge it, and then in reinforcing that I was his physician, that we would be seeing each other again. At our next visit, the

DOI: 10.4018/978-1-7998-4528-7.ch021

patient came in asking if I had a good Christmas holiday. I said yes, I had 2 days off and visited family. The patient was shocked I was able to get to India and back in 2 days, so at least the reference improved.

Chapter 22
Response: “India Is in Asia?”

Warren J. Bareiss
University of South Carolina Upstate, USA

COMMUNICATION AND CONTEXT

Communication is meaningless without context. By that, I mean that meaning is derived through awareness of how messages are conditioned by time and place so that the same message in two different contexts can have two entirely different meanings. What might be humorous in one context can be insulting in another. That is why humor is always a little risky, but the risk is part of the fun. Proffering humor to another person means taking a gamble that the combination of message and context will work in a way that is unexpected, yet appropriate and effective.

Most of the time, when we think of communication context, we are likely to think of the time and place in which communication occurs. On the other hand, context can also be a story in which a communicative act is recounted (Binhammer, 2017; Repede, 2008). In other words, a story about a past conversation embeds one communicative act (the conversation) within another communicative act (the recounting of the conversation).

“India is in Asia?” is a case in point. By recounting a humorous incident, Dr. Tailor frames a conversation with her patient, James, in a particular way to illustrate her point about respecting patients. As a communication scholar, my job is to take a step back, looking at not only what transpired in the examination room, but also how Dr. Tailor constructs that conversation through her story.

In essence, Dr. Tailor’s story is about demonstrating respect toward patients by illustrating her use of humor in response to a *faux pas* made by James. In this chapter, I will analyze many facets of the conversation described, focusing on “face-work” as my principle theoretical emphasis, informed by empirical studies of humor in doctor-patient communication. I will also draw upon narrative theory, specifically dramatism, to analyze how Dr. Tailor has constructed her story in a specific way to make her point.

DOI: 10.4018/978-1-7998-4528-7.ch022

Face-Work

"Face-work" is a communication concept often used to describe interpersonal communication encounters involving sensitive issues, especially when a potentially embarrassing event occurs. Goffman's (1967/2003) description of face-work is generally the starting point for all such research. For Goffman, communication has a ritualized dimension which he describes as "universal human nature" (p. 13). Human nature is revealed through complex rules of communication, varying by place and time, through which we can express ourselves, be understood, and understand one another. Each person brings a sense of identity to every communicative encounter. That identity is a shared sense of self—their "face"—which establishes rules of conduct and expectations among participants. Face involves such factors as desired respect from others, pride in oneself, and the image that one cultivates--whether based in truth, fabrication, or a combination of both (see also, Brown & Levinson, 1987; Cho & Sillars, 2015).

Regardless of time or place, communication rules are remarkably complex and nuanced, depending upon who is communicating with whom, what sorts of things are being discussed, and the context of those discussions (Mahvar, et al., 2020). This complexity sometimes leads to mistakes in rule following which threaten the face of one or more communication participants. "Losing face" results in embarrassment due the public revelation that one's face is, after all, a socially agreed upon artifice (Burton, 2012; Brown & Levinson, 1987; Goffman, 1967/2003).

Following Goffman's line of thinking, what might appear to be a simple conversation between two people really involves two highly sophisticated maneuvers engaged in by both people simultaneously. On one level, there is the give and take of the message sending and receiving within the socially conditioned communicative system. At a deeper, often less conscious level, both people are also continually watching and listening for the other to make a mistake in the process and thereby lose face. This is when face-work takes place.

Assuming that each person in the conversation has the other's interest at heart, both will be ready to save the other's face without hesitation should a *faux pas* occur. Or, at the very least, each participant will be ready at all times to save their own face in such a circumstance. In other words, when a breach occurs that jeopardizes one or the other's face, at least one of the participants is prepared to re-establish the lost face (i.e., to restore equilibrium among participants so that communication can resume (Goffman, 1967/2013). Communication is thus a highly sophisticated system even for those of us with modest formal education, especially when we add to the situation other factors including sensitivity of the topic, social distance, and respective power distance between communicators (Claramita et al., 2020).

At first glance, humor seems to be an easily understood means of face saving. Following a face-losing mistake, one could make a self-deprecating joke (Saunders, 1998, p. 363). For instance, I had a professor in college who sometimes burped when talking with students to which he had a ready joke: "Pardon my pig." This little joke simultaneously revealed the artifice of the serious, learned academic face that had momentarily dissolved, while also relieving tension caused by loss of face through a smile or a laugh by the students.

Humor, however, is not so simple. Humor can be self-denigrating, as in the example above, but it can easily be insulting if delivered as an attack by the other person. Humor can easily miss its target, and not be considered funny. Humor can be offered to the other person, but the cue might be missed or ignored. And humor might be mistaken as being initiated when it was not, leading to an inappropriate laugh. Each of these conditions leads to further loss of face for one or more conversation participants.

Indeed, one might argue that humor is among the more delicate means of face-work (Beach & Prickett, 2017; Glenright et al., 2017; Haakana, 2002).

Face-Work and Humor in Clinical Settings

Like all forms of communication, clinical visits are conditioned by *a priori* rules, boundaries, power dynamics, and anxieties making loss of face a perpetual problem for both patients and healthcare providers. Appropriate responses to loss of face in healthcare settings requires quick thinking, sensitivity, and awareness of contextual expectations and limitations (Little, et al. 2000).

Numerous studies have examined ways that humor is used by both patients and providers in the preservation and re-establishment of face among clinical visits (c.f., Cho & Sillars, 2015; Saunders, 1998; Rhys & Schmidt-Renfree, 2000). As these studies indicate, humor serves specific functions in patient-provider communication, sometimes with multiple functions in play at the same time (Archer et. al, 2019). Typical functions include reduction of power distance between patients and providers, easing tensions in stressful circumstances, establishing friendly relationships, maintaining or challenging a superordinate position, controlling the flow and tone of discourse, signaling mistakes and requesting forgiveness, demonstrating solidarity, minimizing or accepting the seriousness of a situation, and seeking reassurance (Archer et al., 2019; Saunders, 1998).

When we consider humor as a face-saving strategy in clinical visits, it is crucial to inquire about who initiates humor, when and how offers of humor are made, and motivations for doing so. Equally important to the overture is the response. Is the offer accepted, rejected, or ignored? Under what circumstances does reciprocation of humor occur, and when is it not wanted or appropriate? In essence, in clinical visits, who is invited to share in the expression of humor, what is the result, and how does that vary from situation to situation?

Face-Work and Dramatism

Having briefly addressed functions of humor in face maintenance and the functions of humor during clinical visits, I will now turn to narrative form. While Dr. Tailor's example of humor is undoubtedly a face-saving technique made on behalf of her patient, Dr. Tailor communicates that act to us through the use of a story. Like humor and face-work, stories as forms of communication are far more complex than they might first appear. Stories are carefully constructed means of framing events in the past to express meaning in the present (Charon, 2006; Riessman, 1993).

One of the most commonly used methods of analyzing stories is Kenneth Burke's (1969) pentad which itself is derived from Burke's broader theory of dramatism. For Burke, human interactions are like scenes in a play wherein each participant enacts their respective part. In telling stories, we all shape the scenes and parts played to our own advantage so that stories are rhetorical devices through which we reconstruct our particular world views.

Burke's dramatism shares much in common with Goffman's vision of face-work (Bell, 2008). Whereas Goffman argues that participants in a conversation follow a "line," defined as "a pattern of verbal and nonverbal acts by which he expresses his view of the situation" (1967/2003, p. 7), Burke argues that we are all actors playing our parts in roles that are largely pre-written by social custom.

Burke's pentad is generally represented as a five-pointed star with points labeled as "actor," "act," "scene," "agency," and "motive." The actor is the primary character in the story, and the act is what that person does. There are also secondary actors, of course, and they perform their own actions. The scene is where the action takes place. Agency consists of resources available to the actors, and motive is why actors behave as they do (Burke, 1969).

Burke's pentad is featured widely in college classrooms and textbooks as a tool for narrative analysis (Bell, 2008). Less commonly used is Burke's (1961) guilt-redemption cycle, a further elaboration of his dramatistic theory. While the pentad lays out the parts of a story, much like a map shows parts in relations to the whole, the guilt-redemption cycle takes us *through* the story along a temporal dimension. For Burke, stories generally involve some sort of social breach that needs to be made right. Again, this brings us back to Goffman's thinking in which the social breach is the loss of face which needs to be restored—either by the person losing face or by another person in the conversation acting on the first person's behalf—for the flow of communication to continue.

When the breach occurs in the guilt redemption cycle, a kind of pollution disturbs the social setting, calling for restitution via "purification." Purification can occur in one of two ways. One way takes the story toward "mortification" in which the person who performed the breach blames themselves. The other means of purification is to blame someone else, a "scapegoat." Once blame is thus assigned in the story—either to oneself via mortification or to another via scapegoating—the story is resolved via restoration of social order. Restoration again merges well with Goffman's notion of face-work wherein equilibrium is regained through careful face-work (Burke, 1961).

USING FACEWORK AND DRAMATISM TO INTERPRET AN AWKWARD MOMENT IN A CLINICAL VISIT

Face-Saving Humor in Practice

Having established a theoretical background pertaining to face-work, humor, and dramatism, my goal in this section of the chapter is to demonstrate those concepts with respect to "India is in Asia." I will first examine the story through use of the pentad and then illustrate how the narrative parts function with regard to humor, face-work, and the guilt-redemption cycle.

The narrative structure of Dr. Tailor's story is straightforward when examined via Burke's pentad. The scene is an examination room in a Kentucky hospital. At a wider level, the scene also includes the United States in the first two decades of the 21st Century, an era marked by tensions about and reassessment of historical relationships, particularly along the lines of race and class.

Dr. Tailor is the primary actor, and her action—making a little joke—is done with the motivation of avoiding embarrassment of her patient, James. Although James is not the primary actor in the story, his words initiate an awkward, face-risking moment.

Agency is critical to the story because of the customary asymmetrical power dynamic between doctor and patient, accentuated by James's minimal formal education common among the economically disadvantaged population served by the hospital. I should also point out that as narrator, Dr. Tailor maintains her agency over the story because it is she who structures the narrative, telling it from her perspective. Indeed, the actual identity of James is not known, and he is entirely represented entirely through the word choice of Dr. Tailor, a critical point to which I will return later in the analysis.

When we consider this part of the exchange, it's crucial to recall the larger social context—the scene—beyond the confines of the examination room. As I mentioned above, the story takes place in the early 21st Century United States during a time of reconsideration of national values and historical legacy. It is an era in which historical monuments, for instance, are being reevaluated and when patterned police behavior toward people of color is a matter of daily conversation. The fact that Dr. Tailor is Asian is a crucial factor as the tension builds in the story. While we don't know James's race, we do know that James is both confused about Dr. Tailor's Asian identity and also curious as to why he is confused. This is dangerous turf with respect to face-work, given the sensitive nature of the wider socio-cultural contextual factors and possibility of offense.

James is, in effect, now heading toward potential face-losing disaster. If James says too much about what he expects "Asians" to look like, he might make an inappropriate remark pertaining to race which would be awkward for both James and Dr. Tailor. Nevertheless, James is determined to solve the mystery of why he misunderstood what he was told. Tension in the story builds as James proceeds with his inquiry, explaining that he expected to be examined by someone who "looked Asian."

Dr. Tailor tries to resolve the situation by explaining that her family is from India and that India is in Asia. Given that James now realizes that he knows little of world geography, he finally experiences loss of face, albeit entirely unintended by Dr. Tailor. First, James was expecting someone who in his mind was "Asian," and failing in that assumption, he was reminded about his lack of education by a person who is highly educated.

James then moves into face-work mode by repeating what he has just learned as a question, "India is in Asia?" Seeking affirmation of that newly learned fact, James attempts to regain face through mortification: "I didn't learn geography so good." This is a poignant moment in the story when James realizes that his own curiosity led him to lose face in the presence of Dr. Tailor. Note that James didn't blame his school or society, which he could have easily done as a scapegoating maneuver. Rather, he puts the blame for his poor geography skills upon himself: "I didn't learn" as opposed to "I wasn't taught."

Significantly, James is already in the weaker position in the communicative relationship, given the institutionalized roles of doctor and patient. Having admitted his own "guilt," through "mortification," to use Burke's terminology, James has weakened his position further. Had James blamed the educational system in which he was taught, or poverty, or some other external target, he might have saved face on his own, but instead, he put himself completely at the mercy of Dr. Tailor to do the necessary reparative face-work.

At this point, Dr. Tailor shifts gradually into a humorous approach, beginning with a nonverbal cue (a non-judgmental vocal tone) while listing various places constituting Asia. In telling the story, Dr. Tailor doesn't explain her motive for turning to humor at this particular moment. It might have been based on past experience, instinct, or even nonverbal cues that James was communicating. Whatever her reason, Dr. Tailor joked that she and James would regroup for another lesson at James's next visit.

By "[r]eframing the next appointment as a geography lesson," Dr. Tailor skillfully deconstructs and undermines the entire scene. Rhetorically transforming herself into a geography teacher, Dr. Tailor accentuates the social construction of her face as a person with socially recognized, medical expertise. As such, Dr. Tailor makes transparent the entire artifice of role construction, saying, in effect, "A moment ago, I was a doctor, but now I'm a geography teacher." The absurdity of role construction—of patient and doctor—and all the power dynamics, expectations, behavior patterns that come with those roles dissolves by being made transparent. This is the crux of the humor: revelation that the whole scenario in which James and Dr. Tailor find themselves is based on an unspoken arrangement whereby each person agreed to respect the other's carefully constructed face. James accidentally lost his face, whereas Dr. Tailor deliberately transformed hers.

Significantly, the new role that Dr. Tailor adapts through her joke remains an authority figure in the form of a school teacher. To do otherwise, for example, to "play the fool" in a self-deprecating manner might overplay her hand, taking her too far from her established role. As a faux teacher, Dr. Tailor provides the geography lesson that James admittedly is lacking in a way that is neither punitive or embarrassing.

As with humor generally, this is a risky maneuver because James might reject Dr. Tailor's offer of humor. Indeed, James might take the gesture as an insult in which his lack of formal education is emphasized as a point of ridicule. We don't know what James' reaction is because that element is left out of Dr. Tailor's narrative, although given the fact that the point of the story is to illustrate sensitivity, we assume that James was not offended by the gesture.

Finally, to fully understand the face-saving function of Dr. Tailor's joke, we need to consider the importance of its place in the temporal function of the humor. Significantly, Dr. Tailor's joke looks forward to the next appointment, when "we would regroup for another geography lesson at his next visit." The joke projects ahead in time, ensuring that both patient and doctor would meet again on, routine, friendly terms. As such, Dr. Tailor signals that the relationship between herself and James has not been jeopardized by James's misunderstanding. Both faces are thereby restored.

Dr. Tailor's intent was, as she writes, to acknowledge James' error without being disrespectful, but also to reinforce that the doctor-patient relationship remained intact. Both faces were thus preserved so that the relationship could return to the normalcy expected in the circumstances. Had Dr. Tailor not framed her maneuver as humor, she might have lost her face in the exchange by seeming to talk down to or even to scold James, thereby stepping out of the prescribed role of gentle healer. Indeed, without careful face-work on the part of Dr. Tailor, any future relationship would be awkward at best, as the faces of each participant would not be fully clear to the other.

Context and Interpretation

Dr. Tailor's use of humor was without question an act of compassion. Dr. Tailor recognized potential embarrassment in the moment due to James' lack of cultural capital, so she offered a gesture of humor to preserve James's face. By "compassion," I mean that Dr. Tailor put herself into James' position, imagining James' emotions in the moment. To be compassionate in that way, we must be mindful of where the other person is coming from. What resources do they bring to the communicative situation, and how do they use those resources to get their point across while maintaining their sense of identity and respect? What is the face that they want to project?

When James made a rhetorical error on a topic that is particularly sensitive in the broader sociocultural environment, Dr. Tailor demonstrated awareness of the error as well as her ethical responsibility to repair the damage. She did so by offering James a lesson in geography and a joke about meeting again at their next "lesson." Undoubtedly, Dr. Tailor's gesture was meant as a signal of forgiveness and as a mutually beneficial path out of the situation, while maintaining a friendly doctor-patient relationship moving forward. To use a popular adage, for a moment, rather than communicate role to role, Dr. Tailor attempted to communicate with James soul to soul.

On the other hand, as we have seen throughout this chapter, communication is fraught with contradictions, even with the best of intentions. While Dr. Tailor's overture to James evidently repaired the breach in the moment, his framing of the story also leaves out a significant element crucial to any doctor-patient relationship: the patient's point of view.

Dr. Tailor's joke, as described in the story, was offered *to* James, but not necessarily shared *with* James. Communication teachers and scholars would describe the situation as a "linear" model of communication (i.e., one-way with Dr. Tailor as sender and James as receiver; c.f., McCornack, 2016; Shannon & Weaver, 1949). When thinking of communication as a linear process, emphasis is placed primarily on the intent of the message sender rather than on the perceptions and response of the receiver. As du Pre and Foster (2016) note, "one shortfall of this approach is that it tends to support an uneven balance of power. The person assumed to have the most valuable information is often given license to set the tone and terms of an interaction" (p. 14). Framing her offer of humor in this linear way, Dr. Tailor's story leaves significant issues unaddressed: What was James' reaction? Did he laugh or smile? Did he understand Dr. Tailor's gesture on his behalf? If so, did he welcome that gesture? Would James have felt comfortable enough to rebuke Dr. Tailor if he was offended by the remark?

Sometimes, what is not said is as important as what is said. Dr. Tailor's silence regarding James' response emphasizes an important challenge regarding healthcare providers' communication with patients. Compassionate communication is not just being ready and willing to do face-work on behalf of patients, although that readiness and willingness is crucial. Fully compassionate communication is *transactional* communication (Martin, 2011).

Transactional communication requires a two-way flow of information so that the message sender is also a message receiver and vice-verse (Barnlund, 1971; du Pre & Foster, 2016; Martin, 2011; Rushton, et al., 2007). The transactional nature of humor requires not just that the message be sent and received in its respective contexts, but that it be sent and received *effectively*. The only way to judge this is by the receiver's response. In the case at hand, readers will never know what James thought of the geography joke.

As effective communicators, healthcare providers need to continually check to make sure that what they are saying is understood and received in a respectful, non-face-threatening way to ensure that they understand patients' perspectives (Byrd et al., 2020; du Pre & Foster, 2016; Tanveer, et al., 2018). I mentioned at the start of this chapter that humor is a tricky business because meaning coded as humor can be easily misunderstood or missed entirely. Thus we must be careful not to assume that compassionately intended humor is received as intended. Communicating transactionally, we need to continually check for responses that clearly signal "message received."

In writing these words, I am in no way critiquing Dr. Tailor's communication skills with patients. I assume that in the moment, Dr. Tailor did look for signs that James understood and welcomed the joke. Rather, because that part of the exchange is absent from the story, I am taking the opportunity to remind readers of the importance of being an effective partner in multidirectional communication with patients.

IMPLICATIONS FOR MAINTAINING POSITIVE COMMUNICATION WITH PATIENTS

Specific Recommendations Based Upon This Case

Dr. Tailor's use of humor signaled her awareness of potential embarrassment that James might have felt. Her joke was also a demonstration of sensitivity toward James' vulnerability in the moment. Given the analysis presented in this chapter, I offer a few further suggestions, moving toward more awareness of the transactional potential of patient-provider communication:

Recommendation 1: Listen deeply.

Implementation 1: When people speak, the words that they use and the thoughts that they express reflect a lifetime of experiences, good and bad. Most of the time, people don't realize how their current and past circumstances condition what they say right now. When listening to patients, try to understand where they are coming from—not just mentally and emotionally, but also with respect to economic and social conditions. This might require a great deal of patience, and even forgiveness—as in this case study—but will go a long way toward building trust, and thus, richer, more effective communication.

Recommendation 2: Remember that humor is risky.

Implementation 2: Humor can work very well in reducing stress, demonstrating connection, and saving face. On the other hand, well-intentioned humor can be easily misinterpreted as sarcasm, cynicism, and personal insult. This is where the transactional model of communication is essential, bringing us to the next recommendation:

Recommendation 3: Check to make sure that the patient understands your offer of humor.

Implementation 3: Nonverbal responses are particularly revealing: Do patients laugh in response to your joke? If so, does the laugh reveal shared appreciation of the joke, or does it reveal displeasure? Look for body language: Facial expressions and body language will tell you if your sense of humor is appreciated or not. And of course, what do patients say in response to a well-meant offer of humor? Does their verbal response demonstrate both understanding and sharing of the humorous intent?

Recommendation 4: Self-referential humor is likely to be the safest form of humor in a face-working situation, especially when striving to help the patient recover from a *faux pas*.

Implementation 5: Recall that Dr. Tailor's joke referred to herself, not to James. By shifting the attention to herself, Dr. Tailor deflected potential shame felt by James.

A Few Self-Reflexive, Concluding Remarks

As I write the final words of this chapter, I am aware of a certain irony. I have pointed out that Dr. Tailor maintained a rhetorical position of power by framing the story of the humorous incident entirely from her perspective. The irony in writing this chapter is that as author, I am doing exactly the same thing by reframing the story entirely from my own perspective. This chapter, in other words, is yet another layer of context, and just like Dr. Tailor (and James for that matter), I bring my own cultural capital to the situation so that my perspective is conditioned by where I'm coming from.

Through various circumstances that have brought me to where I am today, I have developed some knowledge of communication, face-work, humor, and the importance of context. I have used that knowledge to try to understand Dr. Tailor's use of humor in trying to save her patient from feeling embarrassed. Other communication scholars could look at the same story and the same joke, interpreting them in different ways based on their theoretical perspectives.

Although my interpretation of the specific instance described in this chapter is certainly open to equally valid re-interpretations, I feel safe in concluding that virtually all communication scholars will agree that context informs meaning and that any communicative act reflects many factors conditioned by many contexts. The important thing to remember is that all of us bring our own sets of tools (looking at it positively) or baggage (looking at it negatively) to every communicative situation—whether we are healthcare providers, communication scholars, or patients. As such, we need to always remember to ask two fundamental questions: Where is the other person coming from? Where am I coming from? Answers to these questions remind us to be aware of how our respective positions of power inform appropriate use of communication techniques, including humor, in doing the never-ending of maintaining face, not just for ourselves, but also for those with whom we work on a daily basis.

REFERENCES

Archer, B., Azios, J. H., & Moody, S. (2019). Humour in clinical–educational interactions between graduate student clinicians and people with aphasia. *International Journal of Language & Communication Disorders*, *54*(4), 580–595. doi:10.1111/1460-6984.12461 PMID:30779411

Barnlud, D. C. (1970). Transactional model of communication. In K. K. Sereno & C. D. Mortensen (Eds.), *Foundations of communication theory* (pp. 83–102). Harper & Row.

Beach & Prickett. (2017). Laughter, humor, and cancer: Delicate moments and poignant interactional circumstances. *Health Communication, 32*(7), 791-802. doi:10.1080/10410236.2016.1172291

Bell, E. (2008). *Theories of Performance.* Sage Publications, Inc.

Binhammer, K. (2017). The story within the story of sentimental fiction. *Narrative*, *25*(1), 45–64. doi:10.1353/nar.2017.0003

Brown, P., & Levinson, S. (1987). *Politeness: Some universals of language use.* Cambridge University Press. doi:10.1017/CBO9780511813085

Burke, K. (1961). *The rhetoric of religion: Studies in logology.* University of California Press.

Burke, K. (1969). *A grammar of motives.* University of California Press. doi:10.1525/9780520341715

Burton, L. L. (2012). Defacement: Indigenous patients' experiences in Baja Verapaz, Guatemala. *The Howard Journal of Communications*, *23*(2), 119–135. doi:10.1080/10646175.2012.667723

Byrd, A., Iheagwara, K., McMahon, P., Bolton, M., & Roy, M. (2020). Using multisource feedback to assess resident communication skills: Adding a new dimension to milestone data. *The Ochsner Journal*, *20*(3), 255–260. doi:10.31486/toj.19.0054 PMID:33071656

Charon, R. (2006). *Narrative medicine: Honoring the stories of illness.* Oxford University Press.

Cho, M. K., & Sillars, A. (2015). Face threat and facework strategies when family (health) secrets are revealed: A comparison of South Korea and the United States. *Journal of Communication*, *65*(3), 535–557. doi:10.1111/jcom.12161

Claramita, M., Prabandari, Y. S., Graber, A., & Scherpbier, A. J. J. (2020). Challenges of communication skills transfer of medical students in the cultural context of Indonesia. *The Interdisciplinary Journal of Problem-Based Learning*, *14*(1). Advance online publication. doi:10.14434/ijpbl.v14i1.28594

du Pre, A., & Foster, E. (2016). Transactional communication. In E. Wittenberg & B. R. Ferrell (Eds.), Textbook of palliative care communication (pp. 14-21). Oxford University Press.

Glenright, M., Tapley, B., Rano, J. K. S., & Pexma, P. M. (2017). Developing appreciation for sarcasm and sarcastic gossip: It depends on perspective. *Journal of Speech, Language, and Hearing Research: JSLHR*, *60*(11), 3295–3309. doi:10.1044/2017_JSLHR-L-17-0058 PMID:29098274

Goffman E. (2003). On face-work: An analysis of ritual elements in social interaction. *Reflections, 4*(3), 7-13. (Original work published 1967) doi:10.1162/15241730360580159

Haakana, M. (2002). Laughter in medical interactions: From quantification to analysis, and back. *Journal of Sociolinguistics*, *6*(2), 207–235. doi:10.1111/1467-9481.00185

Little, M., Jordens, C. F. C., Paul, K., Sayers, E., & Sriskandarajah, D. (2000). Face, honor and dignity in the context of colon cancer. *The Journal of Medical Humanities*, *21*(4), 229–243. doi:10.1023/A:1009077209274

Mahvar, T., Mohammadi, N., Seyedfatem, N., & Vedadhir, A. (2020). Interpersonal communication among critical care nurses: An ethnographic study. *Journal of Caring Sciences*, *9*(1), 57–64. doi:10.34172/jcs.2020.009 PMID:32296660

Martin, C. J. H. (2011). Transactional analysis: A method of analysing communication. *British Journal of Midwifery*, *19*(9), 587–593. doi:10.12968/bjom.2011.19.9.587

McCornack, S. (2016). *Reflect & relate: An introduction to interpersonal communication*. Bedford/St. Martin's.

Repede, E. (2008). All that holds: A story of healing. *Journal of Holistic Nursing*, *26*(3), 226–232. doi:10.1177/0898010108323012 PMID:18755883

Rhys, C. S., & Schmidt-Renfree, N. (2000). Facework, social politeness and the Alzheimer's patient. *Clinical Linguistics & Phonetics*, *14*(7), 533–543. doi:10.1080/026992000750020350

Riessman, C. K. (1993). *Narrative analysis*. Sage Publications.

Rushton, C. H., Reina, M. L., & Reina, D. S. (2007). Building trustworthy relationships with critically ill patients and families. *AACN Advanced Critical Care*, *18*(1), 19–30. doi:10.4037/15597768-2007-1004 PMID:17284945

Saunders, P. A. (1998). "You're out of your mind!": Humor as a face-saving strategy during neuropsychological examinations. *Health Communication*, *10*(4), 357–372. doi:10.120715327027hc1004_4 PMID:16370980

Shannon, C. E., & Weaver, W. (1949). *The mathematical theory of communication*. University of Illinois Press.

Tanveer, F., Shahid, S., & Hafiz, M. M. (2018). Impact of doctor's interpersonal communication skill on patient's satisfaction level. *ISRA Medical Journal*, *10*(5), 306–309.

Chapter 23
But Why Were You in a Bar Fight?

Monalisa M. Tailor
Norton Healthcare, USA

An exceeding number of memes, movies, and jokes are dedicated to the notion that getting old is not fun, but it can be funny. For many people, the aging process can be frightening though. They worry that as their body continues to age that they will lose their freedoms.

Working as a GP, I see many geriatric patients who are clearly embarrassed by their illnesses and injuries. It is as though they feel that their body is betraying them by revealing the secret of their real age through their illnesses and injuries. They sometimes enter my office with a new issue acting like a child prepared to be scolded by their schoolteacher, dreading the punishment that will be dealt out.

It is important for patients, especially elderly patients, to understand that when it is time for the hard talks about changing their lifestyle that they should not feel ashamed. The need to change their lifestyle is a product of circumstances beyond their control. While they may still dread the change, separating the shame from the dread is critical for managing their anxiety, and their physician's communication is key in managing those feelings. This is why humor can be an effective tool for relieving this anxiety.

A particular incident that comes to mind was when one of my favorite 88 year old patients came in for an appointment with her daughter. This patient lived on her own, and her daughter lived close by to assist her when needed. This particular visit took place because my patient tripped in her garage and took a fall. Although she was not badly hurt (thankfully), the patient was on blood thinners which meant she had severe bruising, especially on her face with purple circles under her eyes and across her cheeks.

This is one of my geriatric patients that fits the profile described above about having anxiety about her health and age. She wore the awareness of her mortality like a cloak of shame. When she came to see me about this fall, she was even more nervous than usual to hear my assessment while her face was painted purple with bruises. Seeing the nonverbal signs of her nervousness, instead of giving her my usual greeting, I shook her hand and asked, "But why did you get into a bar fight?" She blinked at

DOI: 10.4018/978-1-7998-4528-7.ch023

me...a moment of shock and confusion passed her face and then she was laughing. A simple one-line joke took the edge off and she was able to engage in a calm conversation throughout the appointment with her dignity intact about the implications of this fall for her independence and ability to live alone.

Chapter 24
Response: "But Why Were You in a Bar Fight?"

Alyse Keller
CUNY Kingsbsorough Community College, USA

RELEVANT LITERATURE

Interactions between patients and physicians are a particularly rich communicative occurrence since "interaction is the fundamental instrument by which the doctor/patient relationship is shaped and through which medical care is directed" (Roter & Hall, 2011, p. 55). As a result, close attention to both the verbal and nonverbal exchanges that transpire between patients and physicians are not only important but necessary. Even though the current healthcare system has come a long way from the paternalistic communication practices of its past, we must still take care to understand and analyze best communication practices for both physicians and patients.

In the past doctors were simply trained to save lives, which emphasized, "protocol over emotion" (Davidson, 2016, p. 33). This approach to medical care neglected to focus on what is important in the patient-doctor interaction--the patient. As a result, doctors and healthcare practitioners often disregarded patient autonomy and desires. Eventually a paradigmatic shift emerged within the healthcare system which moved doctors toward a patient-centered ethic of care. Patient-centered care focuses on the person first. The model of patient-centered care considers the person or patient's whole illness experience by "knowing about the patients' life context (family, work, religion, culture, social support, etc.), as well as personal developmental stages (life history and personal and developmental issues)" (Hudon et al., 2012, p. 173).

To practice patient-centered care, healthcare practitioners are called upon to, "create languages which can bridge the gulf between physician and patient" (Bergum & Dossetor, 2005, p.13). Arguably, one such language that can bridge this gulf, is humor. Humor in the context of medical care can be viewed as "an important communication strategy of patients and providers" (Schopf et al., 2017, p. 374). In particular, humor generates positive effects as "humor can help to relax the patient…But, beyond being comforting and supportive, it can be empowering, and promote adjustment and learning" (Penson et

DOI: 10.4018/978-1-7998-4528-7.ch024

al., 2005, p. 656). Humor's ability to comfort and empower are only two of its many properties. Simply put, humor is productive.

Previous work on humor touches upon a variety of topics, but particularly salient to this case is a study on the use of humor in the context of families living with chronic illness and disability (Keller, 2017). Through interviews and immersive field work, data was collected about family communication on maternal Multiple Sclerosis. Through close analysis of interviews and fieldwork, it was established that humor was the most prominent mode of communication in the study's family unit and was being used as a means of communicating the illness and disability experience with one another. This discovery led to an understanding of humor's therapeutic benefits in the family unit, but most of all led to a greater appreciation of its ability to help individuals communicate about and through their experiences. The functions of humor were defined through the four "R's" of humor: Reframing; Resistance; Relief; and Relational (Keller, 2017).

These four "R's" acts as organizational tools to help understand the humor in families coping with disability and chronic illness. They also work as communicative tools to help describe humor's function and explicate its uses. Humor as a form of r*eframing* relies on the shared ability of two or more individuals to redefine a difficult or trying experience into something that brings levity and ease. For instance, in the original study (Keller, 2017) humor was used by family members to redirect conversations about Multiple Sclerosis (MS) that may have been too painful to talk about. It was used to make a difficult experience into something they could laugh about. Humor as a form of *resistance* is the productive means by which one or more can push back against stigma or stereotypes and empathize with a situation rather than sympathize. Again, humor as resistance manifested itself in the study through its ability to resist sadness and redefine the illness experience as more than a "tragedy." Humor as *relational* means that humor can act as the stimulus for stronger relationships and help develop a greater relational sensitivity towards others. And last, humor as a form of *relief* helps to put individuals at ease or take a break from the emotional chaos that may occur due to their illness or a diagnosis. Humor acts as an outlet which can help all individuals process their experiences, and ultimately enabled the family to communicate more effectively about their lived experiences with MS.

Overall these tools emerged from the use of humor and were then used to help explicate the communicative function of humor in families living with chronic illness/disability. While these tools and their definitions are derived from theories of disability humor (Bingham & Green, 2016) and theories of humor (Bethea et al., 2000), they have applications beyond the family context. It's important to expand upon these tools and allow for their broader application. I argue that these same four R's of humor can be reconceptualized anew and applied in the context of Monalisa Tailor's case. The four functions are not only specific to communication that occurs in a family, but also the communication which occurs in the patient/physician encounter. While the roles and encounters may differ, there are several parallels between the communication occurring in families with chronic illness/disability and the aging patient/provider relationship in Tailor's case.

Individuals with chronic illness/disability and aging patients who may feel helpless in the patient/physician appointment, are facing situations that are beyond their control. First, many patients who are aging are already susceptible to being diagnosed with chronic illness or disability as a result of their age. They are likely being treated in ways that are often infantilizing or patronizing and are confronted with the prospect of losing autonomy. This is a possibility, for many, that can be scary and overwhelming. With this in mind, it takes a family caregiver or healthcare provider to help re-configure how to navigate this fearful scenario. And one such way to navigate this terrain is to shift the way one communicates with those who are aging or possess a chronic illness/ disability. Learning how to communicate through this difficult scenario with grace and ease is a skill. Moreover, infusing these scenarios with humor can help to achieve a situation that is mutually beneficial for all involved.

Each of the four "R's" above can be used in the context of the patient/physician case as a lens to view the way humor functions in a transaction. They operate as tools to help redefine the physician/patient encounter and create new ways of communicating through that experience. As I read Tailor's case, "But Why Were You in a Bar Fight?" I find the four R's of humor are present and applicable to this scenario.

APPLICATION TO THE CASE

Humor As Reframing

Monalisa Tailor's encounter is an important example of the use of humor as a form of reframing. Reframing in the context of humor means to use humor to redirect and reshape a specific event or transaction. The impetus for this reframing may vary from context to context but overall is intended to change the tone or direction of the encounter. From the very beginning of this case, Tailor uses humor as a form of reframing to help their patient.

Tailor mentions from the start that "the aging process can be frightening" and "getting old is not fun, but it can be funny." Both of these descriptions imply that the physician is aware that their aging patient is scared coming into the encounter, but there is hope for reconceptualizing how they view the interaction. Further on, Tailor notices the patient's explicit and implicit signs of her fear through, "the nonverbal signs of her nervousness." This is a significant point to assess since the physician is not only relying on the patient's verbal communication but also the non-verbal cues the patient is providing them.

Tailor notes that "separating the shame from the dread is critical for managing their anxiety, and their physician's communication is key in managing those feelings." This is the moment we understand the power the physician has to shift the communication and outcome of an encounter. After noticing the "cloak of shame" the patient wore into the appointment, Tailor is faced with a decision to make communicatively. This is when we are introduced to the physicians' use of humor as one such tool to communicate through the situation. As the patient shows signs of embarrassment and fear concerning their bruises from a fall, Tailor responds with the humorous remark, "But why did you get into a bar fight?"

Obviously, the patient did not get in a bar fight, and Tailor mentions this is not how they would normally communicate to their patient, but this type of humor reframes this encounter from one that can instigate shame to one in which the patient is at ease. Tailor is perceptive and their observations allowed them to take the burden of anxiety off of the patient, redefining the situation. We see a shift right away in the patient's demeanor when, "she blinked…a moment of shock and confusion passed her face and then she was laughing." Laughter creates comfort and a stronger connection between the patient and physician.

Tailor did not reframe this situation on a whim. Rather a close analysis of the patient and the context led to their use of humor as a tool to reframe the appointment. This reframing was done with the best intentions, as Tailor believed it would benefit both the patient and the situation. Not every patient may find the use of humor as relieving or enjoyable. As such it is necessary that physicians engage in the practice of close reading (Charon et al., 2016), to better understand how to communicate with their patients. Close reading in the medical context is the practice of paying close attention to the details of an encounter by listening, observing, and experiencing with one's patient. It will be noted later that there can be ethical and legal consequences for physicians who don't take the use of humor seriously in the context of their encounter. Yet if used properly, humor as a form of reframing is undoubtedly beneficial.

Humor As Relational

Humor also possesses the ability to create and further develop relationships. Building a relationship between patient and provider is nothing new to the medical literature. Yet, using humor as a relational tool is. It is without a doubt, that the preexisting relationship between Tailor and their patient, is what allows humor to help the situation rather than hinder it. Humor not only relies on a sensitive understanding of the patient and context, but can also result in a stronger relationship between patient and provider.

We don't know the backstory on the relationship between Tailor and the patient, yet the few details we do know provide the information that there is a previous relationship, and it is a positive one. For instance, Tailor explains from the start that this is one of their favorite patients. Additionally, Tailor notes that "this is one of my geriatric patients that fits the profile described above about having anxiety about her health and age." These details provide us with an understanding that a previous relationship exists between patient and provider. As a result, the use of humor may be easier to apply because the patient and physician knew each other before this encounter.

It is not only clear that there is a past relationship, but one in which Tailor has attentively listened to their patient. Charon et. al (2016) state, "The consequences of attentive and accurate listening in a clinical practice can include deep companionship between teller and listener, mutual investment, reciprocal clarity, and affiliation" (p.157). Tailor shows us that through their attentive listening and observation skills, a deeper companionship developed between patient and provider, ultimately opening the door for their confident use of humor. Again, just like with humor as a form of reframing, we see that attention to detail and empathic listening skills open the door for a relationship to exist and humor to be used in that relationship.

It is important to accept that the use of humor does not necessarily necessitate a strong previous relationship. Humor can forge relationships in some scenarios or make existing relationships stronger. In this case, we see the credibility between patient and provider shift after Tailor's joke—"A simple one-line joke took the edge off ...with her dignity intact." This shows that humor as a relational tool can help to strengthen a relationship as well. Again, the foundation of this use of humor relies on the physician's ability to learn a patient's story through close reading and good listening skills. Regardless of the scenario, this is a practice that can lead physicians to use humor appropriately and apply it to their practice. With this, humor as a relational tool proves that humor can be used to both strengthen a preexisting relationship or develop a new relationship between patient and provider.

Humor As Resistance

The use of humor as a form of resistance is another tool that is thematically woven throughout this case. Humor is used strategically by Tailor to ease the patient's worries. Humor belies the traditionally paternalistic approach to medicine. Such an approach can frame older or disabled patients, like Tailor's, as less capable. For example, Tailor elaborates, "It is important for patients, especially elderly patients, to understand that when it is time for the hard talks about changing their lifestyle that they should not feel ashamed." Yet, the shame they feel isn't fabricated. This shame is produced and reproduced culturally. It is a shame they likely sense often. With that said, it takes someone or something to resist these patterns of reproduction, and Tailor does exactly that in this case.

To reduce the shame and manage subsequent patient anxiety, Tailor resists the stereotypical treatment of a geriatric patient and infuses the encounter with humor. People with disabilities, and those who are aging, are often treated as fragile and without autonomy. Tailor opposes this construction by treating their patient with dignity and respect. They do so by infusing their communication with humor. The very definition of paternalistic communication is that which strips the patient of independence. At the root of this encounter is the patient's visible fears of aging and losing their independence as a result of said aging. By resisting the "easy" approach and allowing the patient to regain power, the Tailor shows that they acknowledge her fears but won't let that overshadow the patient's needs and rights.

We further see resistance used in this case as a way to eliminate anxiety and remove the "cloak of shame" the patient is metaphorically wearing. Again, the physician has many choices as to how they can approach the patient. One such approach is to communicate with the patient tenderly and with sympathy. Certainly, this isn't a bad choice and can also be viewed as appropriate. Yet, Tailor resists this choice and opts for a resolution that opens up a different conversation and outcome. Instead of ignoring the patient's anxiety and shame, Tailor directly confronts it with the greeting "But why did you get into a bar fight?" They flip the expected sympathy, into empathy and provide power to the patient they might not have otherwise felt.

Tailor's joke and use of humor in this case immediately resist the stereotypical construction of the "weak, elderly" patient and instead redirects how the patient sees themselves and hopefully the direction of the encounter as a whole. It is within this resistance of the expected, that helps generate communication and foster relationships between the patient and physician. Humor is one way to resist.

Humor As Relief

Finally, the use of humor as a form of relief is omnipresent throughout this case. The impetus for Tailor's use of humor was to relieve the patient of the anxiety and fear they felt due to the oft stigmatized aging process. At the start of the case, Tailor notes that "Working as a GP, I see many geriatric patients who are clearly embarrassed by their illness and injuries. It is as though they feel that their body is betraying them…and sometimes enter my office…acting like a child prepared to be scolded by their schoolteacher, dreading the punishment that will be dealt out." This provides a rich description of how high the stakes are for this, and many other patients, and just how apprehensive they feel entering the physician's office.

With this in mind, using humor to reduce tension and help the patient feel a sense of relief is an important tool for physicians to use. After Tailor uses humor in this case, we witness the direct result when they state, "She was able to engage in a calm conversation throughout the appointment with her dignity intact about the implications of this fall for her independence and ability to live alone." There is a direct correlation in this case between humor and feeling relief. The use of humor is what enabled this final sense of relief for the patient and consequently set the stage for the physician to have a more productive conversation with her. Just one, ostensibly simple joke, broke the tension and helped the physician conduct the rest of the appointment.

TAKE AWAY FROM THE CASE

This case shows that "the value of humor resides, not in its capacity to alter physical reality, but in its capacity for affective or psychological change which enhances the humanity of an experience, for both care providers and recipients of care" (Dean & Major, 2008, p. 1088). Destigmatizing the communication surrounding difficult conversations is of the utmost importance for physicians and healthcare professionals. Aging, and often illness, are inevitable parts of the human experience, and communication in both its verbal and non-formal forms help constitute these experiences. By shifting the traditional approach of discussing aging and illness, physicians possess the power to instigate positive change in the lives of their patients. They can do so by changing their communication style. The use of humor then is one such way of making this change.

When humor in the healthcare setting is "delivered with sensitivity and caring, humor is effective, not necessarily because of its content, but because it conveys empathy and recognizes the dignity of the individual" (Dean & Major, 2008, p. 1094). Monalisa Tailor's case study "But Why Were You in a Bar Fight?" shows us exactly that. As we witness in this case, humor functions and can be analyzed through the four R's of humor; as a form of resistance, a way to relieve tension or anxiety, a relational mechanism, and a mode of reframing the experience. Overall, the use of humor in this case, "is not about making the [aging] experience normal, or regular, rather making the experience *a* norm and *a* regular experience" (Keller, 2017).

From this case emerge two recommendations for healthcare workers to use in their own practices moving forward. First, I provide ways healthcare practitioners can ensure humor is used properly and effectively in order to avoid negative ramifications. And second, I provide suggestions for teaching communication and humor as a learned skill.

Recommendation 1

The four R's of humor, which have been applied to this case, also carry with them potentially ethical and legal ramifications in the healthcare context. Undoubtedly studies have shown that when individuals laugh together, they are more likely to trust or like one another (Kurtz & Algoe, 2017; Abramson, 2019). Yet this trust that is developed doesn't occur in a vacuum. With this, physicians must be cognizant of the potential pitfalls and consequences to the use of humor in the healthcare experience, and how to effectively avoid these negative results.

Implementation of Recommendation 1

As Berger et al. (2004) note, physicians need to be conservative in what humor they use and how they use it in the patient-physician encounter. The content of the humor used and how the humor is used are two important components of the application of humor in the patient/physician scenario. Humor applied in the wrong way, to the wrong patient, can result in terrible consequences. These ramifications can include "breach of contract, defamation, trademark infringement, harassment or hostile work environment, and intentional or negligent infliction of emotional distress" (Schweikart, 2020). Worst-case scenarios have even resulted in medical malpractice claims (Schweikart, 2020).

As such, physicians must be wary of the potential pitfalls of using humor in the healthcare setting (Osincup, 2020). One such pitfall is the fact that some patients may simply not be receptive to humor.

Just like all individuals have different senses of humor, the same holds for the use of humor with a patient. Not every patient will process humor the same way. Another pitfall is that physicians may risk offending the patient, depending on the type of humor they use and the jokes they make. Yet again, not all patients will understand humor from the same perspective or lens.

Certainly, this is not to scare physicians away from the use of humor, but rather to place a warning label. As with any communication practice or approach to care, it must be applied and used wisely. As always, good communication is the basis for effective care. I believe for doctors to ultimately achieve effective and satisfying communication for patients they must humanize medicine in the ways we witness Monalisa Tailor do. As this case shows, "humor relies on an understanding of context, a relational sensitivity towards the other and a keen ability to listen" (Keller, 2017). Additionally, there is an importance placed on the physician "to listen, connect with a patient and follow their lead" (Abramson, 2019). With this all healthcare practitioners should approach the use of humor in the patient/physician encounter with empathy, strong listening skills and an understanding of context.

Recommendation 2

Ultimately Tailor's use of humor, in this case, exemplifies a strong use of empathetic, relational, and observational communication skills. This is the type of communication that may come naturally for some, but for others can certainly be taught. With this in mind, I call on medical schools and practicing clinicians to start learning and practicing this type of communication and humor. Humor and communication are both skills that can be taught and refined.

Implementation of Recommendation 2

First, there is a need to improve communication pedagogy, in medical schools so that physicians can effectively communicate with their patients. Medical schools would be wise to hire communication scholars to teach those courses to start implementing a curriculum that takes a more relational and humanistic approach to communication, as evidenced in this case (Amati & Hannawa, 2014; Villigran et al., 2010). These skills are not only necessary in medical schools but also important for doctors to learn as well. Workshops on effective communication skills and humor are important to continuously keep healthcare workers at the top of their game.

Second, in addition to strong communication skills, education on the importance of humor in the healthcare setting is important as well. Arguably, Tailor uses humor in this case very effectively, but not all doctors would necessarily approach this scenario the same way or may not produce the same results. Understanding the nuances of humor in the healthcare setting, and in particular, through the lens of the Four R's of humor, can help physicians to view humor as a productive and pedagogical tool to connect with their patients.

REFERENCES

Abramson, A. (2019, August 26). The power of humor in healthcare. *Elemental.* https://elemental.medium.com/the-power-of-humor-in-healthcare-1bd412254daf

Amati, R., & Hannawa, A. F. (2014). Relational dialectics theory: Disentangling physician-perceived tensions of end-of-life communication. *Health Communication, 29*(10), 962–973. doi:10.1080/10410236.2013.815533 PMID:24345181

Berger, J. T., Coulehan, J., & Belling, C. (2004). Humor in the physician-patient encounter. *Archives of Internal Medicine, 164*(8), 825–830. doi:10.1001/archinte.164.8.825 PMID:15111367

Bergum, V., & Dossetor, J. (2005). *Relational ethics: The full meaning of respect.* University Publishing Group.

Bethea, L. S., Travis, S. S., & Pecchioni, L. (2000). Family caregivers' use of humor in conveying information about caring for dependent older adults. *Health Communication, 12*(4), 361–376. doi:10.1207/S15327027HC1204_3 PMID:11063286

Bingham, S. C., & Green, S. E. (2016). *Seriously funny: Disability and the paradoxical power of humor.* Lynne Rienner Publishers.

Charon, R., DasGupta, S., Hermann, N., Irvine, C., Marcus, E. R., Colón, E. R., Spencer, D., & Spiegel, M. (2016). *The principles and practice of narrative medicine* [Kindle Version]. doi:10.1093/med/9780199360192.001.0001

Davidson, L. G. (2016). Would you like a map? *Departures in Critical Qualitative Research, 5*(1), 23–36. doi:10.1525/dcqr.2016.5.1.23

Dean, R. A. K., & Major, J. E. (2008). From critical care to comfort care: The sustaining value of humour. *Journal of Clinical Nursing, 17*(8), 1088–1095. doi:10.1111/j.1365-2702.2007.02090.x PMID:18321272

Hudon, C., Fortin, M., Haggerty, J., Loignon, C., Lambert, M., & Poitras, M. E. (2012). Patient-centered care in chronic disease management: A thematic analysis of the literature in family medicine. *Patient Education and Counseling, 88*(2), 170–176. doi:10.1016/j.pec.2012.01.009 PMID:22360841

Keller, A. (2017). *Performing narrative medicine: Understanding familial chronic illness through performance* [Doctoral Dissertation, University of South Florida]. University of South Florida Scholar Commons. https://scholarcommons.usf.edu/etd/6876

Kurtz, L. E., & Algoe, S. B. (2017). When sharing a laugh means sharing more: Testing the role of shared laughter on short-term interpersonal consequences. *Journal of Nonverbal Behavior, 41*(1), 45–65. doi:10.100710919-016-0245-9

Osincup, P. (2020). How to use humor in clinical settings. *AMA Journal of Ethics, 22*(7), 588–595. doi:10.1001/amajethics.2020.588 PMID:32744227

Penson, R. T., Partridge, R. A., Rudd, P., Seiden, M. V., Nelson, J. E., Chabner, B. A., & Lynch, T. J. Jr. (2005). Laughter: The best medicine? *The Oncologist, 8*(10), 651–660. doi:10.1634/theoncologist.10-8-651 PMID:16177290

Roter, D. L., & Hall, J. A. (2011). How medical interaction shapes and reflects the physician–patient relationship. In T. L. Thompson, R. Parrott, & J. F. Nussbaum (Eds.), *The Routledge handbook of health communication* (pp. 83–96). Routledge.

Schöpf, A. C., Martin, G. S., & Keating, M. A. (2017). Humor as a communication strategy in provider–patient communication in a chronic care setting. *Qualitative Health Research, 27*(3), 374–390. doi:10.1177/1049732315620773 PMID:26717942

Schweikart, S. J. (2020). Could humor in health care become malpractice? *AMA Journal of Ethics, 22*(7), 596–601. doi:10.1001/amajethics.2020.596 PMID:32744228

Villagran, M., Goldsmith, J., Wittenberg-Lyles, E., & Baldwin, P. (2010). Creating COMFORT: A communication-based model for breaking bad news. *Communication Education, 59*(3), 220–234. doi:10.1080/03634521003624031

Chapter 25
Humor and Mental Health Therapy

Regina Beach
Centerstone, USA

As a therapist, I specialize in working with children and adult trauma survivors. Most of the adults that I work with have been diagnosed with Post-Traumatic Stress Disorder (PTSD). Others have survived a trauma that does not meet all of the criteria of PTSD and have instead been diagnosed with Other Specified Trauma and Stress Disorder. The point here, is that the people I work with have been through something terrible. Talking about these experiences is difficult, often provoking fear and great sadness.

Therapists are trained to be completely professional. It did not take me long to realize through my practice that complete professionalism is not always the most conducive behavior for helping my clients. Smiling and laughing are critical for their mental health. In fact, research shows that smiling, even if it's a forced smile, tricks our brains into releasing serotonin, which actually makes us happier. Smiling or laughing while they relive their traumas in my office is not going to happen unless I make an effort to elevate the mood, and that is the first reason that I incorporate humor into my therapy sessions.

The second reason that I incorporate humor is to gage stress. Most trauma survivors simply do not respond well to direct questions about people and events close to their trauma. Indirect questions, asked in partial jest, are a much less threatening way to begin conversations. For example, if I am meeting with a new client who I know is a rape victim with children, I may not know if those children were intentional creations or the product of rape. Asking directly about the children is not a good way to encourage conversation if the children are a product of rape. If instead, I make a jest about how I don't know how people with children do it all because I barely have time to get myself ready in the morning, that typically generates a smile and begins a discussion about the children that typically results in any necessary disclosure, even in the case that the children are tied deeply to the trauma.

So that is how humor works well in my line of therapy. The goal is not to get a big barrel laugh, but rather a smile or a small chuckle. The goal is to disarm, calm, and reveal points of stress so that conversation and healing can begin.

DOI: 10.4018/978-1-7998-4528-7.ch025

When the call for cases in this book went out, my mind first went to a particular client. This client was a young adult who is transgender, transitioning from male to female, and happened to be polyamorous. For ease of this case, she will be called Amy. At the time we worked together, Amy was steadily in committed relationships with six different women. A running joke between us had consistently been that I did not know how she managed to keep up with six girlfriends as I felt that one required all of the free time I could manage.

Unfortunately, Amy did not have a supportive home environment. She was not yet financially ready to leave home, but was socially pressured to do so. On the day that Amy told me she had been forced from her home through repeated shaming such as the continual use of her "dead name," misuse of pronouns, degradation of her romantic relationships, etc., she was very sad. When she told me about the dramatic events that led to her leaving home without the financial means to secure her own place, my initial reply to her sad story was, "Well, I can see where the six girlfriends will come in handy now." Amy actually laughed out loud and the mood immediately lightened.

In this case, the humor was extremely effective in lifting the mood and allowing Amy to speak more openly. The acute reaction to my joke was not the norm, but I can consistently count on humor as a better probe to seeking for information than direct questioning if used skillfully. It is critical to reiterate here that in the case of counseling, it is incredibly important for the provider to be very cognizant of the words they are using and how those words may be misconstrued in ways that could trigger the client. In the present case, I was able to joke with this female client about the time commitment involved with having a girlfriend without there being any hint of sexism because the client was aware that I too was a woman who had also dated women. Because of this knowledge, I could have confidence that Amy would interpret my repeated quips about not having time for six girlfriends as a reflection of time, not female stereotypes.

Some clients seek therapy because they know that they need to talk to someone…and yet trusting their therapist enough to disclose can be difficult even if they wish to disclose. Many other clients come to therapy by court order or through peer pressure. These clients are even less prone to disclose. Therefore, any jokes that hint at something that might be against their beliefs or directed at them will be more likely to shut them down rather than put them at ease. It is of the utmost priority that jokes that could even hint at sexism, racism, xenophobia, or homophobia be avoided.

The safest jokes are those that are self-deprecating. In the examples I have provided above, the basis of the jokes has been that my clients clearly have much better time management skills than me to balance the relationships that they maintain. Making oneself the target of the humor helps to ensure that no triggers are accidentally stimulated. Yet, the self-deprecating humor should also focus on topics that do not risk your perceived credibility as their therapist. Admitting that one is shy, busy, or afraid of snakes (as examples) does not reflect upon one's skills as a therapist. Making a self-deprecating joke about being a bad student, a procrastinator, or unorganized may threaten one's credibility. Therapists should wield humor as an essential tool but use it wisely.

Chapter 26
Response: "Humor and Mental Health Therapy"

Scott A. Eldredge
Western Carolina University, USA

Elizabeth D. Dalton
Middle Tennessee State University, USA

Candy J. Noltensmeyer
Western Carolina University, USA

LITERATURE REVIEW

Because of the role it plays in relationship dynamics, humor is a fundamentally communicative process. It is embedded within a message sent by an individual with particular motivations to a receiver that must interpret that use of humor within a social context (Lynch, 2002). Individuals who are skilled at using and interpreting humor are seen as more competent at navigating social situations (Graham et al., 1992). Medical encounters are one such social situation in which humor may be strategically employed. In particular, in counseling and psychotherapy interactions as discussed in the case presented here, both patient and therapist must find ways to feel comfortable discussing personal, and often very difficult, subjects. Humor can be used as an effective tool to facilitate these difficult discussions. For example, humor eases tensions, allows unmentionable topics to be discussed, and allows people to relax (Smith & Powell, 1988). In addition, humor may be used to guard against feelings of overwhelming anxiety while, at the same time, allowing the patient to express those anxieties leading to greater resilience and emotional well-being (Dziegielewski et al., 2003; Martin, 2019).

DOI: 10.4018/978-1-7998-4528-7.ch026

Goals As A Communicative Framework In Healthcare

One way to frame patient-provider communication is by examining each party's goals within an interaction. This approach acknowledges that while both patients and providers have goals pertaining to the medical needs of the patient, they also have goals related to the more social aspects of the interaction. Because they are motivated by layers of different goals (Bensing et al., 2003), providers use specific communication behaviors to achieve those goals with the patient, including humor (c.f., Vergeer & MacRae, 1993).

Clark and Delia (1979) break down this goals-based approach by explaining that in any interaction, goals can be classified as task (i.e., focused on achieving the task at hand), relational (i.e., those concerned with developing, maintaining, or even ending a relationship), or identity goals (i.e., those concerned with portraying and preserving our sense of self and how we are perceived by the outside world). For the healthcare provider, primary, task-focused goals are obvious: help the patient and produce the best possible health outcomes for the patient. But other types of goals are not so obvious or explicit. In healthcare, these secondary goals (Dillard et al., 1989) are most often about preserving both the relationship with the patient as well as maintaining the healthcare providers' own sense of identity. For example, providers who communicate in ways that are clear and complete, encourage partnership, share power, and make an effort to understand patient experiences are more likely to encourage trust (a relational goal) in their patients (Thom, 2001; Thom & Campbell, 1997). Identity goals are present for providers as well. In the moment, the provider may not be consciously thinking about this type of goal. After all, why should they care what the patient thinks of them? But it turns out that, not only does the provider care, but these relational and identity goals often supersede the task-oriented goals of ensuring optimal patient health outcomes (Dalton et al., 2020).

Patients have goals too. We have a "face" to protect, and we want to be a "good" patient in the eyes of our providers (Jadad et al., 2003). We don't want to be judged (Ogden et al., 2020), and we don't want to let our doctors down when they tell us we should take medication, do our physical therapy, or work on repairing a relationship at home. But we also want to get better when we are sick, prevent illness, and heal from our traumas. Often, these things are at odds, making disclosure – the sharing of personal information about ourselves – feel difficult or impossible (Greene, 2009). According to the disclosure decision-making model (Greene, 2009), patients must feel safe when disclosing their personal information, they must feel like disclosure will produce positive outcomes, and they must feel like they are able to talk about the issue effectively. All of these factors patients use to decide whether or not to disclose information hinge on the personal or social aspects of the interaction. However, when assessing these factors, additional social dynamics affect how each party may employ particular communication strategies to achieve their relational goals, which, in turn, affect their success in achieving their task goals.

Culture, Identity, Stigma, and Healthcare

There are many challenges individuals may face in meeting their relational, identity and task goals. "We often assume that if our own experience differs from that of our peers, it must by extension be less legitimate" (Garrison, 2018, p. 620). As a result, differing cultural nuances, group affiliation and identity, and stigma all impact the communication strategies both healthcare providers and their patients choose to employ when attempting to build trust, encourage disclosure, and foster a sense of relationship. While there may be a great many cultural nuances relevant to any patient-provider interaction, for the sake of this case we will focus on the LGBTQIA+ culture, specifically Lesbian and Trans culture. The patient in this case identified as a transgender female, while the provider identified as a woman who has dated women. As Belous & Bauman (2017) noted:

For some, sexual identity labels may provide a sense of community with others who identify in the same manner. Labels offer individuals an opportunity to express themselves and represent their personal journey. The same label provides society with the vocabulary necessary to serve as an important component in conversations regarding privilege and power.

While labels might provide community, they can also constrict our behaviors to those we feel help us belong, which could in turn potentially evoke discrimination (Ferguson, 2015). In other words, labels might be placed upon us by others that don't necessarily fit our personal sense of identity. Furthermore, "as gender-variant people cannot anticipate how they will be 'read' by others, many engage with gender deliberately and self-consciously, tailoring their presentation in ways that will enable them to be seen as they desire" (Garrison, 2018, p. 616). This means that gender-variant individuals are faced with a choice: they can adopt a personal style they feel presents an accurate representation of their self and identity or one that will allow them to pass within generally accepted notions of what constitutes male and female gender binaries. These choices to represent themselves in particular ways have implications for the patient when interacting with a healthcare provider. If patients choose not to disclose their sexual identity, important medical information may not be shared with the provider. For example, research has shown lesbian and bisexual women are less likely to use preventative health services (Graham et al., 2011), and gay men are less likely to return to their healthcare providers if they perceived a lack of support when sharing their sexual identity (Cant, 2007).

While culture impacts how patients and healthcare providers navigate their interactions, the LGBTQIA+ community also must often deal with the effects of stigma and marginalization. In a culture where homosexuals often find themselves the targets of discrimination or even the victims of violence because of their sexual orientation, LGBTQIA+ people often fear they will experience unpleasant interactions and receive inferior medical care if they discuss their sexual identity (Klitzman & Greenberg, 2002; Rossman, et al., 2017). When the healthcare provider identifies as part of the same co-cultural group (LGBTQIA+) as the patient, it diminishes (but doesn't negate) the potential for stigmatizing instances to occur within the interaction, at least relating to gender identity and sexual attraction (Noltensmeyer & Meisenbach, 2016). Much like gender and even humor, stigmas are socially constructed and culturally nuanced, making them challenging to negotiate across varied interactions.

How one internalizes those stigmatized identities will impact how one decides to address the stigma when interacting with others (Noltensmeyer & Meisenbach, 2016). A typical physician visit is often marked by sharing very personal and private information regarding health history, current health issues or concerns, family health information, and sexual information and history. Information-sharing of this nature can be a stressful experience for any patient; however, for the patient that identifies as part of the LGBTQIA+ community, these interactions have the added dimension of bringing a stigmatized identity into the conversation. The Stigma Management Communication Model (SMC) identifies several strategies for managing communication in potentially stigmatizing interactions. Strategy selection is personal and determined by several factors. Once an individual recognizes a stigmatizing message, they must then consider "(a) the public's perception of the stigma and (b) the applicability of the stigma to the individual" (Meisenbach, 2010, p. 276). A public stigma refers to the stereotypes that are normalized throughout society while an internalized stigma reflects how an individual experiences a stigmatized condition and internalizes the public stigma into their own identity (Smith & Applegate, 2018). Thus, how an LGBTQIA+ person internalizes the stigmatized aspects of their identity also affects their decisions whether to actively share their sexual orientation with a physician or keep it concealed.

While there may be a variety of communicative strategies employed to express one's culture and identity while also combatting the internal and social effects of stigma, people also use humor to acknowledge public stigma while accepting the applicability to themselves. For example, self-deprecating humor is often used to indicate an individuals' recognition of the stigma and ease the tension for the non-stigmatized (Goffman, 1963; Meisenbach, 2010). Furthermore, we must also consider the impact of multiple stigmas that may not be managed alone, but may compound (much like interest on a home loan; Noltensmeyer & Meisenbach, 2016). Managing compounding stigmas complicate any given interaction as the stigmatized must quickly assess others perceptions on multiple levels while simultaneously assessing the trustworthiness of their interaction partner and determining what information they feel comfortable disclosing. Humor may be employed as a strategy to navigate compounding stigmas.

APPLICATIONS TO CASE

As demonstrated in the current scenario, we see how humor can facilitate communicative goals and create a space where meaning is shared, trust is earned, and disclosures are safe in the face of potentially stigmatized identities or behaviors. First, let's examine the goals as expressed by the therapist in this case study, and situate her description of "skillful" humor within different types of goals.

In order for the therapist to help her client, Amy, heal, it is imperative that Amy open up to her about sensitive, potentially traumatic information about herself. The therapist has an explicit, task-oriented goal of identifying and gauging Amy's points of acute stress, necessitating Amy's self-disclosure. In order to elicit self-disclosure, the therapist uses humor to approach stressful topics in an indirect manner. She points out the importance of elevating the mood, making Amy feel calm and non-defensive, while simultaneously highlighting shared everyday life experiences such as the challenges of parenting, dating, or simply getting out the door in the morning, that make us more alike than different. In addition, being able to laugh together makes us feel connected rather than just occupying shared space in a doctor's office. As illustrated in Amy's case, humor has a way of cracking us open, or providing a kind of back door into the parts of ourselves we keep locked up.

Secondary goals emerge here as well. In the healthcare setting, providers want to be seen as credible, competent professionals that patients can rely upon for quality care. Identity goals associated with healthcare providers include being seen as a "good doctor," responsibly stewarding medical resources, and being a patient advocate (e.g., Scott et al., 2020). In the case of treating Amy, the effective use of humor rests on the therapist's ability to balance her own identity as a credible professional with Amy's sense of comfort. When using humor to elicit disclosure, the therapist refers to a recurring joke about time management in dating that neither targets Amy nor erodes her own abilities to provide professional, therapeutic support for her. While this example highlights the need for some reciprocity in disclosure between therapist and client, the therapist points out that the importance of maintaining the integrity of therapy sessions should moderate the type of information she shares with clients. Time management is a relatively innocuous topic. But situating her difficulty with time management within her personal life as opposed to her professional life as a therapist is what maintains the therapist's professional credibility.

At the same time, it discloses something personal about herself, satisfying the need for reciprocity in building trust.

In terms of relational goals, evidence shows that healthcare providers seek to avoid discordance with patients while building trust, rapport, and solidarity (e.g., Adams, 2017). The therapist knows that Amy will only open up to her if she feels safe enough within their relationship to do so, in line with Greene's (2009) disclosure decision-making model. To create safety and gain trust, her relational goals include downplaying the inherent client-provider power dynamic by using humor in a way that promotes parity rather than emphasizing her elevated professional status. Specifically, the therapist revealed that Amy was aware that the therapist also dated women, thus identifying the therapist as a member of the LGBTQIA+ culture. By outing herself as a member of the stigmatized group, the therapist is able to provide another way to encourage self-disclosure by identifying membership as a point of connection. Her joke about the convenience of having six girlfriends in the context of a traumatic event lands safely within the confines of their shared space as queer women. It does not degrade Amy as a trans woman with an unconventional (as defined by a heteronormative culture) number of romantic relational partners. In addition, the joke allows both Amy and the therapist to share their identities and acknowledge the stigma associated with identifying with the LGBTQIA+ culture. Therefore, she is able to maintain a space where client and therapist are communicating as partners, attaining her relational goal of trust and equality.

While humor is a useful tool that may enhance self-disclosure in a therapeutic setting, it is imperative to consider additional factors that may influence how humor is received. Among these factors is the time it takes to develop the intimacy needed for effective humor use in a relationship. Social penetration theory (Altman & Taylor, 1973) posits that relationships increase in intimacy as a function of enduring, deepening, mutual self-disclosure. An ongoing personal or professional relationship, therefore, provides more time and opportunities to connect and reveal parts of themselves to one another. Time has allowed Amy to reveal her trans identity and the therapist to reveal her lesbian identity, connecting them through the broader LGBTQIA+ community and letting them share jokes about one's dating practices within that group. If one fails to take the time to establish shared identity within a group, a joke will more than likely miss its mark and be perceived negatively (c.f., Ellithorpe et al., 2014).

In addition, their time together has allowed them to establish "running jokes." Running jokes serve as a way to build community and connect with others on a personal level (Demjén, 2016). But these jokes must be perceived as funny to both parties, or the jokes lose their ability to connect people. In this case, the therapist had carefully gauged the depth of their shared identity between them and felt safe in her assumption that Amy would find her jokes humorous. As the therapist relates keeping up with six girlfriends to her own lack of time management, she legitimizes Amy's experience by comparing a stigmatized practice (polyamory) to a non-stigmatized one (poor time management). Amy processes this joke for what it is intended to do because she is aware that the therapist is a part of the LGBTQIA+ community. If Amy was unsure of her therapist's status as a member or ally, she may have responded quite differently to the joke.

PROFESSIONAL RECOMMENDATIONS

For therapists working with trauma survivors, humor and professionalism do not have to be at odds. At its core, this type of practice involves dyadic human conversation, wherein disclosure, social support, information-seeking, and other communication processes can be enhanced by the use of humor. But mental health professionals who use humor therapeutically are often walking a metaphorical tightrope. While balancing attentiveness and self-awareness with their own goals for the encounter, they must be attuned to the risks that lie below that tightrope. Potential communicative pitfalls of humor include: timing that violates the normative pace of relational development, inaccurate assumptions about shared identity, inappropriate disclosures, and the overuse of self-deprecation.

Among the assumptions of social penetration theory (Altman & Taylor, 1973) is that relationships develop in a "normal" way when the depth of disclosure is mutual and gradual. While the client-therapist relationship develops at a faster pace with less mutuality of disclosure (which is expected of the client but not the therapist), this theory still holds lessons for the effective use of humor in these relationships. For example, it may not be "safe" to incorporate humor in initial encounters. Without deeper baseline knowledge of the client, especially in the face of trauma, it is difficult to know what, if any, topics are safe - or at least non-offensive - to discuss humorously. Rather, it is increasing intimacy with the patient over time that reveals where the appropriate and effective spaces for joking and humorous remarks are.

A particular risk in the current case is that the client would not fully see herself as part of the therapist's in-group as the therapist assumes. The fact of dating women is one point of commonality between the therapist and client. However, other layers of the client's identity - namely her transgender status and polyamorous dating preference - are not explicitly shared by the therapist. There is risk that the client would not see herself as being in completely the same "tribe" as the therapist after all. If out-group status is indeed perceived, the joke will not likely be evaluated as positively, and can alienate the receiver. This would be highly detrimental to the therapist-client relationship, impeding trust, disclosure, and the overall ability to achieve therapeutic goals. Therefore, work is required, in the form of thorough information-seeking, listening (at which therapists tend to excel), and putting in the time to develop the relationship with the client. On the other hand, for a provider who seeks to align herself with her client in shared identity - in this case, queerness - self-disclosure, openness, and adequate clarity about who she is as a person and a professional may be necessary communicative steps that are unique to the context of mental healthcare.

Although self-disclosure is no longer seen as a taboo practice in therapy, and is in fact embraced as both a necessary and inevitable part of the practice (Bridges, 2001; Knox & Hill, 2003), self-disclosure on the part of the therapist can be a delicate matter to manage. Aspects of the self the therapist chooses to share with clients should align with the provider's identity goals while also meeting the client's needs; providers, therefore, should engage in self-reflection about who they want to be - as a professional and as a person - in the eyes of their clients. While humor can be an effective conduit of such self-disclosures (Ervin-Tripp & Lampert, 2009), this does not mean that only positive information should be disclosed. If negative information is highly relevant to a conversational partner, disclosing it in a humorous way can enhance perceptions of both competence and warmth (Bitterly & Schwitzer, 2019). In other words, if there is an opportunity to bond over something such as a shared minor bad habit (e.g., nail biting), it may be beneficial to the relationship for the therapist to disclose her bad habit in a humorous way. For more serious disclosures, such as the shared experience of a miscarriage, the therapist should not disclose unless she has already achieved personal resolution on the topic (Knox & Hill, 2003), and humor is likely inappropriate.

In terms of the type of humor used in the present case, the therapist explains that self-deprecating humor is the safest kind of humor in these situations. She points out that keeping herself as the target of her own joke is a way to avoid having the client perceive the humor as aggressive. The risk is that, as she points out, self-deprecation may undermine the perceived professionalism of the therapist. This has been observed in situations where an extreme *amount* of self-deprecating humor erodes credibility (Andeweg et al., 2011), but in this case, the therapist points out that the *topic* of self-deprecation can have a similar effect. This suggests that there are role-bound, regulative rules when it comes to using self-deprecating humor. Specifically, if she undermines the attributes or abilities that qualify her as a therapist - such as her intelligence, experience, or professional organizational skills - this can put her credibility with her client at risk. Therapists, therefore, should ask themselves which aspects of their identities are professionally and personally safe to sacrifice in the process of using humanizing, power distance-reducing, self-deprecating humor.

Ritual humor, the repetitive use of specific jokes and enactments that create pivotal social touchstones (Jensen, 2018), may be another useful tool in the therapeutic context. This type of humor can be used to create a space of dignity when public stigma may threaten an individual's sense of belonging and personhood. Though this has been examined at the cultural and organizational level, this case demonstrates opportunities to discuss the role of ritual humor in interpersonal, patient-provider therapeutic contexts. For mental health care providers, this may involve picking up on safe, lighthearted, and humorous points of commonality between themselves and their clients, as well as generalized observations about the outside world, to which they can occasionally return to ease tension and set a tone for openness in the interaction. By easing tensions around a particular subject matter, the use of the "running joke" helps the therapist identify potential areas of difficulty that the client carries and that warrant further exploration for healing to take place (Sparks et al.,2005). In this case, the therapist has identified Amy's polyamorous relationships as a source of shaming and degradation Amy has experienced at the hands of her family. In sharing this running joke related to their romantic lives, the therapist is able to periodically check-in with Amy on this particular source of trauma to determine healing progress.

For the purposes of this case study, the authors, as communication researchers, have attempted to present a perspective that looks at the use of humor as a strategy within a therapeutic setting. Here, the therapist uses humor to achieve particular task, identity, and relationship-oriented goals that ultimately help the client progress in her healing process. In taking this goal-oriented perspective, it is important to remember that humor within the patient-provider relationship in and of itself is not the end goal; rather, humor is the means to creating a social environment that promotes trust and trustworthiness between healthcare provider and patient. In this way, humor allows therapists and their clients to successfully develop and maintain the social aspects of their relationship that may ultimately determine the effectiveness of the therapeutic interventions.

REFERENCES

Adams, E. T. (2017). *Managing multiple goals in opioid prescription communication: Perspectives from trauma physicians* [Masters Thesis]. Communication, University of Kentucky. doi:10.13023/etd.2017.107

Altman, I., & Taylor, D. (1973). *Social penetration: The development of interpersonal relationships*. Holt.

Andeweg, B., Gagestein, S., de Jong, J., & Wackers, M. (2011). *'Poke fun at yourself': The problem of self-deprecating humor*. First World Engineering Education Flash Week.

Belous, C. K., & Bauman, M. L. (2017). What's in a name? Exploring pansexuality online. *Journal of Bisexuality*, *17*(1), 58–72. doi:10.1080/15299716.2016.1224212

Bensing, J., van Dulmen, S., & Tates, K. (2003). Communication in context: New directions in communication research. *Patient Education and Counseling*, *50*(1), 27–32. doi:10.1016/S0738-3991(03)00076-4 PMID:12767581

Bitterly, T. B., & Schweitzer, M. E. (2019). The impression management benefits of humorous self-disclosures: How humor influences perceptions of veracity. *Organizational Behavior and Human Decision Processes*, *151*, 73–89. doi:10.1016/j.obhdp.2019.01.005

Bridges, N. A. (2001). Therapist's self-disclosure: Expanding the comfort zone. *Psychotherapy (Chicago, Ill.)*, *38*(1), 21–30. doi:10.1037/0033-3204.38.1.21

Cant, B. (2006). Exploring the implications for health professionals of men coming out as gay in healthcare settings. *Health & Social Care in the Community*, *14*(1), 9–16. doi:10.1111/j.1365-2524.2005.00583.x PMID:16324183

Clark, R. A., & Delia, J. G. (1979). Topoi and rhetorical competence. *The Quarterly Journal of Speech*, *65*(2), 187–206. doi:10.1080/00335637909383470

Dalton, E. D., Pjesivac, I., Eldredge, S., & Miller, L. (2020). From vulnerability to disclosure: A normative approach to understanding trust in obstetric and intrapartum nurse-patient communication. *Health Communication*, *0*(0), 1–14. doi:10.1080/10410236.2020.1733225 PMID:32122160

Demjén, Z. (2016). Laughing at cancer: Humour, empowerment, solidarity and coping online. *Journal of Pragmatics*, *101*(0), 18–30. doi:10.1016/j.pragma.2016.05.010

Dillard, J. P., Segrin, C., & Harden, J. M. (1989). Primary and secondary goals in the production of interpersonal influence messages. *Communication Monographs*, *56*(1), 19–38. doi:10.1080/03637758909390247

Drew, S. K., Mills, M. B., & Gassaway, B. M. (2007). *Dirty work*. Baylor University Press.

Dziegielewski, S. F., Jacinto, G. A., Laudadio, A., & Legg-Rodriguez, L. (2003). Humor: An essential communication tool in therapy. *International Journal of Mental Health*, *32*(3), 74–90. doi:10.1080/00207411.2003.11449592

Ellithorpe, M., Esralew, S., & Holbert, L. (2014). Putting the "self" in self-deprecation: When deprecating humor about minorities is acceptable. *Humor: International Journal of Humor Research*, *27*(3), 401–422. doi:10.1515/humor-2014-0070

Ervin-Tripp, S., & Lampert, M. (2009). The occasioning of self-disclosure in humor. In N. R. Norrick & D. Chiaro (Eds.), *Humor in interaction* (pp. 3–27). John Benjamins Publishing. doi:10.1075/pbns.182.01erv

Ferguson, S. (2015, January 14). Labels: Empowering, harmful, or both? *Everyday Feminism*. Retrieved from https://everydayfeminism.com/2015/01/labels-empowering-harmful/

Garrison, S. (2018). On the limits of "Trans enough": Authenticating trans identity narratives. *Gender & Society*, *32*(5), 613–637. doi:10.1177/0891243218780299

Goffman, E. (1963). *Stigma: Notes on the management of spoiled identity*. Prentice Hall.

Graham, R., Berkowitz, B., Blum, R., Bockting, W., Bradford, J., de Vries, B., & Makadon, H. (2011). The health of lesbian, gay, bisexual, and transgender people: Building a foundation for better understanding. Washington, DC: Institute of Medicine.

Graham, E. E., Papa, M. J., & Brooks, G. P. (1992). Functions of humor in conversation: Conceptualization and measurement. *Western Journal of Communication*, *56*(2), 161–183. doi:10.1080/10570319209374409

Greene, K. (2009). An integrated model of health disclosure decision-making. In T. D. Afifi & W. A. Afifi (Eds.), *Uncertainty and information regulation in interpersonal contexts: Theories and applications* (pp. 226–253). Routledge.

Jadad, A. R., Rizo, C. A., & Enkin, M. W. (2003). I am a good patient, believe it or not. *BMJ (Clinical Research Ed.)*, *326*(7402), 1293–1295. doi:10.1136/bmj.326.7402.1293 PMID:12805157

Jensen, P. R. (2018). Undignified dignity: Using humor to manage the stigma of mental illness and homelessness. *Communication Quarterly*, *66*(1), 20–37. doi:10.1080/01463373.2017.1325384

Klitzman, R. L., & Greenberg, J. D. (2002). Patterns of communication between gay and lesbian patients and their health care providers. *Journal of Homosexuality*, *42*(4), 65–75. doi:10.1300/J082v42n04_04 PMID:12243485

Knox, S., & Hill, C. E. (2003). Therapist self-disclosure: Research-based suggestions for practitioners. *Journal of Clinical Psychology*, *59*(5), 529–539. doi:10.1002/jclp.10157 PMID:12696129

Lynch, O. H. (2002). Humorous communication: Finding a place for humor in communication research. *Communication Theory*, *12*(4), 423–445. doi:10.1111/j.1468-2885.2002.tb00277.x

Martin, R. A. (2019). Humor. In M. W. Gallagher & S. J. Lopez (Eds.), *Positive psychological assessment: A handbook of models and measures* (pp. 305–316). American Psychological Association. doi:10.1037/0000138-019

Meisenbach, R. J. (2010). Stigma management communication: A theory and agenda for applied research on how individuals manage moments of stigmatized identity. *Journal of Applied Communication Research*, *38*(3), 268–292. doi:10.1080/00909882.2010.490841

Meyer, J. C. (2000). Humor as a double-edged sword: Four functions of humor in communication. *Communication Theory*, *10*(3), 310–331. doi:10.1111/j.1468-2885.2000.tb00194.x

Noltensmeyer, C. J., & Meisenbach, R. J. (2016). Emerging patterns of stigma management communication among burn survivors and relational partners. *The American Behavioral Scientist*, *60*(11), 1378–1397. doi:10.1177/0002764216657384

Ogden, S. N., Scheffey, K. L., Blosnich, J. R., & Dichter, M. E. (2020). "Do I feel safe revealing this information to you?": Patient perspectives on disclosing sexual orientation and gender identity in healthcare. *Journal of American College Health*, *68*(6), 617–623. doi:10.1080/07448481.2019.1583663 PMID:32897171

Rossman, K., Salamanca, P., & Macapagal, K. (2017). A qualitative study examining young adults' experiences of disclosure and nondisclosure of LGBTQ identity to health care providers. *Journal of Homosexuality*, *64*(10), 1390–1410. doi:10.1080/00918369.2017.1321379 PMID:28459379

Scott, A. M., Harrington, N. G., & Spencer, E. (2020). Primary care physicians' strategic pursuit of multiple goals in cost-of-care conversations with patients. *Health Communication*, *0*(0), 1–13. doi:10.1080/10410236.2020.1723051 PMID:32019346

Smith, R. A., & Applegate, A. (2018). Mental health stigma and communication and their intersections with education. *Communication Education*, *67*(3), 382–393. doi:10.1080/03634523.2018.1465988 PMID:31354181

Smith, C. M., & Powell, L. (1988). The use of disparaging humor by group leaders. *The Southern Speech Communication Journal*, *53*(3), 279–292. doi:10.1080/10417948809372729

Sparks, L., Travis, S. S., & Thompson, S. R. (2005). Listening for the communicative signals of humor, narratives, and self-disclosure in the family caregiver interview. *Health & Social Work*, *30*(4), 340–343. doi:10.1093/hsw/30.4.340 PMID:16323726

Thom, D. H. (2001). Physician behaviors that predict patient trust. *The Journal of Family Practice*, *50*(4), 323–323. PMID:11300984

Thom, D. H., & Campbell, B. (1997). Patient-physician trust: An exploratory study. *The Journal of Family Practice*, *44*(2), 169–176. PMID:9040520

Vergeer, G., & MacRae, A. (1993). Therapeutic use of humor in occupational therapy. *The American Journal of Occupational Therapy*, *47*(8), 678–683. doi:10.5014/ajot.47.8.678 PMID:8352326

Chapter 27
'Just Counting the Threads!'

Trevor Kauer
University of Nebraska, Lincoln, USA

My ambulance and team of EMTs (emergency medical technicians) arrived at the rural home of a 65-year-old woman who had fallen in her bedroom. The patient had hip surgery a week prior, and she could not lift herself up, so she used her medical alert necklace to call for help. I walked into the woman's quaint apartment, walls decorated with antique plates and a calendar featuring kittens playing in a basket of yarn. My team and I walked into her bedroom, she was resting on her left side, propping herself up with her arm. She looked a bit dazed, but who wouldn't after falling unexpectedly on your way to the bathroom?

I set down my bag of medical assessment gear, and asked "What are you doing down there, ma'am?" Without missing a beat, she responded sarcastically, "Oh…just counting the carpet threads." She looked to the ground, picked at the fibers a bit, and then back at me, "Yup, they're all still there!" My team tried not to laugh, the woman was obviously in pain and we didn't want to seem disrespectful or unprofessional. But it's not often you meet a patient with a sense of humor while on the floor in pain. Realizing this woman had a witty and dry sense of humor, I felt it was appropriate to at least chuckle at the joke while we replaced her propped up arm with one of our knees to support her until we could get more equipment in the room. I teased back at her, "You know, we're supposed to stand on the ground, and lay in our beds. That's ok though, I get them mixed up all the time too." She laughed and we proceeded with the medical and trauma assessment. The first task was to get her off the floor, but because of her recent surgery we would need to take full c-spine protocol. In other words, we would need to put a neck brace on her and carefully strap her to a backboard with her hips in a special binder to keep them compressed in case there was any fractures or further injury.

The woman lived on the third floor of her apartment and, as luck would have it, the building didn't have an elevator. That meant the team of us were going to carry her down the stairs to the gurney, which was waiting for us on the ground level. We got her situated on the hard-plastic backboard, trying to pad any voids between her and the board, attempting to make her position somewhat comfortable given the circumstances. With the straps in place, we picked her up and headed towards the stairs.

At this point, the woman seemed a bit apprehensive and scared. She was essentially floating in air, unable to move or look in any direction. None of us were paramedics, so we couldn't give her any pain

DOI: 10.4018/978-1-7998-4528-7.ch027

meds until we met up with a medic unit on the way to the hospital. I tried reassuring her, "Alright ma'am, we going to start going down the staircase now. These two strapping young men are going to carry you, and I'm going to guide them down the stairs." Knowing she cracked a joke earlier, I thought laughter may be the best medicine. I tried to ease the fear I could see in her eyes, "Now, we're going to need your help too. It's going to feel a bit bumpy and like a roller coaster. You are tall enough for this ride, but please keep your arms and legs inside the ride at all times." She smiled, and I could see the tension lift and she seemed a bit calmer.

We reached the bottom of the stairs and placed her on the rolling gurney. We lifted her into the ambulance and were on the way to the hospital, a 45-minute drive away. As I started IV lines and took her vitals, if I could keep her talking she seemed to be more comfortable. We chatted about her cat calendar I noticed earlier (because cats are my favorite pet) and her grandkids who like to help change the months. Once we got to the hospital, we parked the ambulance and started to get ready to move her inside the ambulance bay to the emergency room. We opened the doors, prepared to lift her out of the ambulance on the gurney, and she looked at me with a serious and stern look. "Now, I've already been on the floor today, once was enough!" At first I assumed she was serious, I thought, "after three flights of stairs, she doesn't trust us to lift her out of the ambulance!?!" But then I gathered my gullible nature had fallen for her witty sense of humor again, I laughed and said, "Don't worry, we only drop people on days that end with Y." Amused and giggling we rolled her into through the ambulance bay and through the hospital doors.

Once we got into her room, my team and I transferred her to the hospital bed and said our goodbyes while the hospital staff took over patient care. I've been an EMT providing out-of-hospital patient care for almost six years, and I will always remember this woman's resilience and humor in the face of pain and uncertainty. It was inspiring. People call 911 on their worst days, no doubt an ambulance and emergency room can be terrifying places. Yet, if I can use humor to build trust and rapport with my patients, it puts them at ease while making my job a whole lot more fun!

Chapter 28
Response: "'Just Counting the Threads!'"

Andrea L. Meluch
The University of Akron, USA

REVIEW OF LITERATURE

Scholars have long known the importance of providing supportive communication, or social support, to individuals who are experiencing a health crisis (e.g., Albrecht & Goldsmith, 2003; Cobb, 1976). Albrecht and Adelman (1987) offered one of the first definitions of social support in the communication discipline and defined it as "verbal and nonverbal communication between recipients and providers that helps *reduce* [italics added] uncertainty about the situation, the self, the other or the relationship and functions to enhance a perception of personal control in one's life experience" (p. 19). Central to Albrecht and Adelman's original definition is the idea that social support *reduces* uncertainty. Uncertainty is a key concept to understanding why social support is important in medical situations. Uncertainty is experienced by individuals who lack information about a situation (e.g., Brashers, 2001). Health crises are inherently uncertain because there are many unknowns about how the situation will resolve itself (e.g., duration of illness, outcome after an injury; e.g., Politi & Street, 2011).

Moments when we are experiencing a health crisis are naturally filled with uncertainty. The uncertainty that individuals experience in health crises is related to their stress (Albrecht & Adelman, 1987). However, social support scholars have repeatedly contended that social support can help one *reduce* or *manage* uncertainty and, thus, reduce or manage the associated feelings of stress (Albrecht & Adelman, 1987; Albrecht & Goldsmith, 2003; Cohen & Wills, 1985). Although individuals often consider uncertainty to be a negative experience, health communication scholars have recognized that uncertainty is not necessarily problematic (Albrecht & Goldsmith, 2003). That is, uncertainty in a medical situation can have positive outcomes when an individual can use that uncertainty to envision potential positive outcomes from the situation. For example, if someone is injured and needs to call emergency medical services, the uncertainty of the situation can help the individual to feel hopeful about a positive outcome

DOI: 10.4018/978-1-7998-4528-7.ch028

once they reach the hospital. As such, receiving social support can help individuals to manage (not just reduce) uncertainty when presented with medical crises.

Social support can serve multiple functions for individuals (e.g., Cobb, 1976; Cohen & Wills, 1985; Cutrona & Suhr, 1992). Functions that social support serves include *informational, emotional*, and *instrumental* support (e.g., Goldsmith, 2004). Informational support is defined as "the provision of advice, suggestions, and information that a person can use to address problems" (Heaney & Isreal, 2008, p. 190). Informational support is commonly provided by healthcare providers when patients are looking for more information about their health and/or are seeking advice for how to treat a medical condition. Emotional support is defined as "the provision of empathy, love, trust, and caring" (Heaney & Isreal, 2008, p. 190). Through receiving emotional support individuals may experience a greater sense of belonging (Albrecht & Adelman, 1984; Goldsmith, 2004). Finally, instrumental support is the tangible or material support that individuals can receive, such as helping someone (e.g., shopping, cleaning) or providing goods (e.g., lending money) (Heaney & Isreal, 2008). These functions of social support provide individuals with the help and care they need, especially during health crises.

Although individuals need social support in times of crisis, they often will only be the recipients of supportive communication if they seek it (Thoits, 1995). Specifically, individuals use communication to seek certain types of social support (Xu & Burleson, 2001). For example, a patient who is dealing with a health crisis may signal the need for informational support by asking their healthcare provider specific questions about their condition. As such, receiving social support may require communicating one's openness to supportive offers.

Supportive Communication and Humor

Humor is a key communicative act that allows individuals to release tension, reduce stress, and build connection in an uncertain medical situation (e.g., Carver et al., 1993; Meyer, 2000). Although supportive communication does not always include the use of humor, individuals can use humor in their interactions to provide social support to others (Howland & Simpson, 2014). For example, telling someone a joke when they are sad can help to lighten the mood of the conversation and show that someone is listening and cares. However, using humor does not always allow a person to feel supported and can even diminish the quality of the interaction and/or have the opposite effect if one is trying to be supportive (Howland & Simpson, 2014). Further, the type of humor being used can lead to the recipient feeling supported or not. Positive humor, or humor that includes friendly joking, often helps individuals to feel supported whereas negative humor, or humor that is racist, sexist, or in some way inappropriate, can make individuals feel uncomfortable (Howland & Simpson, 2014). Thus, using humor to provide social support is a complex process that individuals, especially healthcare providers, need to consider carefully.

Healthcare Providers and Social Support

Healthcare providers fulfill a critical role in providing individuals with the support they need to manage health crises. Obviously healthcare providers are charged with giving lifesaving care to patients, but critically they also must provide information to patients and can even provide support that shows concern for patients' emotional needs. Medical and health communication scholarship has consistently demonstrated that patients often receive and/or expect to receive social support from their healthcare providers (e.g., Goldsmith & Albrecht, 2011; Neuling & Winefield, 1988; Sloan & Knowles, 2013). Specifically, patients often expect social support and even seek out certain types of support, such as informational support, from their healthcare providers (Meluch, 2018). Research has indicated that patients may experience health benefits from experiencing social support (e.g., Mills & Sullivan, 1999; Robinson et al., 2011). For example, Mills and Sullivan (1999) examined the relationship between informational support offered by nurses to cancer patients and those patients' health outcomes. They found that informational support was associated with reduced patient anxiety, patients' enhanced sense of personal control, greater patient compliance with suggested medical regimens, and patients' feelings of greater security. Thus, healthcare providers' use of social support is often integrally connected to patient experiences and wellbeing.

Patient-Centered Care and Humor

Communication between patients and their healthcare providers is critical for ensuring that patient-centered care is being practiced. Patient-centered care occurs when healthcare providers' communication is effective in meeting the physiological and psychological needs of patients (Mead & Bower, 2000; Stewart, 2001). Humor can be an effective tool for achieving patient-centered care by providing support to patients during times of health crisis (e.g., du Pre, 1997; Scholl, 2007). For example, Scholl (2007) examined how humor can function to provide better patient-centered care. Specifically, she noted that "through humor, patients can express their feelings and thoughts without the threat of aversive consequences" (p. 159). Scholl's study investigated how humor manifests itself in patient-provider relationships and how it can improve patient-centered care. Through her observations of patients interacting with providers in a nursing unit, she found that humor was used to help make patients comfortable and facilitate a better provider-patient relationship.

Applying Health Communication Concepts to 'Just Counting the Threads!' Case Study

Providing patient-centered care is often a key goal of healthcare providers. Healthcare providers often also recognize the impact that humor can have on helping patients through facilitating high quality patient-centered care. As is evidenced in this present case study, humor can be an integral tool for healthcare providers to develop a quality relationship with patients. Specifically, the case study chronicles how an emergency medical technician (EMT) responds to a patient's crisis through the use of shared humor.

The relationship between EMTs and patients is not as well studied as relationships between other types of healthcare providers (e.g., physicians, nurses) and patients. EMTs are a particularly interesting group of healthcare providers in that they only interact with patients in a crisis and for the short period of time until the patient reaches the hospital. As such, examining how EMTs use humor when interacting with patients and the potential outcomes of these interactions has important implications for better understanding EMT-patient communication.

The narrator of the case study is an EMT who is responding to an emergency call. The case study begins with an EMT arriving at the home of a 65-year-old woman who had fallen and injured herself shortly after having a hip surgery. The EMT narrator explains that upon entering the home of the patient they found the patient on the bedroom floor unable to get up. To help lighten the situation the EMT asks the patient what she is doing on the floor and she responds "Just counting the carpet threads. Yup, they're all still there!" The EMT laughs and begins bantering with the patient while they emergency medical services (EMS) team gets her moved to be transported to the hospital. Throughout transporting the patient to the hospital, the narrator notices how she is nervous and uses humor to help relax the patient. He discusses how patients are fearful when EMS is called and how using humor can help to have a calming effect. The case study concludes with the patient being settled into the hospital and the EMT reflecting on how the patient's use of humor and his in response allowed him to observe the patient's resilience throughout a traumatic experience.

Uncertainty is characteristic of a health crisis where EMS is called. As such, uncertainty is a major component of the present case study. As individuals grapple with the uncertainty they are facing because of their health, they often turn to their healthcare providers to give them comfort by helping them to manage this uncertainty. When EMS is called there is uncertainty about the severity of the injury or illness, the treatment that will be provided, and even the costs associated with the medical services. In the present case study, the patient is clearly nervous about the unclear nature of her injury and needing to rely on EMS to treat her while in transit to the hospital. These feelings of uncertainty can make one feel tense and fearful. However, the use of humor is one way to help release this tension and feel some comfort in a challenging situation.

As evidenced by the case study, humor can be an important resource for patients to achieve a sense of control in the face of a health crisis and for healthcare providers to use to create quality interactions with patients. Specifically, throughout the case study the narrator demonstrates how humor is used by the patient to release tension and build a connection with the healthcare providers attending to her during a very uncertain and scary health crisis. For example, the narrator makes a joke about how moving the patient on a gurney is like a rollercoaster ride. The narrator believes by joking around that it will help comfort the patient when she was scared of being moved down several flights of stairs. Thus, the case study clearly reflects medical literature which shows that healthcare providers and patients can use humor to deal with the stress and tension of health crises and to achieve better connections (e.g., Carver et al., 1993; Meyer, 2000).

The case study also illustrates how healthcare providers can use humor to provide social support to patients during a health crisis. Social support can be integral to patients facing health crises. Further, patients both expect to receive and benefit from social support in healthcare interactions (e.g., Goldsmith & Albrecht, 2011; Mills & Sullivan, 1999; Neuling & Winefield, 1988; Robinson et al., 2011). Patients receive social support that serves different functions to help them manage the uncertainty related to their health crisis (e.g., informational support, emotional support; Goldsmith & Albrecht, 2011). For example, in the case study the narrator provides emotional support to the patient by listening and joking with her as she is transported to the hospital. Through providing supportive communication to the patient, the EMT demonstrates how healthcare providers can help patients to manage the stressors of a health crisis through enacting social support.

The importance of providing patient-centered care is clear throughout the case study. In the case study the patient was injured and required attention from the EMS team. Patient-centered care requires healthcare providers to use effective communication in meeting the physiological and psychological needs of the patient (Mead & Bower, 2000; Stewart, 2001). One way that healthcare providers can achieve effective patient-centered care is by using humor to help patients cope in a crisis (e.g., du Pre, 1997; Scholl, 2007). Further, allowing patients to use humor to address their concerns and show vulnerability can help providers to better meet patient psychosocial needs effectively (Scholl, 2007). In the case study, the narrator and patient mutually use humor in their interactions to both help relieve some of the stress of the situation and to talk about the medical care being provided.

Using humor is a complicated communicative decision in medical settings. Humor can easily be misconstrued and lead to greater communication challenges for healthcare providers. However, when humor is used effectively, as illustrated in the present case study, it can be an efficient communication tool for healthcare providers to better connect with patients to help relieve stress and create a more positive experience. The ways in which the present case study intersects with the health communication literature and the use of humor specifically provide valuable insights into how healthcare providers can utilize humor in a medical crisis. The following section highlights how the lessons related to humor illustrated in this case study can be used by healthcare providers to achieve quality patient-provider interactions.

HEALTHCARE PROVIDER USE OF HUMOR IN HEALTH CRISES

Humor is a complicated communicative act. That is, although humor can have many positive uses, such as helping others to cope with stressors more effectively, humor is not universally benign (Howland & Simpson, 2014). Scholars have distinguished between the positive and negative types of humor and even the functions of humor (Howland & Simpson, 2014; Meyer, 2000). Using humor in medical situations must be carefully considered as humor is not a panacea for achieving connection between healthcare providers and patients (Scholl & Ragan, 2003). As such, the present case study is useful to healthcare providers in understanding how to use humor positively and carefully when interacting with patients experiencing a health crisis. Specifically, the case study shows that the EMT using friendly, positive humor that the patient is responsive to.

Throughout the case study the narrator discusses how he knew that the patient was open to the use of humor because of their initial interaction and how he was able to rely on this knowledge to continue to connect with the patient and calm her during a traumatic experience. Prior research indicates that patients need to be open to the use of humor in a medical encounter for it to be effective (Leiber, 1986; Schultes, 1997). Further, healthcare providers must be careful that their humor is used positively in contrast to aggressively or in sarcastic ways that can make the patient feel worse about themselves or the situation (Buxman, 2000; Leiber, 1986). Thus, healthcare providers can use the present case study as an example of how to approach the use of positive humor. In particular, a key takeaway from this case study for healthcare providers is that they must establish that the patient is open to the use of humor to help manage the stress of a health crisis. Patients who are open to humor may use humor initially, like the patient in the present case study did, or may laugh at a provider's joke. Providers should look for cues, like joking, to know that the patient is open to humor being used. After they have established that the patient is open to humor, they can use humor in ways that frame the situation in a more positive way to achieve connection with the patient.

Use of Humor in the Provision of Social Support

Using humor can be an effective way to provide social support (Howland & Simpson, 2014). Specifically, humor can help an individual manage the stressors of a situation which can be very useful in health crises. Although some individuals are more forthcoming in their support needs, others may seek support in less obvious ways. Using humor to lighten the situation may signal that the individual is looking for support to be offered. Healthcare providers who are interested in being supportive of patients may find that they need to be attentive when patients use humor as this could signal support seeking behaviors that would allow them to better connect with the patient to serve specific emotional needs.

Throughout the case study the narrator discusses how it is very stressful and scary for patients who need to call for emergency help and that the emergency medical services team is responsible for making sure the patient is successfully transported to the hospital for care. Further, the patient uses humor and looks scared at different points, which signals that she needs support. The narrator explains that he tries to use humor to show that he cares about the patient's concerns. Specifically, he is using humor to show his understanding of her fear and uncertainty. He jokes around to prove to the patient that things will work out and that the emergency medical services team is taking care of her. In this way, the EMT's use of humor helps the patient to release tension by reframing the situation as more manageable. As such, another key takeaway from this case study is that through showing patients that they care, and using humor to achieve this supportive communication, healthcare providers are able to help patients manage the uncertainty of a health crisis and feel less fearful as they are given the care that they need.

Use of Humor To Achieve Patient-Centered Care

Today healthcare providers recognize the importance of meeting both the physiological and psychological needs of patients. When patients feel their physiological and psychological needs are met by healthcare providers their providers are achieving patient-centered care. One way to meet patients' psychological needs is through using humor to build connection (Scholl, 2007). Specifically, healthcare providers and patients can use humor to develop quality relationships that allow providers to better meet patient needs. Although emergency medical technicians (EMTs) only work with patients for a short period of time, it is still important for them to respond to patients' physiological and psychological needs and to have quality interactions. The present case study is useful to better understand how EMTs can use humor effectively to provide patient-centered care. That is, although EMTs are responsible for the physiological health of patients in an emergency, they also must consider the psychological health of the patients during a traumatic event. Humor is one way that they can help patients to release tension and feel safe during an intimidating situation and, thus, meet both psychological and physiological patient needs. As such, a third key takeaway from this case study is that healthcare providers may want to use supportive communication, and potentially humor, to meet the psychological needs of a patient even in a health crisis.

Health crises are inherently complicated events that require healthcare providers to communicate effectively with patients. Although the use of humor can be misconstrued, humor can be a useful way to communicate about medical issues. The case study, "Just Counting the Threads!," is one such example of how emergency medical service technicians are able to help patients manage the uncertainty of a health crisis by providing supportive patient-centered care through the use of humor. The case study is useful both practically and theoretically as it chronicles a real-life case that relates to a variety of health communication concepts (e.g., uncertainty, social support, patient-centered care). As such, students, healthcare providers, and scholars can use this case study to help understand humor use in healthcare settings.

REFERENCES

Albrecht, T. L., & Adelman, M. B. (1987). Communicating social support: A theoretical perspective. In T. L. Albrecht, M. B. Adelman, & ... (Eds.), *Communicating social support* (pp. 18–39). Sage.

Albrecht, T. L., & Goldsmith, D. J. (2003). Social support, social networks, and health. In T. L. Thompson, A. Dorsey, K. I. Miller, & R. Parrott (Eds.), *Handbook of health communication* (pp. 263–284). Lawrence Erlbaum.

Brashers, D. E. (2001). Communication and uncertainty management. *Journal of Communication, 51*(3), 477–497. doi:10.1111/j.1460-2466.2001.tb02892.x

Buxman, K. (2000). Humor in critical care: No joke. *AACN Clinical Issues, 11*(1), 120–127. doi:10.1097/00044067-200002000-00013 PMID:11040558

Carver, C. S., Harris, S. D., Noriega, V., Pozo, C., Robinson, D. S., & Ketcham, A. S. (1993). How coping mediates the effect of optimism on distress: A study of women with early stage breast cancer. *Journal of Personality and Social Psychology, 65*(2), 375–390. doi:10.1037/0022-3514.65.2.375 PMID:8366426

Cobb, S. (1976). Social support as a moderator of life stress. *Psychosomatic Medicine, 38*(5), 300–314. doi:10.1097/00006842-197609000-00003 PMID:981490

Cohen, S., & Wills, T. A. (1985). Stress, social support, and the buffering hypothesis. *Psychological Bulletin, 98*(2), 310–357. doi:10.1037/0033-2909.98.2.310 PMID:3901065

Cutrona, C. E., & Suhr, J. A. (1992). Controllability of stressful events and satisfaction with spouse support behaviors. *Communication Research, 19*(2), 154–174. doi:10.1177/009365092019002002

du Pre, A. (1997). *Humor and the healing arts: A multimethod analysis of humor use in health care.* Lawrence Erlbaum. doi:10.4324/9781410602329

Goldsmith, D. J. (2004). *Communicating social support.* Cambridge University Press. doi:10.1017/CBO9780511606984

Goldsmith, D. J., & Albrecht. (2011). Social support, social networks, and health: A guiding framework. In T. L. Thompson, R. Parrott, & J. F. Nussbaum (Eds.), *The Routledge handbook of health communication* (2nd ed., pp. 335-348). Routledge.

Heaney, C. A., & Isreal, B. A. (2008). Social networks and social support. In K. Glanz, B. K. Rimer, & K. Viswanath (Eds.), *Health behavior and health education: Theory, research, and practice* (4th ed., pp. 189–210). Jossey-Bass.

Howland, M., & Simpson, J. A. (2014). Attachment orientations and reactivity to humor in a social support context. *Journal of Social and Personal Relationships, 31*(1), 114–137. doi:10.1177/0265407513488016

Leiber, D. B. (1986). Laughter and humor in critical care. *Dimensions of Critical Care Nursing, 5*(3), 162–170. doi:10.1097/00003465-198605000-00006 PMID:3635471

Mead, N., & Bower, P. (2000). Measuring patient-centeredness: A comparison of three observation-based instruments. *Patient Education and Counseling, 39*(1), 71–80. https://doi.org/10.1016/S0738-3991(99)00092-0

Meluch, A. L. (2018). "Above and beyond": An exploratory study of breast cancer patient accounts of healthcare provider information-giving practices and informational support. *Qualitative Research in Medicine & Healthcare, 2*(2), 113-120. doi:10.4081/qrmh.2018.7387

Meyer, J. C. (2000). Humor as a double-edged sword: Four functions of humor in communication. *Communication Theory, 10*(3), 310–331. https://doi.org/10.1111/j.1468-2885.2000.tb00194.x

Mills, M. E., & Sullivan, K. (1999). The importance of information giving for patients newly diagnosed with cancer: A review of literature. *Journal of Clinical Nursing, 8*(6), 631–642. https://doi.org/10.1046/j.1365-2702.1999.00296.x

Neuling, S. J., & Winefield, H. R. (1988). Social support and recovery after surgery for breast cancer: Frequency and correlates of supportive behaviors by family, friends and surgeon. *Social Science & Medicine, 27*(4), 385–392. https://doi.org/10.1016/0277-9536(88)90273-0

Politi, M., & Street, R. L. (2011). Patient-centered communication during collaborative decision making. In T. L. Thompson, R. Parrott, & J. F. Nussbaum (Eds.), *The Routledge handbook of health communication* (2nd ed., pp. 399–414). Routledge.

Robinson, J. D., Turner, J. W., Levine, B., & Tian, Y. (2011). Expanding the walls of the health care encounter: Support outcomes of patients online. *Health Communication, 26*(2), 125–134. https://doi.org/10.1080/10410236.2010.541990

Scholl, J. C. (2007). The use of humor to promote patient-centered care. *Journal of Applied Communication Research, 35*(2), 156–176. https://doi.org/10.1080/00909880701262658

Scholl, J. C., & Ragan, S. L. (2003). The use of humor in promoting positive provider-patient interactions in a hospital rehabilitation unit. *Health Communication, 15*(3), 319–330. https://doi.org/10.1207/S15327027HC1503_4

Schultes, L. S. (1997). Humor with hospice clients: You're putting me on. *Home Healthcare Nurse, 15*(8), 561–566. https://doi.org/10.1097/00004045-199708000-00013

Sloan, A. G., & Knowles, A. (2013). Improving communication between healthcare providers and cancer patients: A pilot study. *Journal of Communication in Healthcare, 6*(4), 208–215. https://doi.org/10.1179/1753807613Y.0000000040

Stewart, M. (2001). Towards a global definition of patient centred care. *British Medical Journal, 322*, 444–445. https://doi.org/10.1136/bmj.322.7284.444

Thoits, P. A. (1995). Stress, coping, and social support processes: Where are we? What next? *Journal of Health and Social Behavior,* 53-79. doi:10.2307/2626957

Xu, Y., & Burleson, B. R. (2001). Effects of sex, culture, and support type, on perceptions of spousal social support: An assessment of the "Support Gap" hypothesis in early marriage. *Human Communication Research, 27*(4), 535–566. https://doi.org/10.1111/j.1468-2958.2001.tb00792.x

Chapter 29
A Prescription for Humor

Suzy Prentiss
The University of Tennessee, USA

My dad was an expert joke teller who never messed up a punch line; unfortunately, it was a skill I did not inherit from him. Though I cannot recall any of his stock jokes, I do know that sharing them was good for him. Living in a situation where so little was out of his control, Dad suffered from diabetes and heart disease and hypertension and later kidney failure, his attitude and how he shared that with others was still his domain. I think that empowerment was very important for him. I can recall that his "clean" jokes were usually received with hearty laughter and the more questionable ones still went over pretty well. When my dad started infusing humor into his hospital visits, he was in his later years and his jokes were never sexist or racist, so a lot of people let a bad word or a suggestive element slide by. Looking back, I appreciate the grace they showed as he did not intend to offend anyone. It made him extremely happy to make people laugh and smile.

"How about a thick steak and a scotch?" Though that might be an appropriate order at a restaurant, it's probably not so appropriate when medical professionals ask if you need anything before a procedure. Yet those words were a typical retort of my dad. My dad was a storyteller and a jokester who felt that his medical team, from the receptionist to the surgeon, needed a laugh to brighten their day. Sometimes, people loved and appreciated my dad's humor, sometimes my family and I would cringe as we knew his attempt at goodwill fell short. On many occasions I would ask him, "Why?" Why did he tell an off-color (maybe even rude) joke, crude story, or make comments about having "scotch" before any medical procedure, from having a flu shot to a colonoscopy? (By the way, my dad was not a drinker and I never even remember seeing him drink scotch, yet that was his "go to" line.) Though his words may change, the sentiment of his response to my question was always the same, "They see sick people all day and it must be hard and hardly anyone says, 'thank you,' so I try to make them smile." How could I disagree with that logic?

Other times, his humor was not universally well received…at least not immediately. I recall one incident, his last colonoscopy, that epitomized my dad's use of humor with medical professionals. As he aged, it became harder to find good veins for taking blood or connecting an IV. Dad always offered advice for the best place to try and appreciated a job well done. On this day, Dad was getting ready for

DOI: 10.4018/978-1-7998-4528-7.ch029

a colonoscopy and so a technician was trying to get a blood sample and then connect the IV. He was not doing so well. After a few tries, with the young male technician getting visibly stressed (and I think embarrassed), Dad tried to lighten the situation and remarked "it is a good thing you're not a vampire, you can't get any blood." You could tell by his face; he did not find my dad's comment funny. He did not laugh or smile, and he seemed to bristle at the remark. The other people around, though, the nurse and another tech, appeared to find it very funny. They both laughed and smiled and gave the impression they found the remark in good humor. My dad did not seem aware of the tech's discomfort as his head was down and he was concentrating on doing a better job yet from my vantage point on his other side, I could see he was uncomfortable. I recall saying something like, "Dad's veins are hard to find, don't worry," in an attempt to support the tech and redirect the conversation, and I think it worked for a bit. When the doctor entered the room, he had already heard that the "vampire" was having a challenge and seemed to enjoy the story. Though I know Dad was worried about his colonoscopy, this atmosphere of laughter and connection calmed him right down. I am not so sure about the technician, though. A nurse would later share that the technician trying to get blood had "no sense of humor," and his colleagues hoped he would relax and engage with them more. I know that is what my dad intended, yet I wondered if maybe he had hurt his feelings. No one likes to have their work questioned and as a former superintendent of schools who was quite protective of his teachers and staff, my dad knew that. I know for sure that my dad would never intend to be disrespectful or demeaning and yet I also know that the intentions of our communication are not as powerful as the way our messages are received.

A few weeks later we returned for a follow-up visit. I can remember talking to my dad about not giving the tech a hard time and being "nice" if we saw him. Dad asserted that he was "just having fun" and that the tech knew Dad "didn't mean anything" by his comments. I explained that his remarks could have been hurtful despite his intentions. As we walked into that section of the hospital, we caught a glimpse of the technician who also spotted us. Dad hollered "it's the vampire," in his booming, friendly voice. I cringed. Thankfully, the technician broke into a smile and said, "the blood is flowing better." He also asked how Dad was doing and said it was nice to see him. We saw him one more time as we were leaving, and a nurse remarked that he seemed more relaxed and talked with everyone more. That made my dad very happy, and he basically told me that he had been right and that "humor helps."

My dad was always well-intentioned with his humor and genuinely wanted to make people smile and laugh. Sadly, my dad eventually passed away. As my sister and I made phone calls and handled business and legal matters, we were surprised by how many people from his various doctor's offices remarked at how much they enjoyed his visits and his humor and how much they would miss him. Those comments were unexpected though very much appreciated. The way we choose to communicate and engage with others is complicated yet also empowering. My dad did not choose to use humor at anyone's expense but used it, instead, to connect and say, "thank you." I think his story is a good example of how humor can be used in healthcare for a variety of beneficial uses such as making personal connections, alleviating stress, and redirecting nervous energy. As I reflect on my dad's legacy and the lessons he taught us, and wonder why he did what he did, I think now that his humor was as much for himself as those around him. Instead of being a sick, elderly patient with a myriad of health problems, my dad was the friendly and funny gentlemen who made people laugh. When he saw people smile, it reduced his own fears and worries. In that way, it was good medicine for him as a patient and a type of therapy. At the later stages of his life, Dad no longer had many options about his healthcare and that lack of agency and free will was hard for him. His daily routine, diet and level of independence were dictated by his doctors and conditions. His attitude and how he approached his health challenges and interactions with medical professionals were entirely up to him. His use of humor was his coping mechanism, and I am sure many other people use humor in this way, too.

Chapter 30
Response: "A Prescription for Humor"

Susan M. Wieczorek
University of Pittsburgh at Johnstown, USA

POSITIVITY AND AGENCY IN THE MEDICAL CONTEXT

Humor communicates information through the lens of culture, context, and situation. At its core, humor fulfils a heuristic purpose that fundamentally reflects an aspect of "positivity" (Nikopoulos, 2017) through mental shortcuts intended to help connect with others. Although not all jokes result in mutual understanding or shared amusement, they intend to provoke positive affect between at least some of the parties involved. Researchers argue that the effectiveness of this connectivity depends upon similarity of social norms (Dunbar & Mehu, 2008), ability to empathize (Christoff & Dauphin, 2017), the primary use of the ego (Freud, 1961), a stimulus/response/revelation factor (Porteous, 1988), interactional linguistics (Chen, 2016); and even an element of threat to the listener (Lee et al., 2015). Likewise, the use and interpretation of humor depends upon the settings within which these interactions occur; the environments that the participants normally frequent such as work, social, and family settings (Epstein & Joker, 2007); and the demographic characteristics of the participants including their age, profession, gender, and cultural differences (Forabosco, 2009). Together, these factors affect how humor and positivity relate to agency within the hierarchical system of healthcare.

From an ontogenetic perspective, human development involves aspects of agency and humor at the earliest stages of life. Infants begin to mirror their parents' facial expressions, gestures, and sounds in an increasingly more controlled fashion as they learn through reinforcement how not only to respond appropriately to stimuli but also how to produce stimuli that help elicit intentional reactions from others (Kärtner, 2015; LoBue, 2019; Porteous, 1988). Although this control of affective displays begins even prior to language acquisition (Ekman & Friesen, 1971; Gunnery, 2015), younger children learn early on how to give nonverbal or verbal cues that direct the receiver's attention towards hints for interpreting the message (such as an eye twinkle when the sender wants the receiver to realize the message was in

DOI: 10.4018/978-1-7998-4528-7.ch030

jest). Through this naturally acquired process, the intent, delivery, and monitoring of humor primarily lies within the control and skill level of the initiator.

Setting likewise affects the perception, use, and acceptability of humor at all ages. In the medical context, setting plays a particular role due to the number of conflicting forces which often challenge the effectiveness and interpretation of humor. Examples of such influences include the health and cognitive acuity of the patient, the level of urgency of the visit, the patient team (including family, caregivers, and support personnel such as clergy), the healthcare team (including doctors, nurses, and ancillary staff), and the purpose (chief complaint) of the visit. These contextual forces often upstage or alter the perceptions of interactants, sometimes causing misinterpretation of intended messages. Communication becomes challenged when responses, interpretations, and perceptions seem unpredictable or even unexpected due to the variability of this unique context.

The healthcare setting uniquely affects *how* and *why* humor surfaces for medical professionals and patients alike. Although most of the literature analyses humor's redeeming qualities for practitioners in training and development or within patient care, it likewise suggests how patients themselves can use humor as a coping mechanism when dealing with serious illness, anxiety, depression, and challenges with self-esteem (Kuiper et al., 2004; Kuiper & Borowicz-Sibenik, 2005; Yue et al., 2004). By asserting themselves through humor, patients inadvertently demonstrate their willingness to communicate directly with their provider, suggesting their willingness to participate actively in decisions involving their own care. This results in improved self-worth and confidence while allowing for a reduction in uncertainty, confusion, and stress—even when heightened emotions and conflicts exist (du Pré, 1998; Lingard, 2013). Relational bonding between interactants improves through mutually respectful encouragement of communication which has been found to lead to overall feelings of satisfaction and wellbeing (Hardy, 2020; Sousa et al., 2019) as well as a more human perspective of illness and disease (Liu et al., 2017). Overall, humor exists as a primary means for enabling patients to cope with their medical challenges not only in the face of serious injury or death but in facing physical, emotional, and mental struggles on a day-to-day basis as well.

Although humor can act as an equalizing force within the natural hierarchical structure of the medical setting, control generally lies in the hands of the practitioner, the one hired as the medical expert. Patients trust in the knowledge, experience, skill, and recommendations of the healthcare team, but they often do so in a compromising or vulnerable state of mind such as being sedated, unconscious, or simply too sick and in pain to respond. This environment reinforces the paternalistic relationship associated with physician/patient communication (Taylor, 2009) and, in so doing, all too often places the patient outside of the realm of control. When patients initiate humor within the interaction, the equilibrium shifts back in favor of the patient, affording an element of agency and returning to more patient-centered care (Jiang, 2019).

An excellent example of how patients and healthcare professionals take momentary control of the often bizarre situations that take place within this medical context is "gallows humor" which "treats serious, frightening or painful subject matter in a light or satirical way" (Watson, 2011, p. 38). According to Maxwell (2003) and Phua et al. (2005), this strategy provides cognitive and/or behavioral coping in reaction to stress and results in a range of responses from respectful to sarcastic. Although some argue that this form of humor merely provides comic relief from distressful circumstances (Kim, 2015), the potential always exists for someone to become offended by the humor, especially when it is witnessed without awareness of the full context of the situation or when it is conveyed seemingly at the expense of the person towards whom the humor is directed (Abbott, 2014; Epstein & Joker, 2007; Tajfel, 1981). Similarly, in "A Joke Is Just a Joke (Except When It Isn't)," Hodson et al. (2010) argue that social norms also affect the interpretation of in- and out-group jokes and could result in listeners becoming hostile and feeling alienated. In all these cases, overheard joking received out of context can offend the listener and even result in potential ethical considerations as well (Millard, 2015; Piemonte, 2015). Depending upon who is listening and how this information might be interpreted, gallows humor can easily be misinterpreted and result in challenging communication outcomes.

Although research focusing strictly on patient use of gallows humor remains relatively sparce, Gramling and Gramling (2012) noted in their palliative care studies that patients tend to avoid challenging conversations with their doctors out of fear that it might compromise the quality of care by creating a "barrier to self-expression" which presents a "major threat to modern concepts of autonomy" (p. 1170). In effect, patients are often afraid to express themselves out of fear of being stifled or appearing incompetent. Humor may help to break this barrier by serving as an equalizing factor that allows patients—momentarily at least—to be on the same level as their practitioners, encouraging mutual human interaction. They argue, however, this can only be accomplished when the practitioners respond to the patient humor in a respectful, validating manner.

Similarly, Besinier (2016) asserts that humor is "primarily an intersubjective process that people deploy for multiple purposes, including a sense of mutual reassurance, a demonstration that one 'knows ones place,' and a display of ones fundamental good" (p. 78). Humor acts as a bridge between the formalities of medical information exchange and the often more humanistic, emotional, or empathetic exchanges that occur within the complex patient/practitioner interaction. "Knowing ones place" (the traditionally hierarchical aspect of this dyad) becomes less important than "ones fundamental good" (the more equalizing, humanizing aspect). When patients near the end of life (or are suffering at any stage of an illness), autonomy tends to diminish as decision making falls more into the hands of caregivers and practitioners than of patients themselves. Humor acts as a powerful tool for patients to assert themselves dynamically into a conversation even at a time when they feel most vulnerable.

In short, humor's presence in the medical context affords diversion from the seriousness and challenges of an illness, provides patients and practitioners with a method for coping with the situation, initiates an element of positivity within an all-but pleasant environment, and affords users an element of autonomy despite their vulnerability or lack of control over their illness. No matter the illness or magnitude of the problem, the positivity that humor provides empowers patients within the medical interaction, enabling them to participate in decisions involving their own health. It helps to initiate conversation, asserts an element of control, and enables patients to communicate in a natural manner that reveals one's humanity through shared amusement. Humor's positivity facilitates the communication dyad, opens the door for continued conversation, and provides agency in a situation that all but denies one's autonomy.

A wealth of additional research considers how positivity associated with patient-initiated humor provides an outlet and/or a mental objectification of health problems that are for the most part beyond their control. This positivity allows for greater resilience in the face of illness and psychological stress (Venetis et al., 2019). Numerous articles spanning the gamut of health-related topics have noted how humor facilitates patient care and how humor initiated by patients can in fact benefit their satisfaction, coping mechanisms, resilience, and health outcomes. A sample of these include HIV/AIDS (Black, 2012); COVID-19 (Chiodo et al., 2020); hospice, palliative care, home healthcare, and dementia (Clark et al., 2016); cancer (Venetis et al., 2019), anxiety and depression (Falkenberg et al., 2011); suicidal ideation (Lee et al., 2020); neuropsychology (Saunders, 1998), stress-induced trauma (Sliter et al., 2014), pain tolerance (Zweyer et al., 2004), physical home therapy (Low et al., 2014); and substance abuse (Canha, 2016). Although this list is certainly not exhaustive, it demonstrates the expanse and significance of humor research in the care of patients by facilitating communication through positivity, shared decision making, and autonomy within the medical environment.

APPLICATION TO "A PRESCRIPTION FOR HUMOR"

In Suzy Prentiss's endearing portrayal of her father's use of humor during his many interactions with healthcare professionals towards the end of his life, the positivity he shared with all those around him resonated throughout her story. "Dad" as she called him, seemed to delight in his use of "stock jokes" because he not only "never missed a punch line" but he also valued the shared experience of making someone laugh in the midst of a relatively dismal environment. He never seemed to feel defeated—even when the hardest hearts of younger, insecure workers like the novice phlebotomist seemed too consumed by the process of patient care to crack a smile. To Dad, everyone was his equal; and everyone deserved to experience a happy moment in life just as he did. If they did not laugh, he did not take it personally. He simply persisted until he caught a glimmer of pleasure in their eyes. Seeing a mere hint of a smile on someone's face was better than any medicine he could take. As Dad put it, "It made him extremely happy to make people laugh and smile. It made him as happy as it made others." A joke's effectiveness depends on both the sender and receiver. Humor must be shared for it to work. Dad invited everyone to participate in his jest to help divert attention away from the concerns of the moment and to lighten the mood for everyone. Dad's masterful skill of never missing a punch line simultaneously empowered and delighted him. As Suzy put it, "It made him extremely happy to make people laugh and smile."

Equally endearing was Suzy's fear of embarrassment from her father's persistent joking. Taking on an adult-like "responsible" role, Suzy still felt apologetic of how her father behaved, and she wished to silence him. Perhaps the parent/child hierarchy remains long after the teen years as does the embarrassment of not being able to control the words or actions of a loved one. Suzy set herself apart from Dad, fearing that the healthcare worker's judgement might have some reflection on her. Suzy felt accountable for her father's behavior even while Dad dismissed her concerns and persisted despite her cautious objection: "Dad asserted that he was 'just having fun' and that the tech knew Dad 'didn't mean anything' by his comments." One might imagine that as he said this, he implied, "Lighten up, Suzy! Quit trying to discipline me. I know what I am doing. I'm still the adult in the room, the one in control, not you!" She took her place as the obedient child with all the love and respect spilling over in her words, "How could I disagree with that logic?" She couldn't, she knew it, and she lovingly cherished his gutsy persistence all the more.

Indeed, Dad did know what he was doing. He wanted to distract himself from his own fears of getting a colonoscopy, ease the stress of the phlebotomist who seemed to be too nervous to "find" his vein, and calm his own daughter's worry about possible complications from the test. In his own subtle way, Dad took control of the situation by brightening the atmosphere and diverting everyone's attention away from an unpleasant procedure and from the fearful anticipation of a potentiality serious diagnosis. Dad did not want to think about this any more than he wanted others to feel sorry for him or to worry about him. He took it upon himself to ease the tension and to make others smile back at him—a mirroring of human kindness and genuine emotion that he felt everyone needed, including himself.

When Suzy returned to the health facility and cringed upon seeing the same technician, her father persisted hollering, "It's the vampire!" To her relief, the young man joined in the fun as he "broke into a smile and said, 'the blood is flowing better'" and asked how he was feeling this day. Unlike the first encounter when the phlebotomist ignored Dad's invitation to participate in his humor, he validated Dad, recognized his genuine attempt at lightening a tense moment, and shared equally in the amusement. Dad not only improved the stress level of the original encounter, but he also left a memorable impression upon the young phlebotomist who, like his more experienced colleagues, now realized the empowering, patient-centered role that humor plays in patient care. It is safe to say that the next time this young man faced a challenging vein, this funny incident would come to mind. Dad's humor created a positive impact on the worker not only for Dad's particular interaction but likely for all subsequent patients in that worker's future. This small act created a memorable, equalizing bond between the two and served the purpose of lightening their day during a less than ideal circumstance. Dad was right, "humor helps."

In the days and weeks following Dad's passing, this notion became even more evident to Suzy and her family members while interacting with his caregivers concerning business and legal issues. She stated, "...we were surprised by how many people from his various doctor's offices remarked at how much they enjoyed his visits and his humor and how much they would miss him." Indeed, Dad's humor left a lasting impression on all those who knew him. It also provided lasting comfort to Suzy and her sister because their father's legacy continued to hold meaning in the lives of others and to bring memorable joy for years to come in the hearts and minds of those who cared for him. Dad impressed the young phlebotomist and perhaps influenced every subsequent interaction he had with other patients. He learned to laugh and communicate with other patients due to caring for Dad. Likewise, Dad taught everyone he knew that despite the risks of being misinterpreted when telling a joke, the joy of humor leaves a lasting impact on others. Dad mastered the art and benefits of the use of humor in the medical context and he shared his art through example with all he met.

THE MESSAGE FOR HEALTHCARE PROFESSIONALS

This case demonstrates how telling jokes empowered Suzy's father in a world where control increasingly slipped past him as his illness progressed. He could not control the lack of viable veins in his arms, the results of the colonoscopy, or his illnesses including diabetes, kidney failure, heart disease, and hypertension. These only increased in severity with age. One thing he could control was his own wit, his ability to make people smile, and his need to overcome the inevitable path towards his pending death. His humor delighted him as much as it did all those around him. Humor afforded him autonomy, a chance to participate in his own care, a means for engaging when he himself felt so removed from watching himself being acted upon as others cared for his needs. Indeed, "his humor was as much for himself as those around him," "it reduced his own fears and worries," and "it was good medicine for him as a patient and a type of therapy."

Suzy's heartfelt story honored her father's life, his illness, and his contribution to the lives of those who cared for him. Dad's narrative, however, lives on through the stock jokes he told, the human kindness he showed, and the treasured smiles and laughs that live on through everyone's memories. Humor allowed him to face the unknown, to lighten the stressful environment, and to allow Suzy to forget (if only momentarily) about his impending death. If ever there is a time for communicating through human kindness, it is near the end of one's life. Through his illness, Dad communicated hope, resilience, purpose, empowerment, positivity, and control through the sprinkling of humor in his illness narrative.

Much can be learned from this case as it exemplifies the needs of patients within the unique, complex environment of the medical setting. To begin with, medical professionals must be attentive to individual patient needs, especially during periods of depression, anger, anxiety, and hopelessness. Often immediate medical issues overshadow the mental distress that also affects treatment and procedural outcomes. One cannot treat the illness without also treating the person who experiences the illness. They go hand in hand. The importance of treating the whole person should never be overlooked. Yue et al. (2014) discuss this concerning adaptive humor styles which help the initiator of humor to affiliate with others and/or attempt to enhance positively of oneself in other's eyes. This form of humor increases self-esteem and enhances subjective happiness. Again, humor often fulfils patients' need to feel better about themselves and those around them. Recognizing this need can lead to improved understanding and increased support systems to be recommended for the patient.

How funny or sensible patients' jokes may be is not as important as *why* these jokes arise. Being attentive to the needs of the patient and understanding why they are joking provides important information about the condition and mindset of the patient. Perhaps it tells of the patient's current cognitive acuity; but it also indicates an underlying need that may be of critical importance. Humor should never be dismissed as nonsensical, inappropriate, or irrational. Medical professionals should be aware of why the humor arose and should carefully assess how to respond most effectively. Anecdotally, it was personally communicated to this author that a home health nurse of an Alzheimer patient noted that when she clipped his toenails, a piece flew towards her and down the front of her blouse. The man teased, "I can get that for you." Horrified and embarrassed, the wife who was present stated, "He'd never normally say anything like that!" The nurse simply smiled, joking back to him, "No, that won't be necessary." The worker assessed his mental acuity, realized he was harmless, eased the wife's concern, and just made light of the situation.

Additionally, practitioners should make note of the specific moment *when* humor surfaces. Even if patients are unaware of why they are feeling a certain way or what purpose their humor might fulfil, healthcare professionals should pay particular attention to what might be driving patients' humor when it surfaces. As Dad began using gallows humor in referring to the phlebotomist as a vampire, he may have recognized that the technician became stressed (possibly due to his own inexperience or to his superior's presence) and wanted to help him calm down enough to find the vein. The joking might also have occurred due to Dad's own stress levels rising or the pain inflicted upon him from being poked and prodded so much. When patients intuitively initiate humor, a key stimulus may be motivating them to do so. Once identified, healthcare workers can address or compensate for what might be bothering them. Possibly, Dad simply was feeling like an object (a human pin cushion) and not an individual. He may have joked to encourage the technician to treat him more humanely, to recognize him as a person rather than an object, or even just to validate his concerns about upcoming procedures. Recognizing that humor surfaces to fulfil a conscious or subconscious patient goal—no matter how small—should motivate the practitioner to identify the need and facilitate the patient in fulling it.

As a final note, healthcare workers must remember to protect not only the patient but also themselves when encountering inappropriate or misinterpreted humorous exchanges. No one deserves to be physically, mentally, or sexually harmed because of misinterpreted or ill-intended dialogue. Mutual respect and understanding must be maintained for both the patient and the practitioner alike. Effective management of humor assures the safety, integrity, and humanity of all involved.

In short, humor remains a complicated yet potentially helpful aspect of medical communication. Many theoretical, empirical, and anecdotal examples of humor involving patient care demonstrate the power of communal laughter, a pleasant or teasing smile, a witty comment, or a shared story from the past. Humor embraces an element of positivity that is as innate and universal as a baby's smile. It potentially provides agency during challenging moments, brightens stressful times, and allows for connectivity between people of all walks of life as they enter the medical context with the hope of effective, satisfying health outcomes.

REFERENCES

Abbott, R. (2014, April 22). Unconscious patient says doctors mocked him. *Courthouse News*. https://www.courthousenews.com/unconscious-patient-says-doctors-mocked-him/

Besnier, N. (2016). Humour and humility: Narratives of modernity on Nukulaelae Atoll. *Etnofoor, 28*(1), 75–95.

Black, S. P. (2012). Laughing to death: Joking as support amid stigma for Zulu-speaking South Africans living with HIV. *Journal of Linguistic Anthropology, 22*(1), 87–108. doi:10.1111/j.1548-1395.2012.01140.x

Canha, B. (2016). Using humor in treatment of substance use disorders: Worthy of further investigation. *The Open Nursing Journal, 10*(1), 37–44. doi:10.2174/1874434601610010037 PMID:27347254

Chen, L. (2016). Laughter, smiling and their pragmatic/interpersonal functions: An interactional linguistic account. *Concentric: Studies in Linguistics, 42*(2). Advance online publication. doi:10.6241/concentric.ling.42.2.05

Chiodo, C. P., Broughton, K. K., & Michalski, M. P. (2020). Caution: Wit and humor during the COVID-19 pandemic. *Foot & Ankle International, 41*(6), 763–764. https://doi-org.pitt.idm.oclc.org/10.1177/1071100720923651. doi:10.1177/1071100720923651 PMID:32338052

Christoff, M., & Dauphin, B. (2017). Freud's theory of humor. In V. Zeigler-Hill & T. Shackelford (Eds.), Encyclopedia of personality and individual differences (living edition). Springer. doi:10.1007/978-3-319-28099-8_588-1

Clark, C., Nicholas, J., Gordon, E., Golden, H., Cohen, M., Woodward, F., Macpherson, K., Slattery, C., Mummery, C., Schott, J., Rohrer, J., & Warren, J. (2016). Altered sense of humor in dementia. *Journal of Alzheimer's Disease, 49*(1), 111–119. doi:10.3233/JAD-150413 PMID:26444779

du Pré, A. (1998). *Humor and the healing arts: A multimethod analysis of humor use in health care*. Lawrence Erlbaum Associates.

Dunbar, R. I. M., & Mehu, M. (2008). Naturalistic observations of smiling and laughter in human group interactions. *Behaviour, 145*(12), 1747–1780. doi:10.1163/156853908786279619

Ekman, P., & Friesen, W. V. (1971). Constants across cultures in the face and emotion. *Journal of Personality and Social Psychology, 17*(2), 124–129. doi:10.1037/h0030377 PMID:5542557

Epstein, R., & Joker, V. R. (2007). A threshold theory of the humor response. *The Behavior Analyst, 30*(1), 49–58. doi:10.1007/BF03392145 PMID:22478488

Falkenberg, I., Jarmuzek, J., Bartels, M., & Wild, B. (2011). Do depressed patients lose their sense of humor? *Psychopathology, 44*(2), 98–105. doi:10.1159/000317778 PMID:21196810

Forabosco, G. (2009). Cognitive aspects of the humor process: The concept of incongruity. *Humor: International Journal of Humor Research*, *5*(1), 45–68. doi:10.1515/humr.1992.5.1-2.45

Freud, S. (1961). The ego and the id. In *The standard edition of the complete psychological works of Sigmund Freud* (Vol. 19, J. Strachey, Ed. & Trans., pp. 3–66). Hogarth Press. (Original work published 1923)

Gramling, D., & Gramling, R. (2012). Laughing at the dark: Tactical humor for autonomous decision making in serious illness. *Journal of Palliative Medicine*, *15*(11), 1170–1172. doi:10.1089/jpm.2012.0279 PMID:23116272

Gunnery, R., & Ruben, M. A. (2015). Perceptions of Duchenne and non-Duchenne smiles: A meta-analysis. *Cognition and Emotion*, *30*(3), 501–515. doi:10.1080/02699931.2015.1018817 PMID:25787714

Hardy, C. (2020). Humor and sympathy in medical practice. *Medicine, Health Care, and Philosophy*, *23*(2), 179–190. doi:10.100711019-019-09928-0 PMID:31637581

Hodson, G., Rush, J., & MacInnis, C. C. (2010). A joke is just a joke (except when it isn't): Cavalier humor beliefs facilitate the expression of group dominance motives. *Journal of Personality and Social Psychology*, *99*(4), 660–682. doi:10.1037/a0019627 PMID:20919777

Jiang, S. (2019). Pathways linking patient-centered communication to health improvement: A longitudinal study in China. *Journal of Health Communication*, *24*(2), 156–164. doi:10.1080/10810730.2019.1587110 PMID:30849289

Kärtner, J. (2015). The autonomous developmental pathway: The primacy of subjective mental states for human behavior and experience. *Child Development*, *86*(4), 1298–1309. doi:10.1111/cdev.12377 PMID:25930102

Kim, J. (2015, February 26). Should health care providers joke about patients? Medical gallows humor can help providers cope, but at what cost? *Psychology Today*. https://www.psychologytoday.com/us/blog/culture-shrink/201502/should-health-care-providers-joke-about-patients

Kuiper, B., & Borowicz-Sibenik, M. (2005). A good sense of humor doesn't always help: Agency and communion as moderators of psychological well-being. *Personality and Individual Differences*, *38*(2), 365–377. doi:10.1016/j.paid.2004.04.015

Kuiper, N., Grimshaw, M., Leite, C., & Kirsh, G. (2004). Humor is not always the best medicine: Specific components of sense of humor and psychological well-being. *Humor: International Journal of Humor Research*, *17*(1), 135–168. doi:10.1515/humr.2004.002

Lee, C. Y., Chiang, Y. C., Li, A., Li, X., Wu, Y. T., Lin, Y. J., Zhao, Y., & Zhang, X. (2020). Influence of humor expression on suicidal ideation among adolescents: Mediating effects of depressive emotion and positive emotion. *BMC Psychiatry*, *20*(1), 421. doi:10.118612888-020-02814-7 PMID:32842996

Lee, J. Y., Slater, M. D., & Tchernev, J. (2015). Self-deprecating humor versus other-deprecating humor in health messages. *Journal of Health Communication*, *20*(10), 1185–1195. doi:10.1080/10810730.2015.1018591 PMID:26020507

Lingard, L. (2013). Language matters: Towards an understanding of silence and humour in medical education. *Medical Education*, *47*(1), 40–48. doi:10.1111/medu.12098 PMID:23278824

Liu, Y. P., Sun, L., Wu, X. F., Yang, Y., Zhang, C. T., Zhou, H. L., & Quan, X. Q. (2017). Use of humour in medical education: A survey of students and teachers at a medical school in China. *BMJ Open*, *7*(11), e018853. doi:10.1136/bmjopen-2017-018853 PMID:29187417

LoBue, V. (2019). *9 months in, 9 months out: A scientist's tale of pregnancy and parenthood*. Oxford University Press. doi:10.1093/oso/9780190863388.001.0001

Low, L., Goodenough, B., Fletcher, J., Xu, K., Casey, A., Chenoweth, L., Fleming, R., Spitzer, P., Bell, J., & Brodaty, H. (2014). The effects of humor therapy on nursing home residents measured using observational methods: The SMILE cluster randomized trial. *Journal of the American Medical Directors Association*, *15*(8), 564–569. doi:10.1016/j.jamda.2014.03.017 PMID:24814320

Maxwell, W. (2003). The use of gallows humor and dark humor during crisis situations. *International Journal of Emergency Mental Health*, *5*(2), 93–98. PMID:12882095

Millard, W. B. (2015). Gallows humor, fearmongering continue to spread. *Annals of Emergency Medicine*, *65*(2), 21A–22A. doi:10.1016/j.annemergmed.2014.12.022 PMID:25756100

Nikopoulos, J. (2017). The stability of laughter. *Humor: International Journal of Humor Research*, *30*(1), 1–21. doi:10.1515/humor-2016-0062

Phua, D., Tang, H., & Tham, K. (2005). Coping responses of emergency physicians and nurses to the 2003 severe acute respiratory syndrome outbreak. *Academic Emergency Medicine*, *12*(4), 322–328. doi:10.1197/j.aem.2004.11.015 PMID:15805323

Piemonte, N. M. (2015). Last laughs: Gallows humor and medical education. *The Journal of Medical Humanities*, *36*(4), 375–390. doi:10.100710912-015-9338-4 PMID:26062447

Porteous, J. (1988). Humor as a process of defense: The evolution of laughing. *Humor: International Journal of Humor Research*, *1*(1), 63–80. doi:10.1515/humr.1988.1.1.63

Saunders, P. A. (1998). "You're out of your mind!": Humor as a face-saving strategy during neuropsychological examinations. *Health Communication*, *10*(4), 357–372. doi:10.120715327027hc1004_4 PMID:16370980

Sliter, M., Kale, A., & Yuan, Z. (2014). Is humor the best medicine? The buffering effect of coping humor on traumatic stressors in firefighters. *Journal of Organizational Behavior*, *35*(2), 257–272. doi:10.1002/job.1868

Sousa, L., Marques-Vieira, C., Antunes, A. V., Frade, M., Severino, S., & Valentim, O. S. (2019). Humor intervention in the nurse-patient interaction. *Revista Brasileira de Enfermagem*, *72*(4), 1078–1085. doi:10.1590/0034-7167-2018-0609 PMID:31432968

Tajfel, H. (1981). *Human groups and social categories: Studies in social psychology*. Cambridge University Press.

Taylor, K. (2009). Paternalism, participation and partnership—The evolution of patient centeredness in the consultation. *Patient Education and Counseling*, *74*(2), 150–155. doi:10.1016/j.pec.2008.08.017 PMID:18930624

Venetis, M., Chernichky-Karcher, S., & Lillie, H. (2019). Communicating resilience: Predictors and outcomes of dyadic communication resilience processes among both cancer patients and cancer partners. *Journal of Applied Communication Research*, *48*(1), 49–69. doi:10.1080/00909882.2019.1706098

Watson, K. (2011). Gallows humor in medicine. *The Hastings Center Report*, *41*(5), 37–45. doi:10.1002/j.1552-146X.2011.tb00139.x PMID:21980898

Yue, X. D., Liu, K. W.-Y., Jiang, F., & Hiranandani, N. A. (2014). Humor styles, self-esteem, and subjective happiness. *Psychological Reports*, *115*(2), 517–525. doi:10.2466/07.02.PR0.115c18z6 PMID:25153846

Zweyer, K., Velker, B., & Ruch, W. (2004). Do cheerfulness, exhilaration, and humor production moderate pain tolerance? A FACS study. *Humor: International Journal of Humor Research*, *17*(1), 85–119. doi:10.1515/humr.2004.009

Chapter 31
Breaking Up Is Hard to Do: A Humorous Strategy to Help De-Escalate and Terminate the Patient/Provider Relationship

Carrie H. Cox
Western Kentucky University, USA

Stephen A. Cox
Murray State University, USA

Diagnosed four years ago, I knew I was starting a "fight" against a terrible disease. What I did not realize is that I was also starting long-term relationships with three committed physicians—three relationships I needed to live but, eventually, wanted to live without.

With another exhausting semester happily ended, my husband, Steve, and I were driving to attend an academic conference when my phone rang. It was Amanda from Vanderbilt Medical Center. "Hi Carrie. This is Amanda at Vanderbilt Breast Center I'm calling to tell you the biopsy results are back from the pathologist. I'm sorry to say they came back positive. You do have breast cancer. We will need to see you next week. I've scheduled your appointments for Wednesday morning starting at 9:30. You will meet with the three physicians on your care team: the surgeon—Dr. Sweeting, the oncologist—Dr. Rexer, and the plastic surgeon—Dr. Higdon." In shock and disbelief, I naively responded, "Well, let me look at my calendar to see if that works for me…"

I quickly learned that cancer is never convenient. The avalanche of doctor appointments, tests, procedures, and treatments would not neatly accommodate my calendar. My schedule of "things-to-do" for family, work, and myself would no longer take precedence; I was no longer in control. My appointment preferences were inconsequential to my committed physicians' shared goal of saving my life and keeping me "cancer free."

Patient/provider relationships contain a "love/hate" dynamic—medical patients love being healthy but hate to "go see the doctor." Patients typically control the initiation and longevity of these medical

DOI: 10.4018/978-1-7998-4528-7.ch031

relationships by voluntarily seeking and keeping appointments. Patients desire to acquire treatment, restore health, and stop seeing their physicians as quickly as possible! As a cancer patient, I wanted it resolved as quickly as possible, to stop seeing these three physicians, and to resume my unfettered routine.

But cancer doctors know they treat complicated, deadly diseases that offer no quick-fixes or guarantees. Cancer treatment requires long-term, committed relationships between physicians and patients. Thus, Drs. Sweeting, Rexer, and Higdon insisted seeing me far more often, over a much longer span of time, than I ever imagined. Since starting my breast cancer fight, I have had five surgeries and a mind-boggling "72" doctor's appointments and counting! This does not include additional radiation treatments and physical therapy sessions! Although declared "cancer free" early in the process, follow-up appointments with each physician continue as they work to monitor and preserve my health. These three physicians provide the lens through which I view my cancer and the team with whom I fight it. But when will this fight be over; when can I finally say goodbye to these three physician relationships and move on?

Each physician had me at "hello!" They all exuded the compassion, attentiveness, and confidence I needed my physicians to demonstrate. I should have known they wanted a long-term relationship when they first handed me a thick, three-ring binder irresistibly titled, "Breast Cancer Treatment Information" packed with explanations, Q&A, contact information, and comforting "We will take great care of you" promises and testimonials. I immediately became an eager relational partner desperate for their individual attention and skilled hands. I admit it; I led them on. I willingly showed up to every appointment and disrobed when they told me to. Nothing suggests, "We're in a relationship" quite like a willingness to be naked in front of someone. And yes, out of medical necessity, they all touched me! But my husband was always present; we were all comfortable with this arrangement.

Healthcare requires medical providers to face the naked-truth and carefully treat each unique patient. Breast cancer required that I abandon my conventional modesty and be exposed to necessary treatments. And the life-or-death gravity of cancer caused me to initially cling to these relationships and the hopefulness each physician conveyed. We were in this fight together; these relationships were consequential to my survival.

Although surgeons are notoriously meticulous, serious professionals, Dr. Sweeting's disarming warmth and approachability masked those requisite traits inviting comfortable conversation so she could understand both "Carrie" her cancer patient, and "Carrie and Steve," the couple she was helping. We always reciprocated her warmth with sincere interest in her as a person, not just as a surgeon. Thus, she was always happy to see us as we mutually shared updates about family and life events prior to discussing my health. Over time, our mutual self-disclosures deepened our patient/provider relationship.

Steve and I have always needed humor and laughter in our marriage, especially during trying circumstances. Thankfully, each of these physicians understood it was our coping mechanism. Indulging us much as a friend would, Dr. Sweeting always played along, amused as Steve and I teased one another or made sarcastic jokes to diminish the gloom of my cancer:

Sweeting: "How are you feeling today, Carrie? How's your pain?"

Carrie: "Okay. It's not too bad."

Steve: "Honestly, Carrie won't complain even if it hurts. She's tough; she's very long-suffering."

Carrie: "Yes I am! Being married to Steve has prepared me for the pain of a double mastectomy!"

Sweeting: "I see your reconstructive surgery is scheduled for next month."

Carrie: "I was always a 'straight A student' when it came to boobies. I don't know what it will be like to finally fill out a bra."

Sweeting: "What size do you want your implants to be?"

Carrie: "Oh, Steve asked Dr. Higdon to turn me into a 'double-D'!"

Steve: "I did not say that!!! NO...but could he!?!? Really??? Just kidding..."

But six months ago, my feelings about seeing these three wonderful physicians started to change and Steve knew it. My once acute survival instinct and desperate need to see my physicians had subsided into ambivalent feelings of obligatory, relationship drudgery as Steve and I were headed to yet another follow-up appointment with Dr. Sweeting. Why would seeing this precious woman who helped save my life now feel like drudgery?

As Steve and I began our hour-long drive to Vanderbilt, we looked at each other and wearily said, "Here we go again." Steve asked me if I knew how long these follow-up appointments would continue - "How much longer do we have to do this? Can't they just see you once a year? You're feeling good. It's been well over three years. When will they stop needing to see you?" I replied, "Honey, I really don't know. You've been at almost every appointment. What do you remember them saying?" s we talked, we remembered being told, "We'll be seeing you for a while," but a specific timeframe defining "a while" eluded us. Clearly, it was time we ask these doctors, "Why do you keep holding on?" and tell them, "We're ready to move on!"

As a communication professor who studies "organizational assimilation" (i.e., anticipatory socialization, organizational encounter, metamorphosis, and employee exit; Jablin, 2001), Steve looked at it as an organizational relationship that needed an "exit conversation." He needed to initiate this conversation to discuss a timeline for de-escalating and terminating these interpersonal, patient/provider relationships (Knapp, 1978). As he drove, Steve quietly pondered how to initiate the "We need to talk..." talk! Breakups are always difficult. How do you tell your life-saving doctors, "We're tired of this relationship, but you keep insisting that we see each other!" Because Dr. Sweeting knows us well, our typical use of humor may soften it while also reassuring her of our endless appreciation for all she has done.

As we reached the end of the appointment, Steve took the opportunity to humorously ask Sweeting if or when we could stop seeing one another:

Sweeting: "Do you have any other questions?"

Steve: "Dr. Sweeting, Carrie and I have been talking. You know...we've been seeing you now for over three years. Wow, that's long! That's a long time to be SEEING someone (head nodding). Now, don't get us wrong. NO doubt! Seeing you has been SOOOO good for us...and we're pretty sure it's been good for you, too. Right (big smile, head nodding)??? But we're starting to ask, "How much longer does she want to keep seeing us?" I mean, we know THIS RIGHT HERE is pretty great...and it's HARD to let go of a gooood thing...we understand. But maybe it's time for us to talk about it. Now, we're not pushing you away; no, no, no! We love you! But let's face it. We're all adults here. We know THIS has always been an 'open relationship' (wink). WE KNOW you've been seeing other patients. And honestly (deep sigh)...we've been seeing other physicians. Now, we totally respect YOU will be making that call; that is NOT ours to make. You're the doctor! But when you're ready to let go...you just let us know."

Sweeting: "Ooooh, that's good! That's real good! That's hilarious (shaking her head and laughing)."

It worked! Dr. Sweeting appreciated and laughed at the humor. It started the conversation we needed to gain clarity on a timeframe when we could say goodbye. Fully empathizing with our uncertainty, Dr. Sweeting explained the medical reasons why each physician will continue monitoring my health and for, approximately, how much longer. While these patient/provider relationships will not be ending soon, at least we have started the de-escalation and, funny thing, we all feel very good about it.

REFERENCES

Jablin, F. M. (2001). Organizational entry, assimilation, and disengagement/exit. In F. Jablin & L. Putnam (Eds.), *The new handbook of organizational communication: Advances in theory, research, and methods* (pp. 732–818). Sage. doi:10.4135/9781412986243.n19

Knapp, M. L. (1978). *Social intercourse: From greeting to goodbye*. Allyn and Bacon.

Chapter 32 Response: "Breaking Up Is Hard to Do: A Humorous Strategy to Help De-Escalate and Terminate the Patient/Provider Relationship"

Ryan Goke
North Dakota State University, USA

Maranda Berndt
The Pennsylvania State University, USA

LITERATURE REVIEW

When transitioning into the workplace, employees experience three stages: *anticipatory socialization, organizational assimilation,* and *organizational exit* (Jablin, 1987).

1. *Anticipatory Socialization*: The time of uncertainty for newcomers before they are immersed in the organization's culture.
2. *Organizational Assimilation:* The process through which the organization socializes the employee and attempts to instill their goals, values, and norms.
3. *Organizational Exit*: Employees leave the organization, resulting in turnover.

The stages of the relationship that healthcare patients experience with their medical teams mirror the organizational assimilation process of employees in the workplace. Newcomers have certain expecta-

DOI: 10.4018/978-1-7998-4528-7.ch032

tions of the treatment process, relational roles, and hospital norms that they must reconcile once they encounter reality. Additionally, the relationships developed between doctors and their patients undergo a similar transformation as patients are admitted, treated, and eventually no longer need their services. In both contexts humor is used as an invaluable tool. Humorous discourse is conceptualized as a "communicative process that constructs new shared meaning out of ambiguity" (Lynch, 2002, p. 443). In this way, humor is used to make sense of ambiguous exchanges. In the organizational environment humor provides a sense of identity and sensemaking for new hires (Heiss & Carmack, 2012). In healthcare, humor can alleviate stress and burnout in medical professionals (Joshua et al., 2005) and aid in patient recovery (Johnson, 2002).

Anticipatory Socialization

Before entering the workplace, prospective employees have already developed (often unrealistic) expectations and beliefs about the organization (Jablin, 1987). Large discrepancies between expectations and reality can shock newcomers and make their transition difficult. Similarly, patients form expectations of the treatment process, the relationship they prefer with their physician, and their level of involvement in healthcare decisions even before their first appointment. The first encounter between patient and doctor will attempt to reconcile those expectations. In fact, doctor-patient communication is designed to establish a strong interpersonal relationship, facilitate the exchange of information, and include patients in decision making (Platt & Keating, 2007).

The use of humor in the initial interaction helps establish the physician-patient relationship by breaking the ice and developing trust (Joshua et al., 2005). It also cultivates a sense of familiarity and helps facilitate difficult conversations. For example, physicians may use humor to help establish a sense of equality with their patient and reduce the formal power distance between them (Berger et al., 2004). Patients may also use humor to distance themselves from the fear of their illness and the negativity that accompanies the diagnosis and treatment (Beach & Prickett, 2017; Francis et al., 1999).

Assimilation

Assimilation is the process through which the organization socializes employees to conform to its values and norms, containing two parts: *encounter* and *metamorphosis* (Jablin, 1982). Expectancy violations during the encounter phase can be effectively addressed using empathetic humor by veteran workers (Heiss & Carmack, 2012). Humor is particularly useful as an information-seeking tool for newcomers because it allows them to solicit information with low risk to their image. In healthcare, patients assimilate to their role and the treatment procedure through a similar process by negotiating their preferences with those of the doctor and asking questions for clarity. Unfortunately, questions and information-seeking behaviors can be viewed as disruptive or annoying to doctors despite being a necessary part of the assimilation process (Grunloh et al., 2018).

Organizations ensure stability through a hierarchy that assigns roles with accompanying behavioral expectations (Vandenberghe et al., 2017). Once employees accept these roles and expectations, they have reached metamorphosis (Jablin, 1987). Upon diagnosis, patients begin a similar journey toward metamorphosis as they accept their prognosis and participate in their treatment. Each patient processes bad news differently and requires varying levels of information and support, just as employees have different needs as they assimilate to the organization. To accommodate the individual needs of their patients, physicians should assess the environment and ensure that their emotional support and delivery of the bad news are appropriate (Sastre et al., 2011). Additionally, they must be cognizant of how their patients process information, adjusting the level of information disclosed and its source of delivery to account for these needs (Adamson et al., 2018).

The hierarchy of power in an organization influences the communication between superiors and subordinates (Bisel et al., 2012) just as the power distance in the doctor-patient relationship affects their communication, perceptions, and expectations (Grunloh et al., 2018). Because of their medical expertise, doctors carry a disproportionate amount of power. When doctor and patient values or treatment preferences do not align, the doctor is often tasked with convincing the patient of the best option, regardless of personal preferences (Grunloh et al., 2018). In the organization, employees decide which information is pertinent to pass on to their superior, filtering content and manipulating the message (Jablin, 1987). Similarly, patients determine which information is pertinent to share with their doctor to help with diagnosis.

Exit

Eventually, the final stage of assimilation will be reached by employees and they will leave the organization. Sometimes this is their choice, other times it is forced through termination. Humor can induce shock and be difficult to understand if used incorrectly (Priego-Valverde, 2009), potentially contributing to an employee's decision to leave. Offensive humor used by superiors may undermine the benefits of a positive humor climate and increase employee perceptions of exclusion (Tremblay, 2017).

Similarly, patients eventually reach the end of their tenure, ideally through remission in their illness. It is important for patients to see their treatment through to the end and not terminate the relationship with their physician prematurely. The decision to continue treatment is influenced by the patient's satisfaction with their physician (Fallowfield & Jenkins, 2004). However, even satisfied patients will eventually require less interaction with their doctor as they complete the treatment process. Once a patient is no longer in need of acute treatment from their physician they may begin the post stage follow-up care. Follow-up care is necessary to allow early detection of a possible recurrence (Collins et al., 2004). Research has found that breast cancer survivors often experience depression and anxiety immediately following radiation treatments (Deshields et al., 2005), highlighting the importance of continuing doctor-patient interactions on some level even after going into remission. Follow-up care provides additional psychological support and rehabilitation for patients who need it (Collins et al., 2004). However, there may be a point where patients feel they would like a change to follow-up care, or to terminate it.

When it comes to terminating relationships Knapp (1978) discusses three functions of leave-taking behaviors in interpersonal relationships: (1) summarizing the substance of the discourse; (2) signaling the impending decreased access between the communicators; and (3) signaling supportiveness. Knapp (1978) states that most relationship farewells include a recollection of the history of the relationship. From there, it is often stated that there is going to be an absence from someone in the party for a while. Signaling supportiveness can communicate that even though the current relationship may be over, there is a possibility for a future relationship of some kind. For patient-physician relationships, if there is a possibility of the need for future care, it is important for the patient and physician to be in agreement. The mutual withdrawal is an example where both parties come to an agreement that the relationship can end. Along with that, the patient may express their want for a temporary termination, where they hope for the possibility of reopening the relationship in the future, if necessary (Hayes-Bautista, 1976).

APPLICATION

Carrie's journey through her cancer treatments reflects the experience of employees as they adjust to their new environment. The journey begins with uncertainty as they anticipate the socialization process and begin assimilating, gradually becoming more comfortable and familiar with the treatment or organizational process through metamorphosis. Eventually, Carrie reaches the end of her tenure and begins to separate herself, transitioning toward an exit.

Anticipatory Socialization

Much like an incoming employee, Carrie experienced large amounts of uncertainty during her first encounter with the healthcare team that would be responsible for her treatment. In this stage Carrie made judgements about her doctors and reconciled her anticipatory expectations with reality. The first interactions with Dr. Sweeting were critical to establish a positive doctor-patient relationship and for Carrie to feel more at ease (Goold & Lipkin, 1999). If she viewed her team as competent, supportive, and positive she would have greater trust in their abilities. Because chronic cases like cancer require ongoing treatment and frequent interactions with their doctors, it is especially important for these patients to have a strong relationship with their doctor.

Much like an incoming employee, Carrie was expected to conform to the expectations and values of the hospital. The assimilation process erodes any sense of autonomy and individuality, which is why cancer patients often experience feelings of anxiety and loss of autonomy during and after their treatment (Deshields et al., 2005). They have little say in what must be done. Establishing a strong relationship with the doctor can mitigate the stress and uncertainty of the situation. Carrie clung to the relationships with her doctors and looked to them for hope. They were what pushed her through the treatments and helped her stay informed. Because they answered her questions and provided her and her husband with emotional support, she was confident in their abilities as physicians and trusted them throughout the treatment process.

Assimilation

During assimilation Carrie would forge group affiliations and process expectations through observation and information seeking, much like a new employee (Heiss & Carmack, 2012). Cues from others can help indicate the type of role and relationship that is expected with superiors, which is why Carrie would look to her doctors for guidance. Dr. Sweeting was warm and approachable, putting Carrie and Steve at ease and always making sure to get to know them as individuals, not just as her patients. Dr. Sweeting also disclosed information about herself as an individual, which deepens the relationship and provides more opportunities to establish trust and personal connections (Beach et al., 2004). Since bedside manner is often used by patients to judge the general competence of their physician (Hall et al., 1981), Dr. Sweeting strengthened the trust Carrie and Steve had in her professionally through these interactions. She also remained patient-centered, including them in the decision-making process and taking time to answer their questions so that they can make an informed decision together (Randall & Wearn, 2005).

Carrie's doctors used a paternalistic approach at the start of her treatment, acting on her behalf from a perspective of obligatory beneficence (Cody, 2003). She had limited say in what types of treatments she underwent or even when her appointments were scheduled. Her limited freedom is mirrored by new employees who also have limited autonomy and are heavily supervised. However, as they assimilate toward metamorphosis, they acquire more freedom and comfort in performing tasks. During the early stages, Dr. Sweeting took charge and had a plan. However, despite having more power because of her expertise (Hoerger et al., 2013), she provided Carrie and Steve with a binder of information, reassured them, and made time to answer all their questions. These behaviors influenced their satisfaction with the quality of care (Hall, 2006) despite limited input. For some patients, this is enough inclusion for them to feel comfortable and increase their confidence in the doctor (Goold & Lipkin, 1999).

New employees with limited autonomy can employ humor as a sense making tool as they adjust to the workplace in the same way Carrie and Steve used humor as a coping mechanism to make sense of their situation and help them adjust (Heiss & Carmack, 2012). They had a history of employing humor in their marriage and their everyday lives, so it was a large part of their sense-making process. The doctors responded positively to their use of humor, even encouraging it and joining in occasionally. This led to a stronger rapport being established between the five of them (Scholl, 2007). Dr. Sweeting accounted for Carrie and Steve's preferred communication style, tailoring it to their individual needs, which encouraged them to trust her and open up more (Joshua et al., 2005). Additionally, it allowed the doctors to view Carrie and Steve as more than just patients and helped them feel equal. Eventually, Carrie and Steve used humor as a form of information-seeking to determine how much longer they would have to remain in this relationship (Wanzer et al., 2005). Not only was this tactic effective and consistent with the tone of their relationship with the doctors, it also reduced tension and confrontation while having "the talk."

Exit

Just as the organizational hierarchy assigns roles with behavioral expectations, the expertise of Dr. Sweeting creates a power distance that makes it difficult for Carrie and Steve to bring up their desire to terminate the relationship (Grunloh et al., 2018). In the traditional paternalistic view of the relationship that was used early on in Carrie's treatments it would not be appropriate for them to suggest a change that was not prescribed by Dr. Sweeting. Typically, physicians employing a paternalistic approach tend to discourage patient input. This perspective grants the physician ultimate power and say, without having to answer to their patients. Because the dynamics gradually shifted toward a patient-centered approach, and because of the trust and dynamic of the relationship Carrie and Steve have established with Dr. Sweeting, they have the opportunity to voice their concerns without upsetting her (Scholl, 2007). However, some doctors view additional questions or propositions as a violation of trust or a threat to their authority (Grunloh et al., 2018). Therefore, Carrie & Steve could still be concerned with how Dr. Sweeting might react and the effect it might have on their relationship.

Despite the possibility that Dr. Sweeting might view their suggestion to terminate the relationship negatively, using humor as a way to reduce tension and soften the blow provided a way for them to bring up their concerns in a less confrontational and offensive way (Joshua et al., 2005). At this point Carrie and Steve have reached the metamorphosis stage of the relationship, having internalized the expectations of their situation and gained a better understanding of the relationship with Dr. Sweeting. Therefore, they also have a better understanding of which behaviors and strategies are appropriate and will reduce tension. Steve and Carrie use humor to deploy three leave-taking behaviors. They summarized the history that they have had with Dr. Sweeting and stated their desire to not see her as often, but signal supportiveness for what has developed in their relationship (Knapp, 1978). Dr. Sweeting laughed at the humor and received it appropriately, which is important for this tactic to successfully reduce potential tension

(Granek-Catarivas et al., 2005). She responded by giving Carrie and Steve an update on the treatment process, which is important for patients to feel involved in their care (Randall & Wearn, 2005).

TAKE-AWAYS

Because patients experience relational development with their doctor similarly to the way newcomers assimilate to the organization, there are some key organizational practices that will help facilitate a smooth termination of the relationship. It is important to keep in mind that cancer patients form relationships with their treatment teams out of necessity, so their encounter phase may be abrupt and intrusive. Practitioners must understand that these relationships are temporary and occur out of necessity, often against the will of the patient. Therefore, it is particularly important that patients feel welcomed and reassured of their uncertain situation. Engaging them in humorous discourse is one way to do this because it provides a less threatening avenue for information seeking and reduces the power distance between doctors and patients. In the same way that employees become more efficient and autonomous as they assimilate to the organization, patients become more proficient and adept at successfully engaging their doctor as they move toward exiting the relationship.

Metamorphosis in the organizational environment transforms employees into productive and self-sufficient individuals that have internalized the goals and values of the organization. Clear boundaries are established to help guide employees through this process. Similarly, practitioners should help guide patients through the transformative process of treatment, helping them accept their situation and work through it. That process should include a clear definition of roles, responsibilities, and co-constructed vision. It should also include the use of humor to provide patients with a channel for seeking information that is low risk and allows them to cope. Humor allows a patient to make light of their lack of knowledge in a way that preserves their reputation but also allows them to gather the missing information. Over time patients should become more independent and more comfortable with their doctor. Patients look to their physician to help guide them through their treatment and to establish their respective roles in the process. They also look to their physician for cues on the use of humor and the level of openness and disclosure in their relationship. Because of their expertise, medical professionals carry a disproportionate amount of power and can inadvertently discourage input and questions from patients. When patients are uncomfortable approaching their doctor, it can make it more difficult for them to bring up questions or concerns that they have. Using humor to forge a relationship with open communication and reduced tension helps alleviate the power structure and increase the patient's confidence in terminating the relationship when it is time for them to exit.

The imbalances of power in doctor-patient relationships must be negotiated through clear communication, just as they are in organizational relationships. Not all patients prefer or understand humor in the same way and those individual differences must be accommodated. The satisfaction of patients with their doctor is related to their satisfaction with their interactions, in the same way that satisfaction of newcomers to an organization relies on their communication satisfaction with superiors and coworkers. Physicians help set the tone of the relationship and how humor is used because of their superiority. Because doctors are especially prone to overestimate their communication abilities, and because patients and doctors might have different perceptions of appropriate humor, doctors must take particular care to ensure that they accommodate the communication and humor preferences of their patients. The power imbalance in the doctor-patient relationship makes it difficult for the patient to establish highly salient channels of communication or voice their preferences. If they are not careful, doctors might use humor that their patients do not understand or find inappropriate. Patients may be reluctant to correct their doctor or express their preferences, leading to greater dissatisfaction that they keep to themselves. Therefore, doctors must pay careful attention to the type of humor that their patients use and what they prefer. Even though the relationships between doctors and their patients are temporary, it is still important to accommodate their humor preferences so that everyone is on the same page.

Because humor is ambiguous and co-constructed, doctors and patients must take extra care to ensure they are on the same page when it is used between them. Humor is a tool that can help newcomers assimilate to the environment but, if used inappropriately, can deter them from feeling accepted. In the same way, patients can feel included or excluded from the treatment process depending on how humor is used. When discussing difficult or uncomfortable subjects, patients can use humor as a way to distance themselves, occasionally using humor that can be perceived as harsh. It is important for doctors to dissect why patients use humor so that they can further understand their intended meaning behind it. Additionally, engaging patients in their humor can encourage them to discuss the difficult subjects they are attempting to avoid, presenting it in a less threatening way. In the case of a terminal illness, humor can be used by patients as a way to regain control in a context where all their power has been stripped away. Again, it is important for medical professionals to understand their patient's use of humor and co-construct its meaning in their dialogue. When engaging patients with humor, medical staff must ensure that patients understand the humor, that it is appropriate, and that they appreciate it.

As with all organizational assimilation processes, the final phase requires the individual to exit. For healthcare patients, their exit should occur once they have finished their treatment and are no longer dependent on the relationship with their physician. The use of humor throughout the relationship allows the patient to feel more comfortable when approaching the exit phase. Using humor in the exit stage of the relationship as an information seeking tactic is particularly effective because it lowers the risk of offending the superior and reduces tension in the situation. Having already established humorous discourse as a relational norm increases the likelihood of a patient employing it in the exit phase. If a patient has not had an active role in their treatment decisions or has not been informed by their doctor of their updated condition it can be difficult for them to know whether they are approaching the exit stage or continuing to assimilate. Being stuck in an indefinite stage of metamorphosis can be frustrating to patients. Humor is an effective tool to bridge the gap between the frustration that they feel and the information they are trying to find out. Informing them of the process and what remains reduces uncertainty, increases trust, and establishes a common understanding of the end goal.

Based on these implications, we summarize by recommending that practitioners consider the following when interacting with their patients:

1. Use humor intentionally to break down power distances with patients and help them feel comfortable approaching you.
2. Look for cues from the patient that signal a willingness to participate and an appreciation for humor.
3. Play along and engage in the patient's use of humor.
4. When using humor to help assimilate the patient, be sure they are "in" on the joke.
5. Avoid using humor that could be demeaning, derogatory, or belittling to the patient.

REFERENCES

Adamson, M., Choi, K., Notaro, S., & Cotoc, C. (2018). The doctor-patient relationship and information-seeking behavior: Four orientations to cancer communication. *Journal of Palliative Care*, *33*(2), 79–87. doi:10.1177/0825859718759881 PMID:29514545

Beach, W. A., & Prickett, E. (2017). Laughter, humor, and cancer: Delicate moments and poignant interactional circumstances. *Health Communication*, *32*(7), 791–802. doi:10.1080/10410236.2016.1172291 PMID:27420294

Berger, J. T., Coulehan, J., & Belling, C. (2004). Humor in the physician-patient encounter. *Archives of Internal Medicine*, *164*(8), 825–830. doi:10.1001/archinte.164.8.825 PMID:15111367

Bisel, R. S., Messersmith, A. S., & Kelley, K. M. (2012). Supervisor-subordinate communication hierarchical mum effect meets organizational learning. *Journal of Business Communication*, *49*(2), 128–147. doi:10.1177/0021943612436972

Cody, W. K. (2003). Paternalism in nursing and healthcare: Central issues and their relation to theory. *Nursing Quebec*, *16*(4), 288–296. doi:10.1177/0894318403257170 PMID:14596114

Collins, R. F., Bekker, H. L., & Dodwell, D. J. (2004). Follow-up care of patients treated for breast cancer: A structured review. *Cancer Treatment Reviews*, *30*(1), 19–35. doi:10.1016/S0305-7372(03)00141-5 PMID:14766124

Deshields, T., Tibbs, T., Fan, M. Y., Bayer, L., Taylor, M., & Fisher, E. (2005). Ending treatment: The course of emotional adjustment and quality of life among breast cancer survivors immediately following radiation therapy. *Supportive Care in Cancer*, *13*(12), 1018–1026. doi:10.100700520-005-0801-z PMID:15800768

Fallowfield, L., & Jenkins, V. (2004). Communicating sad, bad, and difficult news in medicine. *Lancet*, *363*(9405), 312–319. doi:10.1016/S0140-6736(03)15392-5 PMID:14751707

Francis, L., Monahan, K., & Berger, C. (1999). A laughing matter? The uses of humor in medical interactions. *Motivation and Emotion*, *23*(2), 155–174. doi:10.1023/A:1021381129517

Goold, S. D., & Lipkin, M. Jr. (1999). The doctor-patient relationship: Challenges, opportunities, and strategies. *Journal of General Internal Medicine*, *14*(1), S26–S33. doi:10.1046/j.1525-1497.1999.00267.x PMID:9933492

Granek-Catarivas, M., Goldstein-Ferber, S., Azuri, Y., Vinker, S., & Kahan, E. (2005). Use of humour in primary care: Different perceptions among patients and physicians. *Postgraduate Medical Journal*, *81*(952), 126–130. doi:10.1136/pgmj.2004.019406 PMID:15701747

Grunloh, C., Myreteg, G., Cajander, A., & Rexhepi, H. (2018). "Why do they need to check me?" Patient participation through ehealth and the doctor-patient relationship: Qualitative study. *Journal of Medical Internet Research*, *20*(1), 1–14. doi:10.2196/jmir.8444 PMID:29335237

Hall, J. A., Roter, D. L., & Rand, C. S. (1981). Communication of affect between patient and physician. *Journal of Health and Social Behavior*, *22*(1), 18–30. doi:10.2307/2136365 PMID:7240703

Hayes-Bautista, D. E. (1976). Termination of the patient-practitioner relationship: Divorce, patient style. *Journal of Health and Social Behavior*, *17*(1), 12–21. doi:10.2307/2136463 PMID:1270781

Heiss, S. N., & Carmack, H. J. (2012). Knock, knock; Who's there? Making sense of organizational entrance through humor. *Management Communication Quarterly*, *26*(1), 106–132. doi:10.1177/0893318911414914

Hoerger, M., Epstein, R. M., Winters, P. C., Fiscella, K., Duberstein, P. R., Gramling, R., Butow, P. N., Mohile, S. G., Kaesber, P. R., Tang, W., Plumb, S., Walczak, A., Back, A. L., Tancredi, D., Venuti, A., Cipri, C., Escalera, G., Ferro, C., Gaudion, D., ... Kravitz, R. L. (2013). Values and options in cancer care (VOICE): Study design and rationale for a patient-centered communication and decision-making intervention for physicians, patients with advanced cancer, and their caregivers. *BMC Cancer*, *13*(188), 1–14. doi:10.1186/1471-2407-13-188 PMID:23570278

Jablin, F. M. (1982). Organizational communication: An assimilation approach. In M. E. Roloff & C. R. Berger (Eds.), *Social cognition and communication* (pp. 255–286). Sage Publications.

Jablin, F. M. (1987). Organizational entry, assimilation, and exit. In F. M. Jablin, L. L. Putnam, K. H. Roberts, & L. W. Porter (Eds.), *Handbook of organizational communication: An interdisciplinary perspective* (pp. 679–740). Sage Publications.

Johnson, P. (2002). The use of humor and its influences on spirituality and coping in breast cancer survivors. *Oncology Nursing Forum*, *29*(4), 691–695. doi:10.1188/02.ONF.691-695 PMID:12011915

Joshua, A. M., Cotroneo, A., & Clarke, S. (2005). Humor and oncology. *Journal of Clinical Oncology*, *23*(3), 645–648. doi:10.1200/JCO.2005.09.064 PMID:15659513

Knapp, M. L. (1978). *Social intercourse: From greeting to goodbye*. Allyn and Bacon.

Lynch, O. H. (2002). Humorous communication: Finding a place for humor in communication research. *Communication Theory*, *12*(4), 423–445. doi:10.1111/j.1468-2885.2002.tb00277.x

Platt, F. W., & Keating, K. N. (2007). Differences in physician and patient perceptions of uncomplicated UTI symptom severity: Understanding the communication gap. *International Journal of Clinical Practice*, *61*(2), 303–308. doi:10.1111/j.1742-1241.2006.01277.x PMID:17263717

Priego-Valverde, B. (2009). Failed humor in conversation. In N. R. Norrick & D. Chiaro (Eds.), *Humor in interaction* (pp. 165–186). John Bejamins Publishing Company. doi:10.1075/pbns.182.08pri

Randall, T. C., & Wearn, A. M. (2005). Receiving bad news: Patients with haematological cancer reflect upon their experience. *Palliative Medicine*, *19*(8), 594–601. doi:10.1191/0269216305pm1080oa PMID:16450876

Sastre, M. T. M., Sorum, P. C., & Mullet, E. (2011). Breaking bad news: The patient's viewpoint. *Health Communication*, *26*(7), 649–655. doi:10.1080/10410236.2011.561919 PMID:21598151

Scholl, J. C. (2007). The use of humor to promote patient-centered care. *Journal of Applied Communication Research*, *35*(2), 156–176. doi:10.1080/00909880701262658

Tremblay, M. (2017). Humor in teams: Multilevel relationships between humor climate, inclusion, trust, and citizenship behaviors. *Journal of Business and Psychology*, *32*(4), 363–378. doi:10.100710869-016-9445-x

Vandenberghe, C., Bentein, K., & Panaccio, A. (2017). Affective commitment to organizations and supervisors and turnover: A role theory perspective. *Journal of Management*, *43*(7), 2090–2117. doi:10.1177/0149206314559779

Wanzer, M., Booth-Butterfield, M., & Booth-Butterfield, S. (2006). "If we didn't use humor, we'd cry": Humorous coping communication in health care settings. *Journal of Health Communication*, *10*(2), 105–125. Advance online publication. doi:10.1080/10810730590915092 PMID:15804903

Chapter 33
"So, You're Not a Witch?"

Brigitte C. Fosque
Triad Essence Energy and Wellness, USA

R. W. Fosque
Triad Essence Energy and Wellness, USA

Brigitte C. Fosque (owner) and R. W. Fosque are healthcare providers of Triad Essence Energy & Wellness in Greensboro, NC. Triad Essence Energy & Wellness is an alternative medicine provider, primarily focusing on reiki and reflexology services. Reiki is a type of energy work in which a client's chi, or life force, is charged and their chakras are aligned. Reflexology is the application of pressure to specific trigger points in your hands and feet that correspond with the health of other internal body functions. Now, some of you may have just read those explanations and thought they sounded strange, implausible, or downright uncomfortable. This case is written about how humor works in that journey of skepticism to open-mindedness.

Brigitte and R. W. came to discover alternative healthcare with quite separate mindsets. Brigitte was a student of religion and spirituality in college, so when friends invited her to attend a reiki training course, she was very openminded and happy to go. R. W., however, with a background in civil engineering and drafting would have never considered going to such a class if Brigitte had not signed him up for the training without warning.

R. W. sat in his surprise reiki training class with no clue what was in store, a little apprehensive because Brigitte had promised that if he sat through just one class and hated it, he didn't have to go back, meaning there was a good chance he was going to hate whatever was coming. As the instructor began talking about laying healing hands on the sick to let healing energy flow into them, R. W. uncomfortably thought that his teacher had a Jesus complex. The instructor then began walking the class through a series of symbols that they were to draw in the air over clients before beginning their healing hands work. This seemed ridiculous to R. W., who began to suspect that he may have been signed up for a magic class as a joke. He was uncomfortable and very ready to leave, but he had promised Brigitte he would stay for all of one session. It was not until the very end of the evening when R. W. lost his skepticism. When the instructor asked him if he finally felt a shift in energy, R. W. had to chuckle and admit

DOI: 10.4018/978-1-7998-4528-7.ch033

that, "Yeah…I did." He had to laugh because he was out of reasons to resist, no matter how crazy it had all seen moments ago.

In the years since R. W. was introduced to reiki, it has certainly gained credibility as hospitals such as Johns Hopkins and Duke Health begin incorporating it into their integrated medicine recommended treatments and trainings (Duke Health, 2019a, 2019b; The Johns Hopkins Hospital, n.d.). Yet, the idea of energy work, pressure points, or any form of alternative medicine can still be met with doubt, skepticism, and resistance by many. That reluctance to accept potential treatments is perhaps what traditional and alternative medicine have most in common as a practice. It's that moment when a patient/client is told what the healthcare practitioner wants them to do for the sake of their own health and the discomfort that follows which require the same treatments. This suggestion from a traditional medicine practitioner may sound painful or burdensome while the suggestion from the nontraditional medicine practitioner may sound strange or uncomfortable. Here, it is the job of the healthcare practitioner to find the source of the discomfort in order to get the client to accept the treatment. They will know they have found and addressed the discomfort when they get the chuckle. It was no coincidence that when R. W. lost his skepticism that he chuckled; that is the normal reaction to acceptance in such cases.

Hannah Gadsby (2018) explains that humor is actually the relief of tension. She posits that a master comedian knows how to build tension and discomfort and then release it at just the right moment to receive a laugh. That moment when the discomfort is relieved is when people will naturally begin laughing. That is the moment healthcare providers are searching for in the journey to get patients to accept their treatment plan. That moment when the tension is released, they smile, and they can begin to accept a new possibility.

Most of Brigitte and R. W.'s new clientele comes from recommendations. That does not mean that all new clients come in with open minds though. Doing alternative medicine, specifically energy work, in the Southern U.S., Brigitte and R. W. are met with much skepticism, especially from the deeply religious community. New patients are prone to asking questions such as:

1. Is this witchcraft?
2. Is this Satanic?
3. Does this conflict with religious beliefs?

In fact, a new client who was a pastor once asked R. W. if he believed that the source of reiki was "a Satanic underworld type of source." The answer to all of the above questions is, of course, *no*. That simple "no" is enough for many new clients. For others though, accepting alternative medicine treatment is an involved process that requires a lot of Q&A. Having watched R. W.'s own journey through skepticism, Brigitte and R. W. know that it is not their job to convince a new patient, but rather to patiently answer questions without creating any pressure until the client has run out of reasons not to try. They know that the patient is out of reasons to resist when they see the chuckle. That chuckle is the indication that the client is open to treatment.

Although Brigitte and R. W.'s primary tactic is patient listening, they have also decorated their office to put their patient's most frequent concern at ease: a perceived disconnect between energy work and Christianity. The walls of their office are adorned with Bible verses. The doorways have Christian crosses hanging above them. This is a nonverbal message to the clientele that reiki, though certainly not traditional medical practice, does not conflict with Christian beliefs, but also that the practitioners likely hold the same religious beliefs as these patients in the Southern U.S. Typically, when new clients notice these artifacts, there is a visible relaxation, especially in their posture.

Overall though, the humor comes in to play waiting for that chuckle. Most new patients do not believe that reiki or reflexology is a real treatment when they first come to the clinic. The chuckle represents that the internal war is over, and the client has convinced themselves that they are going to move forward with treatment, no matter how crazy they may rationalize it being. You may imagine it being similar to the moment when someone convinces themselves to jump out of a plane for the first time. They may still think the idea is nuts, and they're laughing at the ridiculousness of their own behavior, but nonetheless they are ready to give it a try.

REFERENCES

Duke Health. (2019a). *Reiki: Level one*. Available at: https://dukeintegrativemedicine.org/programs-training/professionals/reiki-level-one/

Duke Health. (2019b). *Reiki: Level two*. Available at: https://dukeintegrativemedicine.org/programs-training/professionals/reiki-level-two/

Gadsby, H. (Writer), & Olb, J. & Parry, M. (Directors), & Bruzzese, F. (Prod.). (2018). Nanette [Netflix Special]. Los Gatos, CA: Netflix.

The Johns Hopkins Hospital. (n.d.). *Reiki*. Available at: https://www.hopkinsmedicine.org/integrative_medicine_digestive_center/services/reiki.html

ADDITIONAL READING

Armstrong, M., Flemming, K., Kupeli, N., Stone, P., Wilkinson, S., & Candy, B. (2019). Aromatherapy, massage and reflexology: A systematic review and thematic synthesis of the perspectives from people with palliative care needs. *Palliative Medicine*, *33*(7), 757–769. doi:10.1177/0269216319846440 PMID:31060455

Baldwin, A. L., Vitale, A., Brownell, E., Kryak, E., & Rand, W. (2017). Effects of reiki on pain, anxiety, and blood pressure in patients undergoing knee replacement: A pilot study. *Holistic Nursing Practice*, *31*(2), 80–89. doi:10.1097/HNP.0000000000000195 PMID:28181973

Joyce, J., & Herbison, G. P. (2015). Reiki for depression and anxiety. *Cochrane Database of Systematic Reviews*. Advance online publication. doi:10.1002/14651858.CD006833.pub2 PMID:25835541

McVicar, A., Greenwood, C., Ellis, C., & LeForis, C. (2016). Influence of study design on outcomes following reflexology massage: An integrative and critical review of interventional studies. *Journal of the Australian Traditional-Medicine Society*, *22*(9), 237–239. doi:10.1089/acm.2016.0015 PMID:27463943

Smith, C. A., Levett, K. M., Collins, C. T., Dahlen, H. G., Ee, C. C., & Suganuma, M. (2018). Massage, reflexology and other manual methods for pain management in labour. *Cochrane Database of Systematic Reviews*, *3*. Advance online publication. doi:10.1002/14651858.CD009290.pub3 PMID:29589380

Thrane, S. E., Maurer, S. H., Ren, D., Danford, C. A., & Cohen, S. M. (2017). Reiki therapy for symptom management in children receiving palliative care: A pilot study. *The American Journal of Hospice & Palliative Care*, *34*(4), 373–379. doi:10.1177/1049909116630973 PMID:26858170

Chapter 34
Response: "'So, You're Not a Witch?'"

Michelle Epstein Garland
University of South Carolina Upstate, USA

REVIEW OF RELEVANT LITERATURE

Humor in health contexts can take many shapes and forms, can be effective or ineffective, and can serve as a stand-alone tool or a tool related to other perceptions and behaviors. For the above case study, we see humor used as a tool and as an outcome, though predominantly an outcome. What this means is that particular concepts and theoretical frameworks serve as the communication behaviors enacted in hopes of achieving the outcome of humor. This is likely vastly different in perspective than the use of humor in the other case studies included throughout this text. The concepts and theoretical frameworks most relevant to this case study are uncertainty management, social judgment theory, and listening. Throughout this response, the concepts and frameworks will be defined and explained from a research and literature standpoint, and they will be applied to the case study presented. Finally, implications and guidance for the use of humor in reiki, reflexology, or other alternative medicine will be provided.

Humor

Humor in health contexts is typically centered on the use of humor in developing and maintaining the provider-patient interpersonal relationship (e.g., Tanto-Beck, 1997). From an interpersonal standpoint, humor can aid in building a number of interpersonal-related variables, such as trust, satisfaction, rapport and the like. Moreover, humor can reduce interpersonal tensions, as can be expected when experiencing or being introduced to reiki, reflexology, or other alternative medicines for the first time. In this case, humor is typically used to diffuse tensions in uncertain situations. As described here, and likely as you see in responses throughout this book, humor can precede a number of interpersonal outcomes as well as serve as an intermediary between humor and those outcomes. For example, humor could lead to practitioner-patient relational satisfaction or practitioner-patient disclosure could lead to humor which

DOI: 10.4018/978-1-7998-4528-7.ch034

could lead to trust. In this case study, however, humor is seen as an outcome itself, which will be further discussed in the application section.

Despite the majority of health-related humor research being centered on the role of provider or practitioner humor, Sala et al. (2002) found that patients used humor to a greater degree than practitioners. While humor can be used for many reasons, Schöpf et al. (2017) identified categories of humor use. The category most relevant to this case study is relationship-protecting humor. Such humor is used to "deal with situations that cause negative emotions such as embarrassment, anxiety, or discomfort," (p. 380). This parallels the findings of Lefcourt and Martin (1986) who identified humor as a coping strategy or defense mechanism.

This case study is centered on health outside of traditional medicine and is seen as interweaving spirituality. While humor has not often been explored in conjunctions with spirituality and health, Carson (1989) clearly aligns health, spirituality and humor. "Humor is transcendent – it momentarily removes one from an isolated personal state to join in surprise at the ludicrous situations of human beings," (p. 198). It is arguable that the patients or clients, when engaging with reiki, reflexology, or other alternative medicine for the first time, may in fact find the situation itself ludicrous.

Uncertainty Management

Uncertainty Reduction Theory (URT), first posed by Berger and Calabrese in 1975 is a theoretical framework that explains the process of reducing uncertainty in new relationships. Since that time, the framework has been utilized across a variety of interpersonal communication contexts. At the core of URT are key concepts of verbal communication, nonverbal warmth, self-disclosure, reciprocity, information seeking, similarity, liking, and shared networks:

- Verbal communication refers to the verbal messages delivered. In a health setting, this could be content messages about what to do during a session, such as take a deep breath or close your eyes, or messages about session follow-up or what should be done at home.
- Nonverbal warmth refers to the messages delivered through gestures, body movement, facial expression, eye contact and the like that encourage connection. In a health setting, this could be direct eye contact when the patient or client is talking, to indicate active listening, or leaning forward while the patient or client is talking, to indicate interest.
- Self-disclosure refers to sharing personal information with another, while reciprocity refers to the sharing of personal information between parties similar in quality and quantity. For example, this could be the provider or practitioner talking about what they did over the weekend and the client or patient responding with their weekend activities.
- Information seeking refers to processes used to gather information. While information seeking can take a number of forms, which will be discussed later, an example would be a patient or client asking for information about medication side effects or clarity regarding treatment options.
- Similarity refers to perceived commonalities between parties. For example, a provider or practitioner may put the patient or client at ease by sharing personal experience with a similar ailment or health challenge.
- Liking refers to feelings of preference, esteem, or approval. In a health context, providers or practitioners are often seen as more likeable when they are relatable and genuine. Shared networks refers to common acquaintances or personal/professional connections. For example, in a health

context, shared networks may be the referral doctor or friends that are also patients of the provider or practitioner.

The URT theoretical framework explains how each of these concepts are correlated with, or related to, reducing uncertainty. Generally speaking, as verbal communication, nonverbal warmth, self-disclosure, reciprocity, information seeking, similarity, liking, and/or shared networks increase, uncertainty decreases.

Four strategies are central to the information seeking process of uncertainty reduction (Berger, 1979, 1987): passive, active, interactive, and extractive.

- The passive process refers to seeking information through listening or watching the communicative interactions of others.
- The active process refers to seeking information through questioning, or otherwise gathering information from, a third party.
- The interactive process refers to seeking information through direct communicative interaction.
- The extractive process, which was added to the strategies later (Ramirez et al., 2002), refers to seeking information through online sources.

Consider the following hypothetical scenario: Alex is struggling with migraines. Alex has done some online research not only about the migraines but also trying to find the best provider, looking at reviews and researching the provider's background and experience (extractive). When arriving for the initial appointment, Alex watches how the care professionals interact with other clients (passive) and asks those in the waiting room about their experiences with the provider (active). Finally, Alex is called back and is able to interact with the provider in person (interactive). Through these processes, Alex is able to reduce uncertainty about the provider, the clinic, and the treatment, which will impact how effective the provider is with providing Alex the best treatment.

Social Judgment Theory

Social Judgment Theory (SJT), first proposed by Sherif (1936), is a theoretical framework of influence for exploring the perceptions one makes when presented with a persuasive message; does it align with what the person already believes or not? Within SJT are concepts of latitudes of acceptance, latitudes of noncommitment, and latitudes of rejection. The latitudes of acceptance include arguments or positions with which the person agrees or considers worthy of consideration. The latitudes of noncommitment include arguments or positions with which the person is either indifferent or unsure of where they stand. The latitudes of rejection include arguments or positions with which the person disagrees or considers unreasonable. Additionally, SJT identifies the anchor, which is the place in which the person currently stands on the latitudes spectrum based on the information given. In the healthcare context, the practitioner or provider seeks to communicate in a way that moves the anchor into the latitudes of acceptance, or if it is already in that latitude, keep it there. The strategies for communication regarding anchor movement are varied and complex. However, it is important for the provider or practitioner to try to determine where the anchor of the patient or client resides in order to determine the extent to which persuasive messages are needed.

How does this relate to humor? Consider the following scenario: Riley is dealing with extreme stress. A close friend has told Riley about reiki. Riley is skeptical about the practice but decides to go by the facility for more information. In speaking with the practitioner, Riley opens up about feelings of doubt and discomfort as Riley is unsure if reiki aligns with or contradicts Riley's religious beliefs. The practitioner recognizes that reiki falls within Riley's latitude of noncommitment, and the practitioner knows that any response given could move Riley's anchor toward the latitude of rejection or the latitude of acceptance. To ease the discomfort and open communication about how reiki might align with Riley's religious beliefs, the practitioner decides to use humor as an influence strategy. By using humor, the practitioner is able to build rapport with Riley and move the anchor toward the latitude of acceptance and resulting in an appointment.

Listening

Listening, particularly active listening, is a key component of competent and effective communication in any context. Listening, when enacted effectively, can minimize miscommunication. While many models for listening exist, the HURIER model of listening (Brownell, 1985) is widely used and application in the health context. HURIER stands for hearing, understanding, remembering, interpreting, evaluating and responding. *Hearing* typically refers to the passive, physiological process of capturing sound stimuli. However, for the HURIER model, hearing goes a step further to highlight the importance of focusing and concentrating on that stimuli. Second, the listener should *understand* the stimuli, which means the listener should decode what is being heard. Communication scholars loosely define decoding as the receiver's role of attaching meaning to the message that has been received. Third, the listener should work to *remember*, which means the "what" has been heard should be retained. It is in retaining the message that the listener is able to act on what has been heard. Fourth, the listener should *interpret*, which means the listener should not only consider what has been heard but also the context of the message. Who said it? In what environment? With what tone? These are just a few of many questions that should be asked when a listener is interpreting a message. In this stage, the listener is trying to determine any underlying meaning or assumptions that may impact the interpretation of the message. Fifth, the listener should *evaluate* what has been heard, understood, remembered, and interpreted. In this stage, the listener is critically analyzing and making judgments about the message, which means evaluating not only the verbal content but also the relational content of the message, the relationship between the communicators and the like. Finally, the listener should *respond*, or provide feedback. This stage is left out of many listening models but is arguably the most telling stage of listening. It is through feedback, or responding, that the original speaker can determine in the message sent was accurately communicated. Feedback can be verbal or nonverbal, intentional or unintentional. At its core, feedback is any discernible response from a receiver. In the health context, with the patient or client as the speaker, feedback will indicate to the provider or practitioner whether or not the patient or client understands the diagnosis, treatment options, next steps, etc. Without such feedback, assumptions of understanding and effective communication are made, and in the health context, such assumptions can be life threatening.

APPLICATION

Throughout the case study, we see terms such as "ridiculous," "a joke," "crazy," and "nuts" when describing original patient perceptions of reiki or reflexology treatment. In each of these cases, a natural response would be a laugh, or chuckle. However, instead of seeing the chuckle as a sign of "skepticism" or "internal war," which the case authors acknowledge the patients or clients often experience, the chuckle is seen as "release of tension" or sign of acceptance. It is likely that such conclusions are drawn from nonverbal indicators, such as relaxing of posture or shoulders; relaxing of jaw muscles; a deep, slow release of breath; unclenching of hands; uncrossing of arms; just to name a few. It is the combination of the chuckle and nonverbal indicators that likely lead to the conclusion of release of tension or sign of acceptance.

In following the chronology of the case narrative, additional applications are found. First, in the narrative of R. W. and his view of reiki, we see that his anchor was originally in the latitude of rejection, but by the end of the class, his anchor had moved to the borderline between latitude of noncommitment and latitude of acceptance. The case study reads, "he was out of reasons to resist." We do not know from the narrative exactly what was said in the class to move his anchor, but we know his anchor did in fact move. As the case study authors later state, "it is the job of the healthcare practitioner to find the source of the discomfort in order to get the client to accept the treatment." For the authors, they feel they have achieved their goal when they get the chuckle.

Second, the case study authors state that most of their "new clientele comes from recommendations." This indicates an element of shared networks, which falls under the umbrella of uncertainty management. Because current clients are sharing their experiences with others, the other manages uncertainty through shared networks. In this way the current client connects the new client with the practitioner and reduces uncertainty in the process. By doing so, such a client is likely closer to the "chuckle" than a client without the shared network because their uncertainty has not been managed to the same degree.

Third, the authors describe a communication interaction that would align with the Sherif's (1936) work on Social Judgement Theory. They state it is the job of the practitioner "to patiently answer questions without creating any pressure until the client has run out of reasons not to try." It is important to note, however, that this may not occur in the first session. Depending on the placement of the anchor upon first engagement, as well as individual characteristics, the time and effort it will take to get to "the chuckle" will vary.

Fourth, as stated in the case study, "Brigitte and R. W.'s primary tactic [for reducing patient anxiety and uncertainty] is patient listening." What they are likely referring to is the HURIER model process. The practitioner must *hear* what the patient of client is saying, *understand* the needs and concerns of the patient and client, *remember* these needs and concerns while *interpreting* the assumptions that undergird the concerns, *evaluate* the best approaches to addressing the concerns and assumptions, and then *respond* in a way that indicates care, concern, value, and support. Listening is needed by the practitioner to best reduce the uncertainty and anxiety of the patient or client, again, to bring them closer to "the chuckle."

Finally, the authors describe the office as decorated to put the patient at ease – Christian crosses on the doorways and Bible verses adorning the office. The artifacts can serve as a source of nonverbal warmth as well as serve as a tool to reduce uncertainty and anxiety for patients or clients, specifically in regard to challenges to belief systems. These indicate to the patient or client an element of similarity, for those who are Christians. Nonverbal warmth, again, encourages connection, as per uncertainty management. For Christians patients or clients, seeing symbols that are familiar and central to their beliefs put them at ease. The messages, through the artifacts, signal that the patient or client is in a safe place that recognizes and appreciates their belief systems. Such messages can bring the patient closer to "the chuckle," as the authors note the visible relaxation of the patients.

ADVICE TO PRACTITIONERS

Laughter, which the authors describe as "the chuckle," can be an indicator of humor. However, providers should be cautious when interpreting a laugh, or chuckle. As Martin (2008) points out, while laughter can be an involuntary response of amusement, it can also be faked. Moreover, a laugh is not always a sign of amusement or some other positive emotion. For some, a laugh can be a defense mechanism in an awkward or uncertain situation or a sign of ill intent. So, while the chuckle can be an indicator of acceptance, as indicated by the case study authors, context clues such as facial expression, gestures, body movement, eye contact, and the like should not be ignored when interpreting meaning. For example, if the patient or client chuckles but is sitting with arms crossed over the chest and avoiding direct eye contact, it is likely that the chuckle is indicating something other than acceptance or approval. More likely, in this case, the chuckle would signal nervousness or skepticism. The nonverbals will help the practitioner or provider determine if there is an underlying serious message that is being covered up or disguised by the patient or client.

To take it a step further, the case study describes humor, or "the chuckle," as "the relief of tension" and "the indication that the client is open to treatment." While "the chuckle" can be an indicator, it does not stand alone as an indicator of such outcomes. Healthcare providers must be cognizant of the fact that listening goes beyond interpretation of a message sender's words. The interpretation phase of the HURIER model includes factoring the meaning placed on words by tone of voice, body posture, facial expression, and any other nonverbal cues a person might offer. In this case, the healthcare provider described the use of these active listening skills to interpret "the chuckle," but healthcare providers should be vigilant to always listen to their patients holistically. For example, if a patient says that they "understand" the information provided to them about their health, but their nonverbal behaviors indicate confusion, it is the healthcare provider's job to note the confusion beyond the words and address it with communication strategies such as providing additional information, providing reassurance, or affirming the patient's role in treatment and decision making.

Nonverbal communication also includes the artifacts that adorn the treatment facility such as the Christian décor in this case. While creating similarity leads to positive results, a few words of warning are needed. Likely, not all patients or clients will be Christians, so artifacts indicating acceptance of other faiths and belief systems should not be excluded. Additionally, if the message of the treatment center is that the energy or other alternative medicine work is spiritual but not religious, such symbols of religion may be contradictory. It is important to evaluate the costs and benefits of each artifact chosen for the treatment center. Healthcare providers must be aware of their patient group and design a meeting space that will put them at ease. For example, a pediatrician should have an office designed as much as possible to be a place that a child feels secure and at home in, to signal to them that this is not a place to be afraid of. Toys, cartoons, candy, and fun photos would be artifacts that a pediatrician could use the way these case authors have used their Christian artifacts.

Perhaps the most notable takeaway for healthcare professionals in this case is their role in moving patients on the latitude of acceptance. Reducing, or managing, uncertainty should be a main goal of any practitioner. "Reducing uncertainty to an acceptable level is necessary for smooth, coordinated, and understandable interactions to occur and for individuals to have a sense of control over their environment and outcomes" (Goldsmith, 2001, p. 515). The goal in healthcare is to have the patient or client comply. Patient compliance refers to "the extent to which a person's behavior (in terms of taking medications, following diets, or executing life style changes) coincides with medical or health advice" (Haynes et al., 1979, pp. 1-2). One reason for non-compliance, as found by Becker and Rosenstock (1984), is the patient's perception of whether or not the treatment will be effective. By reducing uncertainty, the perception toward acceptance can begin to be shifted, moving the anchor toward latitude of acceptance.

If the treatment or approach already lies within the latitude of acceptance, few persuasive messages will be needed. If the treatment or approach lies within the latitudes of rejection, it will be important to determine how important the issue is to the client or patient. If it is important, the patient or client will have larger latitudes of rejection, and therefore will require significantly more persuasion. The goal will be to present messages that move the anchor toward the latitude of acceptance in steps, aiming for a position just within the latitude of acceptance. Large jumps toward acceptance are unrealistic and the attempt may cause the patient or client to fall deeper into latitudes of rejection. Based on the work of Sherif and colleagues (1965), the messages that are the most persuasive are those most discrepant from the anchor of the patient but still fall within the patient's latitude of acceptance or noncommitment. In this task of moving patients down the latitude of acceptance, humor should be considered when developing persuasive messages as humor can play an integral role in successful persuasion when created with the audience and environment in mind. Humor can help to build rapport and trust between providers and patients (Tanto-Beck, 1997), which helps nudge patients towards acceptance of providers' messages.

Taken together, humor has a place in reiki, reflexology, or other alternative medicine. It is a tool for creating and maintaining interpersonal relationships, and, in this case, an outcome of interpersonal interaction and intrapersonal changes. However, the chuckle, like most everything in human communication, can have many meanings. Therefore, practitioners should consider contextual factors and additional communication concepts and frameworks when making sense of their interactions with patients or clients. A chuckle can be more than just a chuckle.

REFERENCES

Becker, M. H., & Rosenstock, I. M. (1984). Compliance with medical advice. In A. Steptoe & A. Matthews (Eds.), *Health care and human behavior* (pp. 175–208). Academic Press.

Berger, C. R. (1979). Beyond initial interaction: Uncertainty, understanding, and the development of interpersonal relationships. In H. Giles & R. N. St. Clair (Eds.), *Language and sociology* (pp. 122–144). Basil-Blackwell.

Berger, C. R. (1987). Communicating under uncertainty. In M. E. Roloff & G. R. Miller (Eds.), *Interpersonal processes* (pp. 39–62). Sage.

Berger, C. R., & Calabrese, R. J. (1974). Some explorations in initial interaction and beyond: Toward a developmental theory of interpersonal communication. *Human Communication Research, 1*(2), 99–112. doi:10.1111/j.1468-2958.1975.tb00258.x

Brashers, D. E. (2001). Communication and uncertainty management. *Journal of Communication, 51*(3), 477–497. doi:10.1111/j.1460-2466.2001.tb02892.x

Brownell, J. (1985). A model for listening instruction: Management applications. *The ABCA Bulletin, 48*(3), 39–44. doi:10.1177/108056998504800312

Carson, V. B. (1989). *Spiritual dimensions of nursing practice*. Saunders.

Goldsmith, D. J. (2001). A normative approach to the study of uncertainty and communication. *Journal of Communication, 51*(3), 514–533. doi:10.1111/j.1460-2466.2001.tb02894.x

Haynes, R. B., Taylor, D. W., & Sackett, D. L. (1979). *Compliance in health care*. John Hopkins University Press.

Lefcourt, H. M., & Martin, R. A. (1986). *Humor and life stress: Antidote to adversity*. SpringerVerlag. doi:10.1007/978-1-4612-4900-9

Martin, R. A. (2008). Humor and health. In V. Raskin (Ed.), *The primer of humor research* (pp. 479–521). Mouton de Gruyter. doi:10.1515/9783110198492.479

Ramirez, A. Jr, Walther, J. B., Burgoon, J. K., & Sunnafrank, M. (2002). Information-seeking strategies, uncertainty, and computer-mediated communication: Toward a conceptual model. *Human Communication Research, 28*(2), 213–228. doi:10.1111/j.1468-2958.2002.tb00804.x

Sala, F., Krupat, E., & Roter, D. (2002). Satisfaction and the use of humor by physicians and patients. *Psychology & Health, 17*(3), 269–280. doi:10.1080/08870440290029520

Schöpf, A. C., Martin, G. S., & Keating, M. A. (2017). Humor as a communication strategy in provider-patient communication in a chronic care setting. *Qualitative Health Research, 27*(3), 374–390. doi:10.1177/1049732315620773 PMID:26717942

Sherif, C. W., Sherif, M., & Nebergall, R. E. (1965). *Attitudes and attitude change: The social judgment-involvement approach*. W. B. Saunders.

Sherif, M. (1936). *The psychology of social norms*. Harper.

Tanto-Beck, W. (1997). Humor in nursing practice: A phenomenological study. *International Journal of Nursing Studies, 34*(5), 346–352. doi:10.1016/S0020-7489(97)00026-6 PMID:9559383

Chapter 35
"I Have Abs!?"

Jennifer Thompson
Kernersville VA Clinic, USA

If anyone had told me when I was 18 years old that I would ultimately become a Registered Nurse, I admit I would not have believed it. Nursing was never on my radar. So, when what initially started as a passing idea (a small blip) became my career of choice (the radar screen in vivid technicolor showing a direct hit), I had no idea what was in store. Namely, that I would learn more from evaluating the symptoms of my friends and family members than I ever would from my actual patients. This sometimes causes problems in that my ability to control my amusement at certain questions and situations fall way short of the mark. Thankfully, some of those friends and family members have the ability to not only share in my amusement but to embrace it when it is discovered that what is thought to be a life-threatening medical concern is anything but.

It was a normal day that included a normal phone call with the person I would consider my best friend. In the course of the conversation, she indicated that she had an upcoming doctor's appointment that she was a little nervous about. When I asked why, she told me that she had noticed a "hard lump" on her stomach. It wasn't painful, necessarily, just there, and she thought she had noticed it growing slightly over the course of a few weeks. So, as a matter of concern, she made an appointment to have it "checked out."

There is some background information that must be explained before continuing with this story. Firstly, she has a history of some back concerns, namely a fairly moderate-to-severe case of scoliosis. She treats this by taking part in yoga, structural therapy, and regular massages. Medication is used only as a last resort and, for obvious reasons, in preparation for air travel. Secondly, at the time of this story, she had had 27 benign tumors removed over the last 11 years, with the largest being 0.9 cm in diameter. This lump was much larger, stretching across her entire abdomen under her ribs. The fact that she had informed me of the upcoming doctor's appointment BEFORE actually going was somewhat of a red flag for me. In her desire to not alarm me, I usually find out about medical appointments AFTER they have already taken place. Finally, she has always been very "in tune" with her body; thus, stating that she was "nervous" for the upcoming appointment indicated yet another cause for concern.

DOI: 10.4018/978-1-7998-4528-7.ch035

So, as the concerned friend that I am, I immediately drove the mile to her home to check out this "lump" that had appeared and was causing my friend such distress. Putting the proverbial nursing cap on and trying to set aside my own feelings of anxiety, I began to perform a modified nursing assessment. Questions began to flow in my quest for information. I asked all of the typical nursing questions: "Does it hurt? Does it affect your movement? Does it change with movement? Have you had a fever? Have you been nauseous, plagued with vomiting, constipation, or diarrhea?" The answer to these was always "no," so this provided some small piece of comfort.

The next part of the assessment was, in retrospect, quite humorous. My friend and I are huggers; that is how we greet each other and say goodbye. However, it is there that physical contact usually stops. Being the touchy-feely type of friends is never something we have been accused of. So, having received negative answers to my questions thus far, I deemed it time to perform a small, focused, hands-on assessment. Placing my hand on the general area of her concern while she was laying down, I didn't feel anything out of the ordinary. Honestly, I could not palpate a lump of any sort. So, I had her stand up with straight posture, and had yet to feel anything at all. I achieved the same result when I had her bend at the waist and straighten.

After my little mini-assessment, I informed her that I could not find anything that I would deem a "lump." Needless to say, this caused some concern on both of our parts. She took my hand and said, "it's right there!" By this time, I had a very curious suspicion that was working its way to the forefront of my consciousness. I told her to put my hand where she knew the "lump" to be, which she did, and then asked here to bend over again. When she had done so, I removed my hand and placed hers on the offending area and asked her to bend again, which she did. She confirmed that she could feel the "lump" as she was standing straight but it disappeared as she bent over. At this point, I began to become amused. When questioned, I took great delight in informing my friend that what she was feeling was, in fact, her abdominal muscle. She had developed "abs!"

Of course, her initial response to this was disbelief and doubt, and I do believe the phrase "no way!" was expelled from her very academic lips (she does have a PhD). After discussion regarding the fact that she did not indulge in strenuous exercise of ANY sort, I brought up the fact that she does, in fact, participate in stretching and yoga on a regular basis. For her, the benefit of the discipline was not limited to increasing the flexibility of her back but also in the strength and prominence of her abdominal muscles. Since she had never had "abs" before, she did not recognize that what she thought was a "lump" was actually an incredibly well-defined muscle.

I don't think I could have shocked her more if I had told her that an atomic bomb had gone off in her living room. Much laughter followed from both of us.

Looking back, this should be a lesson to everyone. Humor and laughter are extremely powerful weapons in a human being's arsenal. They have the ability to both comfort and soothe, and to change the mental status of a person almost immediately. In the world of health and medical care, the ability to laugh and stay positive is an invaluable trait. I challenge anyone who thinks differently to spend a day seeing patients in the shadow of a nurse in a doctor's office or hospital and then attempt to devalue the benefit of humor and/or laughter in a medical setting. The operative word in that sentence was "attempt."

Chapter 36
Response: "'I Have Abs!?'"

Laura E. Miller
The University of Tennessee, USA

THEORETICAL CONSIDERATIONS

Though laughter and health (and, in particular, poor health) may not always be conceptualized simultaneously, they are connected in significant ways. A great deal of literature on how individuals cope with stress has emerged in recent decades. Stress and uncertainty have become norms in everyday living. From health scares, to neighborhood crime, to natural disasters, to financial crises, to global pandemics, to everything in between, the management of stress has emerged as a salient topic for people in all walks of life. As Jen Lancaster notes in her recent (and hilariously written) book, *Welcome to the United States of Anxiety* (2020):

Despite all indicators pointing people toward happiness and contentment, so many of us are paralyzed by angst and weighted down with unnamed dread, largely because we've been conditioned to believe that danger lurks around every corner. (pg. 13)

As a result, and as an attempt to provide recommendations for stress management, various theoretical models shedding light on individuals' patterns of coping and resilience have been developed (Holahan et al., 1996). Each perspective considers the strategies and actions people engage in when faced with a major life stressor.

Stress and Coping Theories

Lazarus and Folkman's (1984) theory of stress and coping has made a significant contribution to the literature on coping with stressors. According to Lazarus and Folkman (1984, 1991), coping is what an individual does cognitively and behaviorally to manage stressful demands (Folkman et al., 1986). Stress, according to this theory, is an interaction between the demands placed on an individual and the availability of his or her coping resources. Not surprisingly, then, variation in coping exists, due in part to individuals' appraisals of a stressor. According to Lazarus and Folkman (1984):

DOI: 10.4018/978-1-7998-4528-7.ch036

Although certain environmental demands and pressures produce stress in substantial numbers of people, individual and group differences in the degree and kind of reaction are always evident. People and groups differ in their sensitivity and vulnerability to certain types of events, as well as in their interpretations and reactions. (p. 22)

Under this framework, the coping process can be described as the behavioral and cognitive efforts to deal with stressors. Such coping strategies have been classified as either problem-focused or emotion-focused (Lazarus & Folkman, 1984). Problem-focused coping confronts the problem, emphasizing what can be done to minimize stress. Emotion-focused coping involves the regulation of emotional distress. Behaviorally, individuals may attempt to actively cope with a stressor (e.g., approach coping). Cognitively, individuals may distance, detach, escape, or avoid information in order to distract themselves from the stressor (e.g., avoidance coping).

According to this theorizing, appraisals and coping influence one's emotional response to life stressors (i.e., finding a lump). Thus, coping can be a way to manage demands, and stressors may be appraised and interpreted differently by different people (Folkman & Lazarus, 1988; Lazarus & Folkman, 1984). For example, individuals may assess a stressor by the harm at stake (primary appraisal; the lump could be malignant) and the availability, and adequacy, of coping resources (secondary appraisal; available social support from a friend who also happens to be an RN). As a result, coping efforts vary from individual to individual, in part, because individuals' reactions to stressors vary. This exact same sentence is in the paragraph below that starts with "For example." It should be removed here, as it is out of place.

A great deal of research on coping focuses on individuals' perspectives, overlooking the interdependence of coping efforts (Goldsmith, 2009). More recent literature, however, has expanded this approach to consider how stress and coping is managed together by close relational partners (Lyons et al., 1998; Revenson et al., 2005). As Afifi et al. (2006) note, "Family members respond and adapt to stress based on their interactions with other family members" (p. 383). Thus, an additional theoretical approach emphasizing the social nature of stress and coping is presented next.

Communal Coping

The interpersonal and health literatures demonstrate that people cope in relationships, and a theoretical approach highlighting this interdependence is communal coping. Introduced by Lyons et al. (1998), communal coping involves "group problem-solving efforts" (p. 583). Although the notion of communal coping can occur with couples, it also extends beyond the dyad to include large community and social units. As such, individuals in close relationships, families, and communities communally cope when they experience, and manage, a stressor together. Thus, communal coping involves the perception of stressors as *our* problems. For example, the RN thinking that *my best friend's tumor affects my life, too, and is our problem,* exemplifies communal coping. Instead of a purely individualistic orientation to coping, in which strategies are initiated to manage individual well-being, relational approaches to coping reflect strategies used to minimize *others'* stress (Coyne & Fiske, 1992). In other words, theorizing on communal coping suggests that individuals cope in ways they perceive to be adaptive not only for their own needs, but also for their partner's needs. Research generally posits that taking a communal perspective improves relational functioning when a partner is ill (Coyne & Smith, 1991; Kayser et al., 1999). That is, according to Acitelli and Badr (2005), couples who appraise the illness as something they will manage *together* are more satisfied with their relationship rather than couples who adopt a more individualistic approach.

Theories of relationship-focused coping, such as communal coping (see also dyadic coping; Revenson et al., 2005) recognize that one partner's stress and coping affects the other. In this sense, one's partner and relationship may simultaneously be a source of support and stress. Responding to, and attempting to manage, a partner's stress places demands on one's own emotional and behavioral resources. Coyne and Smith (1991) refer to this process of interdependent coping as "grappling with each other's presence and emotional needs" (p. 405); this description highlights the possibility that relationships may be a source of both comfort and distress. Such dynamics also may be at play in the current case.

For example, it is possible that the patient does not typically tell the RN about her doctor's appointments because she does not feel emotionally capable of managing how her friend would cope with that information. It is also possible that the patient is hoping to shield the RN (who likely experiences frequent health-related stressors due to the nature of her job) from additional anxiety. Both possible scenarios might prompt the patient to engage in avoidant-focused coping behaviors, such as not disclosing doctor's appointments until after they have passed. As such, the patient illustrates that coping decisions (e.g., avoidant or approach coping) are made based on the perceived needs of the individual *and* their close relational partners. The following paragraphs delineate another set of theories aimed at exploring individuals' coping efforts through uncertainty reduction and management.

Uncertainty Theories

Uncertainty is a common human experience (Berger & Calabrese, 1975) and can arise because of individuals' inability to foresee the future and explain the past (Berger & Bradac, 1982). People also may be uncertain because they perceive a need for more information (Brashers, 2001); thus, more information often decreases uncertainty. Uncertainty also may stem from too much information (Brashers et al., 2002). For example, gaining inconsistent information can heighten uncertainty and add complexity to decision-making processes (Babrow et al., 1998). Uncertainty can also exist when individuals experience ambiguous, inconsistent, complex, or unpredictable events (Berger & Bradac, 1982). Given that the context of healthcare is highly ambiguous and unpredictable, health-related conversations and experiences are often fraught with uncertainty.

According to Berger and Bradac (1982), there are at least two kinds of uncertainty that can be discerned in interactional events. First, cognitive uncertainty refers to individuals' ambiguity about their own, and others' beliefs. For example, the patient in the current case study may question what her friend is thinking as she performs the body scan. Second, behavioral uncertainty concerns the predictability of individuals' own, and others' behaviors. For instance, the same patient described above may question what she should ask her friend in relation to the apparent lump. Thus, uncertainty exists when explanatory and predictive information about themselves and others is lacking. Previous research has adopted various assumptions of uncertainty; such assumptions have been developed by theorists interested in exploring nuanced experiences of uncertainty. Each of the relevant theories are presented and described in the following paragraphs.

Uncertainty Reduction Theory

Many researchers have viewed uncertainty from the perspective of uncertainty reduction theory (URT; Berger & Calabrese, 1975). A major assumption of uncertainty reduction theory is that people are driven to reduce uncertainty about themselves and others; thus, they are motivated to communicate in order to reduce their uncertainty. That is, this perspective views uncertainty as an unpleasant state that can be reduced through communication and information seeking. Originally applied to initial interactions and developing relationships, URT has more recently been applied to more established relationships (Parks & Adelman, 1983) and organizational contexts (Kramer, 2004).

Uncertainty Management Theory

Other scholars have adopted the assumptions of uncertainty management theory (Brashers, 2001). This framework challenges the previous assumption that uncertainty always produces anxiety, asserting that uncertainty experiences vary from person to person. Brashers argued that,

Although people quite often do want to reduce complexity and ambiguity in their lives, perhaps as a prerequisite to decision making, planning, or predicting the behavior of others, there are other times when uncertainty allows people to maintain hope and optimism or when tasks can be performed despite, or because of, uncertainty. (p. 478)

Thus, according to the theory, uncertainty can be negative, but is not uniformly appraised negatively. For example, maintaining or increasing uncertainty can preserve a patient's psychological well-being if certainty about a prognosis is likely to produce distress. Through this lens, uncertainty can be appraised as a resource contributing to the survival or management of a variety of situations, including health-related stressors.

Social Support Theories

An additional coping model is that of social support. A great deal of research has explored how social support can help people cope with stress (Sarason et al., 1990). This body of research has linked social support to a variety of positive effects, including physical health, psychological well-being, and social functioning (Elal-Lawrence & Celikoglu, 1995; Wortman, 1984). More specifically, social support has been linked to more positive adjustment to a variety of stressors, including chronic illness within the family (Revenson et al., 2005), death of a loved one (Parkes, 1972), divorce (Cobb, 1976), and employment termination (Cobb, 1974). Furthermore, social support may improve physical health, through a reduction in stress and increased compliance with medical recommendations (Bauer et al., 2017).

Scholars studying social support have distinguished two types of social support: enacted support and perceived support (Sarason et al., 1990). Enacted social support has been defined as "what individuals say and do to help one another" (Goldsmith, 2004, p. 13), whereas perceived support has been defined as "the perception that support generally is (or would be) available when needed" (Goldsmith, 2004, p. 14). Examples of enacted social support in the context of healthcare include offering advice related to a diagnosis (informational support), delivering food to a patient's home (tangible support), and showing empathy about prolonged diagnostic symptoms (emotional support; Goldsmith, 2004). Emotional support has often been associated with positive outcomes for patients (Nipp et al., 2016), such as improved coping and self-esteem during times of stress.

Conceptualizing Humor As A Coping Strategy

Taken together, each of the aforementioned theories highlight the importance of stress and uncertainty management, particularly in the context of health. People inevitably face a myriad of health challenges throughout their lifetimes (whether it be a personal health crisis or that of a loved one), and learning facilitative management strategies becomes even more important with age. The literature also points to an additional means of coping that has been related to positive outcomes: humor. Specifically, patients, loved ones, and healthcare providers alike have described health-related humor as a coping outlet. In his review piece, Bennett (2003) describes humor in health contexts "as a means of narrowing interpersonal gaps, communicating caring, and relieving anxiety associated with medical care" (p. 1258).

Research similarly suggests that people who use humor as a coping strategy have lower levels of distress (Bennett, 2003), overall greater life satisfaction (Booth-Butterfield et al., 2014), and more social support (DuPre, 1998). Health-related humor can relieve tension and allows people to 'let off steam' in otherwise challenging circumstances. For example, one couple in Miller's (2009) study described how they coined a humorous phrase that helped them cope with cancer:

In fact, we had a fun little saying – 'Oh, just go to Lowe's, get a ladder and get over it.' And every time we would say that to each other, we would just start laughing, and it was kind of like, poof, it would just dissipate everything – it was kind of a good thing. (p. 121)

Similarly, young adult cancer survivors in Iannarino's (2018) study described using humor as a blogging strategy to facilitate coping. Such strategies aimed to promote camaraderie among fellow patients ("I started it…as a way to reach people in the same boat and hopefully let them know that they have a shipmate. Aye, Aye, mateys!"; pg. 1238) and to cope with taxing treatment regimens ("Imagine being stuck in a tube with aliens bombing it from the outside and robots screaming in your ear for an hour"; pg. 1238). Humor is also a useful strategy for healthcare providers: high humor-oriented providers report more coping efficacy (Booth-Butterfield & Booth-Butterfield, 1991) and fewer malpractice claims (Levinson et al., 1997). Intersecting conceptualizations of both coping and humor, the previously cited literature draws clear connections between the facilitative role humor may have on healthcare and illness-related conversations. The following paragraphs practically apply this work to the case study at hand.

PRACTICAL CONSIDERATIONS

Literature on coping, uncertainty, social support, and humor can easily be applied to real-world health contexts. Indeed, Beach and Prickett (2017) argue that many poignant cancer-related coping and support situations are managed through the use of humor and laughter. More relevantly, humor appeared to help the characters in the case cope with the uncertainty surrounding the apparent lump. Delineated below are specific applications of the three aforementioned bodies of theoretical work (stress and coping, uncertainty, and social support) to the current case.

Application of Stress and Coping Theories

The current patient case offers a clear example of *approach-focused coping,* which was previously defined as behaviors aimed at actively coping with the stressor. In this sense, the patient finds the lump and actively engages in behaviors to confront the problem (i.e., makes a medical appointment and seeks out the RN for an informal check-up). The case also indicates, however, that she does not usually reach out to her friend before medical appointments, which shows that she may engage in *avoidant-focused coping* under some circumstances. This behavioral fluctuation aligns with Lazarus and Folkman's (1984) theorizing in that one's coping preferences may fluctuate across the lifespan, across disease stage, and across various medical circumstances.

As previously mentioned, the patient in the current case may also have engaged in *avoidant-focused coping* to protect her friend (the RN) from the uncertainty associated with her tumors. Often, as Brashers and colleagues (2002) theorize, avoiding information can be an uncertainty management strategy – sometimes people may avoid information to manage their own uncertainty, other times people may avoid information because they perceive it will manage others' uncertainty (e.g., to protect close relational partners from worrying about the health stressor). In some cases, however, such avoidance may be ineffective, particularly when relational partners have mismatched preferences for information (or avoidance).

For example, some participants in Miller's (2014a) dyadic study described the inherent challenge relational partners face in negotiating coping styles and communicative preferences. In that study, one wife described this relational dilemma: "I wish he would open up…But I've tried to give him chances where he could…I think I would feel a lot more comfortable with it if I could talk to him about a lot of things" (p. 916). Her husband, on the other hand, described the motivation behind his avoidant coping: "I mean, part of being supportive was not to show fear or great concern over what she was gonna go through because she was having a little bit of a problem dealing with it herself. So it was useless to – would have been no help for her had I shown any fear or grave concern" (p. 917). In this example, the husband's avoidant-focused coping created more anxiety for his wife. Similar to these quotes, it is possible that in the current case, the patient's avoidant-focused coping may in fact increase the RN's anxiety. Indeed, the RN mentions the patient's protective motivations: "In her desire to not alarm me, I usually find out about medical appointments AFTER they have already taken place." Thus, the current case and aforementioned examples demonstrate that coping preferences (e.g., *avoidant* or *approach coping*) do not always align and that these discrepancies can create relational dilemmas, such as increased anxiety for one or both parties.

In addition to employing theoretically relevant coping strategies, the case study patient also mirrors Lazarus and Folkman's (1984) appraisal process. To illustrate, the patient emotionally responds to a health stressor (finding an ambiguous lump). She then assesses the stressor by its potential for harm (*primary appraisal*; a malignancy). She also may assess the stressor through a *secondary appraisal,* or through the lens of the social support available to her. Due to the availability of a best friend, who also happens to be an RN, she may cope better than a patient whose secondary appraisal reveals no available support networks.

Application of Uncertainty Theories

An in-depth analysis of the case brings the characters' uncertainty reduction and management strategies to the surface. Take, for example, the patient's behavior related to her illness uncertainty: she has a history of having benign tumors removed, so she has had ample time to hone her uncertainty management skills. Specifically, she has a pattern of telling her friend (the RN) about medical appointments AFTER they occur. This is clearly an effort to manage her own and/or her friend's uncertainty. Research suggests that the *avoidance* of certain conversations can be a way to manage one's own, and others', uncertainty about challenging topics (Miller, 2014b). Thus, the patient's historical choice to avoid such interactions until after she is certain about her diagnostic results demonstrates an avoidant uncertainty *management* strategy. Conversely, by choosing to seek medical information and counsel from her friend the RN, she is utilizing an uncertainty *reduction* strategy, possibly thinking to herself, "I am more nervous about this lump than I have been with the previous 27 lumps, and I would like more information to reduce my anxiety."

Just as the patient employed theories of uncertainty throughout the case, the RN also made strategic attempts to reduce her uncertainty. Based on the ambiguity of the lump, the RN chose to engage in a classic uncertainty reduction tactic: information seeking. She drove to her friend's house and performed a modified nursing assessment. When the answers to her initial assessment were inconclusive, she chose to continue her quest for uncertainty reduction by engaging in a hands-on assessment. Ultimately, it was through this assessment that the lump (abs!) was discovered. In this case, the RN's information seeking efforts paid off by reducing her own, and her friend's, health-related uncertainty.

Application of Social Support Theories

Lastly, the case study at hand highlights various types of social support and its relevant relational and coping outcomes. After appraising her situation and determining her need for support, the patient illustrates the importance of *perceived support*: support that is perceived to be available when needed. The patient perceived that her friend, the RN, would be a source of available support and that she was accurate in this perception given that her friend indeed showed up at her doorstep. Moreover, the RN demonstrates numerous examples of *enacted support*. Namely, she provided information related to the patient's lump and health status (*informational support*), drove to her house to perform an informal bodily assessment (*tangible support*), and joined the patient in a good laugh about the surprising discovery of abs (*emotional support*). Just as the social support literature suggests, the perceived and enacted support in this case facilitated the patient's (and the RN's) ability to cope with the health stressor.

HEALTHCARE CONSIDERATIONS

The current case and the related literature offer important implications for healthcare providers. Specifically, the case describes humor as an "invaluable trait" when it comes to health-related conversations. Yet, many communication scholars recommend against the usage of universal advice that is meant to encompass all types of people, in all circumstances (Goldsmith et al., 2008). Thus, healthcare providers will want to carefully assess the patient's situation and all related interactional variables prior to the use of humor in medical settings. Normative recommendations (c.f., Goldsmith, 2004) for engaging in humor within the healthcare setting, in other words, what works for most people, most of the time, are delineated below.

RECOMMENDATIONS RELATED TO MULTIPLE GOALS

People often experience multiple interactional goals, and it is important to understand the ways communication can help (or hinder) one's accomplishment of such purposes. Normative recommendations seek to explain how interactants can best achieve satisfying outcomes, and goals greatly influence interactional effectiveness. Theories of multiple goals (Dillard, 1990) suggest that conversational goals such as relationship (i.e., "how close is our relationship?"), identity, (i.e., "who are we to each other?"), and task (i.e., "what tangible goal are we hoping to accomplish?") influence the receipt and interpretation of messages. Relevant to the case at hand, it is likely that such conversational goals impacted both characters' perceptions of humor in the given context. In the current case, the character's realization that "I have abs!" was a positive one that was met with relief and laughter. Healthcare providers should consider, however, that humor may not be as welcome a distraction when/if the task goal of a conversation is to disclose the malignancy of a lump. Additionally, how might the specifics of the case (and its associated conversational goals) shift if the patient was no longer considered to be a best friend, but rather a stranger (i.e., relational goal)? In these altered scenarios, the specific goals and message features (such as the tone of the conversation, the specific language choices, the timing of the message, etc.) all may influence the appropriateness of the humor response.

Moreover, not all attempts at social support are perceived as supportive, and the same could be said for humor. In the current case, the RN was providing support to her friend; however, this enacted support may not be perceived as supportive by a patient with whom she had no prior relationship. The RN mentions that she often interacts with her friends and family about health-related issues, showing that she likely has a plethora of experience joking around with close relational partners, but possibly not in the traditional patient context. Thus, goals, dyadic contexts, and relational histories influence the way humor messages will be perceived and interpreted. A normative approach (Goldsmith, 2004) would recommend that healthcare providers reflect on the multiple goals threaded throughout their interactions in order to assess the appropriateness of humor messages in various contexts and with different patients.

Recommendations Related To Message Features

As previously discussed, adaptive coping, uncertainty management efforts, and support preferences vary based on individual and context. The case explicitly states that, "Humor and laughter are extremely powerful weapons in a human being's arsenal. They have the ability to both comfort and soothe, and to change the mental status of a person almost immediately." Yet, a normative approach (Goldsmith, 2004) would suggest that there are better and worse ways to engage in any communicative behavior (including humor). Moreover, understanding multiple, conflicting meanings can broaden our understanding of why well-intentioned communicative behavior is sometimes perceived in undesirable ways (Goldsmith, 2004). It goes without saying that what is perceived as humorous to one person may be perceived as insensitive to another. What is interpreted as lighthearted by some, might inadvertently increase uncertainty in others. Indeed, not all participants in Bethea et al.'s (2000) study found humor to be a useful way to convey their family caregiving experience. Therefore, healthcare providers would be prudent to attend to the specific message features that may make humor more (or less) effective.

Exploring specific communicative styles shows that message features, or how one goes about communicating, can make a difference and broadens our knowledge of better and worse ways to use humor (or not). A normative perspective would argue that different ways of talking may be more or less related to desirable outcomes. Some message features also may be better at achieving multiple interactional goals, such as conveying concern for a partner, while achieving tasks such as emotional support and uncertainty management. Other features may be more or less satisfying depending on the couple and the conditions under which talk occurred (i.e., such as the timing of the conversation). In terms of case at hand, The RN waited to use humor until she was certain of the benign nature of the lump. It is possible, for example, that if she led the conversation with humor, the patient may not have deemed it as welcoming. This message feature points to the conditional functionality of humor: if certain conditions are met, humor may be more satisfying. The literature, then, would suggest that humor may be effective in some healthcare settings, under some circumstances; and providers should consider features such as *when* humor is occurring to offer initial normative recommendations.

CONCLUSION

Coping, uncertainty, stress, and emotions may all be words that come to mind when we conceptualize health. However, as Wanzer et al. (2005) argue, we can learn how to manage such distress by adopting facilitative strategies:

We cannot avoid all aversive situations. We often make our living in environments filled with distress-producing stimuli. The critical feature then becomes how we are able to use communication to cope with those stressors and remain reasonably productive and happy. Effectively encoded and communicated humor appears to be a positive strategy both socially and in task settings. (p. 105)

In addition, we can begin to consider normative perspectives, which assert that there are better and worse ways of communicating humor in healthcare settings. If, when engaging in humorous communication, healthcare providers are able to focus on (a) what was said (the message itself), (b) how it was said (the message features), (c) and under what conditions it was said (the conversational goals), we can start to better understand why some attempts at humor are more effective than others. Analyzed through broad coping theories, the current case study provides important recommendations for communicating humor in medical settings. Taken together, the literature and the specifics of the case are consistent with normative approaches and demonstrate that attending to multiple goals and message features may be a more satisfying (and appropriately humorous!) way to communicate.

REFERENCES

Acitelli, L. K., & Badr, H. J. (2005). My illness or our illness? Attending to the relationship when one partner is ill. In T. A. Revenson, K. Kayser, & G. Bodenmann (Eds.), *Couples coping with stress: Emerging perspectives on dyadic coping* (pp. 121–156). American Psychological Association. doi:10.1037/11031-006

Afifi, T. D., Hutchinson, S., & Krouse, S. (2006). Toward a theoretical model of communal coping in postdivorce families and other naturally occurring groups. *Communication Theory*, *16*(3), 378–409. doi:10.1111/j.1468-2885.2006.00275.x

Babrow, A. S., Kasch, C. R., & Ford, L. A. (1998). The many meanings of uncertainty in illness: Toward a systematic accounting. *Health Communication, 10*(1), 1–23. doi:10.120715327027hc1001_1 PMID:16370987

Bauer, M., Lee, S., Tossone, K., Lazebnik, R., & Lazebnik, N. (2017). Patterns of social support and compliance with ultrasound study in teen pregnancy. *Journal of Pediatric and Adolescent Gynecology, 30*(2), 299–331. doi:10.1016/j.jpag.2017.03.113

Beach, W. A., & Prickett, E. (2017). Laugher, humor, and cancer: Delicate moments and poignant interactional circumstances. *Health Communication, 32*(32), 791–802. doi:10.1080/10410236.2016.1172291 PMID:27420294

Bennett, H. J. (2003). Humor in medicine. *Southern Medical Journal, 96*(12), 1257–1261. doi:10.1097/01.SMJ.0000066657.70073.14 PMID:14696878

Berger, C. R., & Bradac, J. J. (1982). *Language and social knowledge: Uncertainty in interpersonal relationships*. Arnold.

Berger, C. R., & Calabrese, R. J. (1975). Some explorations in initial interaction and beyond: Toward a developmental theory of interpersonal communication. *Human Communication Research, 1*(2), 99–112. doi:10.1111/j.1468-2958.1975.tb00258.x

Bethea, L. S., Travis, S. S., & Pecchioni, L. (2000). Family caregivers' use of humor in conveying information about dependent older adults. *Health Communication, 12*(4), 361–376. doi:10.1207/S15327027HC1204_3 PMID:11063286

Booth-Butterfield, M., Wanzer, M. B., Weil, N., & Krezmien, E. (2014). Communication of humor during bereavement: Intrapersonal and interpersonal emotion management strategies. *Communication Quarterly, 62*(4), 436–454. doi:10.1080/01463373.2014.922487

Booth-Butterfield, S., & Booth-Butterfield, M. (1991). Individual differences in the communication of humorous messages. *The Southern Communication Journal, 56*(3), 32–40. doi:10.1080/10417949109372831

Brashers, D. E. (2001). Communication and uncertainty management. *Journal of Communication, 51*(3), 477–498. doi:10.1111/j.1460-2466.2001.tb02892.x

Brashers, D. E., Goldsmith, D. J., & Hsieh, E. (2002). Information seeking and avoiding in health contexts. *Human Communication Research, 28*(2), 258–271. doi:10.1111/j.1468-2958.2002.tb00807.x

Cobb, S. (1974). Physiological changes in men whose jobs were abolished. *Journal of Psychosomatic Research, 18*(4), 245–258. doi:10.1016/0022-3999(74)90005-1 PMID:4459457

Cobb, S. (1976). Social support as a moderator of life stress. *Psychosomatic Medicine, 38*(5), 300–314. doi:10.1097/00006842-197609000-00003 PMID:981490

Coyne, J. C., & Fiske, V. (1992). Couples coping with chronic illness and catastrophic illness. In A. P. Stephens & J. Crowther (Eds.), *Family health psychology* (pp. 129–149). Hemisphere. doi:10.4324/9781315800837-9

Coyne, J. C., & Smith, D. A. F. (1991). Couples coping with a myocardial infarction: A contextual perspective on wives' distress. *Journal of Personality and Social Psychology*, *61*(3), 404–412. doi:10.1037/0022-3514.61.3.404 PMID:1941511

Dillard, J. P. (1990). A goal-driven model of interpersonal influence. In J. P. Dillard (Ed.), *Seeking compliance: The production of interpersonal influence messages* (pp. 41–56). Gorsuch Scarisbrick.

DuPre, A. (1998). *Humor and the healing arts: A multimethod analysis of humor use in health care*. Erlbaum.

Elal-Lawrence, G., & Celikoglu, P. (1995). Social support and psychological well-being in breast cancer patients. *Health & Social Care in the Community*, *3*(1), 1–7. doi:10.1111/j.1365-2524.1995.tb00001.x

Folkman, S., & Lazarus, R. S. (1988). Coping as a mediator or emotion. *Journal of Personality and Social Psychology*, *54*(3), 466–475. doi:10.1037/0022-3514.54.3.466 PMID:3361419

Folkman, S., Lazarus, R. S., Dunkel-Schetter, C., DeLongis, A., & Gruen, R. J. (1986). Dynamics of a stressful encounter: Cognitive appraisal, coping, and encounter outcomes. *Journal of Personality and Social Psychology*, *50*(5), 992–1003. doi:10.1037/0022-3514.50.5.992 PMID:3712234

Goldsmith, D. J. (2004). *Communicating social support*. Cambridge University Press. doi:10.1017/CBO9780511606984

Goldsmith, D. J. (2009). Uncertainty and communication in couples coping with serious illness. In T. D. Afifi & W. A. Afifi (Eds.), *Uncertainty, information management, and disclosure decisions: Theories and applications* (pp. 203–225). Routledge.

Goldsmith, D. J., Miller, L. E., & Caughlin, J. P. (2008). Openness and avoidance in couples communicating about cancer. *Communication Yearbook*, *31*(1), 62–115. doi:10.1080/23808985.2007.11679065

Holahan, C. J., Moos, R. H., & Schaefer, J. A. (1996). Coping, stress resistance, and growth: Conceptualizing adaptive functioning. In M. Zeidner & N. S. Endler (Eds.), *Handbook of Coping: Theory, research, applications* (pp. 24–43). Wiley.

Iannarino, N. T. (2018). "My insides feel like Keith Richards' face": A narrative analysis of humor and biographical disruption in young adults' cancer blogs. *Health Communication*, *33*(10), 1233–1242. doi:10.1080/10410236.2017.1350909 PMID:28825504

Kayser, K., Sormanti, M. E., & Strainchamps, E. (1999). Women coping with cancer: The influence of relationship factors on psychosocial adjustment. *Psychology of Women Quarterly*, *23*(4), 725–739. doi:10.1111/j.1471-6402.1999.tb00394.x

Kramer, M. (2004). *Managing uncertainty in organizational communication*. Erlbaum.

Lancaster, J. (2020). *Welcome to the United States of anxiety: Observations from a reforming neurotic*. Little A.

Lazarus, R. S., & Folkman, S. (1984). *Stress, appraisal, and coping*. Springer.

Lazarus, R. S., & Folkman, S. (1991). The concept of coping. In A. Monat & R. S. Lazarus (Eds.), *Stress and coping: An anthology* (pp. 189–206). Columbia University Press.

Levinson, W., Roter, D., Mullooly, J., Dull, V., & Frankel, R. (1997). Physician-patient communication: The relationship with malpractice claims among primary care physicians and surgeons. *Journal of the American Medical Association, 277*(7), 533–559. doi:10.1001/jama.1997.03540310051034 PMID:9032162

Lyons, R. F., Mickelson, K. D., Sullivan, M. J. L., & Coyne, J. C. (1998). Coping as a communal process. *Journal of Social and Personal Relationships, 15*(5), 579–605. doi:10.1177/0265407598155001

Miller, L. E. (2009). *Cancer survivorship: Couples' communication and adjustment after treatment is complete* [Doctoral Dissertation, University of Illinois at Urbana-Champaign]. IDEALS Dissertation Publishing. http://hdl.handle.net/2142/87548

Miller, L. E. (2014a). Communication dilemmas in the context of cancer: Survivors' and partners' strategies for communicating throughout survivorship. *Issues in Mental Health Nursing, 35*(12), 914–923. doi:10.3109/01612840.2014.934939 PMID:25426747

Miller, L. E. (2014b). Uncertainty and information seeking in cancer survivorship. *Health Communication, 29*(3), 233–243. doi:10.1080/10410236.2012.739949 PMID:23682727

Nipp, R. D., El-Jawahri, A., Fishbeing, J. N., Eusebio, J., Stagl, J. M., Gallagher, E. R., Park, E. R., Jackson, V. A., Pirl, W. F., Greer, J. A., & Temel, J. S. (2016). The relationship between coping strategies, quality of life, and mood in patients with incurable cancer. *Cancer, 122*(13), 2110–2116. doi:10.1002/cncr.30025 PMID:27089045

Parkes, C. M. (1972). *Bereavement: Studies of grief in adult life.* International Universities Press.

Parks, M. R., & Adelman, M. B. (1983). Communication networks and the development of romantic relationships: An expansion of uncertainty reduction theory. *Human Communication Research, 10*(1), 85–107. doi:10.1111/j.1468-2958.1983.tb00004.x

Revenson, T. A., Kayser, K., & Bodenmann, G. (2005). Introduction. In T. A. Revenson, K. Kayser, & G. Bodenmann (Eds.), *Couples coping with stress: Emerging perspectives on dyadic coping* (pp. 3–10). American Psychological Association. doi:10.1037/11031-000

Sarason, B. R., Sarason, I. G., & Pierce, G. R. (1990). Traditional views of social support and their impact on assessment. In B. R. Sarason, I. G. Sarason, & G. R. Pierce (Eds.), *Social support: An interactional view* (pp. 9–25). Wiley.

Wanzer, M., Booth-Butterfield, M., & Booth-Butterfield, S. (2005). "If we didn't use humor, we'd cry": Humorous coping communication in health care settings. *Journal of Health Communication, 10*(2), 105–125. doi:10.1080/10810730590915092 PMID:15804903

Wortman, C. B. (1984). Social support and the cancer patient: Conceptual issues and methodological issues. *Cancer, 53*(10), 2339–2360. doi:10.1002/cncr.1984.53.s10.2339 PMID:6367944

Chapter 37
Four-Thirty on a Friday

Shana Ratner
University of North Carolina at Chapel Hill, USA

My first time seeing Ms. S was also my second day on the faculty as a general internist. As we built our bond, I helped her manage her medical problems and worked with her to stay healthy. We worked on her heart, and she quit smoking. We kept her updated with screenings. She waited for me during my 3-month maternity leave after I had my second child.

One day, she came in for a routine follow-up visit. It happened to be 4:30 on a Friday, the end of a packed day and week. I had been zooming around all day—not unusual for a busy primary care provider, academic, and mom of two kids under 3-years-old.

I began to talk with her as I usually did about her care: “Any questions or concerns you have today? How have you been doing with your medication? How is your family?” She went to answer, but then paused and looked at me quizzically. “Doctor, have you had a hard day?” she asked with a glint in her eye. I asked myself, “How does she know?” I thought I was doing a good job of being present and listening. I wondered what was conveying my frazzle.

“Look down,” she laughed.

When I looked down, I saw what she saw: On my feet were two black shoes. However, on my feet were two VERY different black shoes. The left shoe was black with a silver, square buckle. The right shoe was black with brass interlacing circles.

The two of us began to laugh and laugh. I don’t remember if she or I said it first, but we exclaimed, “Mama got dressed in the dark!”

I left that appointment with a smile on my face, refreshed despite a hard and busy week. I walked over to the nurses’ station and showed my team nurse my feet. She looked down, paused, and began to howl with laughter, tears streaming down her face.

Ms. S. was getting older. She came to see me more frequently to help manage her medical conditions. When I asked her each time how she was, she told me what was new, and then she would proceed to say, “Ok, let’s see your shoes.” “Ok. Let’s see your earrings.” And finally, “How are your babies?”

DOI: 10.4018/978-1-7998-4528-7.ch037

If I passed the test of matching shoes and earrings, we could then proceed to work together on her health goals. She took a few steps forward and a few steps back. Neither of us was perfect, but we were doing our best.

As she aged, she began to bring more family members to the visit for support. She would introduce each new family member to me by telling them the story of that day. If I came in with a medical student or resident, which I often did, she would make sure that they knew exactly why she was asking her doctor to see her shoes. I can't count the number of times we shared this story. Sometimes, she would tell it. Sometimes, I would tell it. Each new introduction brought a retelling. We would bond, laugh, and connect again.

A few years later, we found that she had developed cancer. This situation was certainly no laughing matter. She started chemotherapy. When she had a question about chemotherapy, she would call my office to ask my opinion before ringing her oncologist. When she was hospitalized for complications of chemotherapy, I would sit by her hospital bed. Her family greeted me warmly. Usually, she knew who I was. Sometimes, she did not. I sat there and held her hand and told her I would continue to be there for her. If she was not alert enough to check my shoes, her daughters did it for her.

After too many hospitalizations and the continued growth of her cancer, she came to me to talk. She wanted to really talk. Before we discussed the reason for her visit, we went through our dance, the checking, the laughter, the reminiscing.

Then, she told me that she did not want to do chemotherapy anymore and was ready for hospice care. She wanted to dance. She wanted to spend time with her grandchildren and great-grandchildren. She did not want to spend her time in the hospital. We made a plan for hospice care. We hugged. We cried.

She started that visit with our story. We laughed before we cried. We were doctor and patient but, more importantly, we were two imperfect individuals sitting together doing our best.

Chapter 38
Response: "Four-Thirty on a Friday"

Michael J. Hoppmann
Northeastern University, USA

Carey Noland
Northeastern University, USA

INTRODUCTION AND THEORY

Introduction

Famed medical author and surgeon Atul Gawande often shares his opinion of what would make medicine, an endeavor in which failure is "so easy, so effortless" (Gawande, 2007, p.4) better. He aptly identifies many of the challenges providers encounter: daunting expectations, the need to cope with illness and allow people to "lead a life as long and free of frailty as science will allow" (p. 5). The amount of information medical professions must learn is both vast and incomplete, their profession rife with uncertainty and ambiguity. The expectation is that they do their work "humanely, with gentleness and concern" (p. 5). It is no wonder those in the medical profession suffer from burnout, fatigue and depression. It would be easy to become pessimistic, jaded, and disconnected. Not only do patients expect perfection from medical providers, but physicians hold similarly high standards for themselves and their colleagues: almost all new resident physicians expect that they will never make a medical mistake during the course of their long career (Noland & Carl, 2006), yet most do. A study found that 84.3% of medical doctors in England made a medical mistake, with devastating results for both patient and provider. The providers experienced increases in stress, anxiety, sleep disturbance, and lower professional confidence. Most became anxious about the potential for future errors. Society holds physicians to a high standard of perfection, both professionally and physically. There is no room for error in medicine.

DOI: 10.4018/978-1-7998-4528-7.ch038

Dress to Impress

The high standards we hold physicians to include their personal appearance. Professional appearance is of the utmost importance. A highly publicized study found that what medical doctors wear may matter more than what doctors (and even patients) might think (Petrilli et al., 2018). In this study, just over half of the 4,062 patients surveyed in the clinics and hospitals of 10 major medical centers said that what physicians wear is important to them — and more than one-third said it influences their satisfaction with their care. They rated the providers on how knowledgeable, trustworthy, caring and approachable the physician appeared, and how comfortable the attire made the patient feel. The majority of respondents favored formal attire with a white coat, followed by scrubs with a white coat, and formal attire without a white coat.

Achieving a professional appearance is taught in medical school and supervised closely during physician's internships and residential training. What physicians wear is important to patients, influencing not only their satisfaction with their doctor, but their perceptions of competence.

Being a Doctor is Stressful

Job satisfaction is defined as "a pleasurable or positive emotional state from the appraisal of one's job or job experiences" (Locke, 1976, p. 1304). There are three main appraisals that people make when evaluating their jobs: cognitive (evaluative), affective (or emotional), and behavioral (Hulin & Judge, 2003). Sadly, most doctors report low levels of job satisfaction and happiness with their work. In Sandeep Jauhar's "Doctored," he reports that only 6 percent of doctors are happy with their jobs and they commit suicide at twice the rate of the general population. Over half are unsure they would recommend the practice of medicine to young people. More concerning than a lack of happiness is physician burnout. Burnout is a prolonged response to chronic emotional and interpersonal stressors on the job. It is defined by the three dimensions of exhaustion, cynicism, and inefficacy (Maslach, 2001). According to the Centers for Disease Control and Prevention (2008), a significant correlation exists between exposure to occupational stressors and the onset of various physical, emotional, and mental health problems—all of which can affect quality of life, provider productivity, quality of interpersonal communication, and may lead to professional burnout. Keidel (2016) views burnout as a syndrome that includes physical exhaustion, a negative job attitude and negative self-concept, and a general loss of concern for patients or clients. The provider who is experiencing burnout may feel more tired than usual and low in personal energy.

Benign Violations as the Essence of Using Humor

Attempts to understand what makes human communication funny are about as old as the study of rhetoric and poetry itself. And since humor is so central to successful persuasive communication, it comes as no surprise that many of the greatest thinkers in the history of rhetoric (such as Aristotle, Cicero, Quintilian and Campbell) also feature prominently in the theory of humor. Traditional humor models have tended to emphasize one of three aspects as central to making people laugh: 1) A feeling of superiority over others, 2) A perception of incongruence in what is said and done, 3) or the creation of relief and escape from an uncomfortable situation (Morreall, 2020). These so-call superiority, incongruence and relief theories of humor are certainly not without merit, but each of them has serious shortcomings. In this analysis we will concentrate on one of the most recent humor models instead, the so-called Benign Violation

Theory (BVT). The BVT originates in the work of Veatch (1998). Veatch claims that for a situation to be perceived as humorous, there must be 1) a violation of a subjective moral principle, which 2) does not threaten the overall normality of the situation, and 3) the violation and the normality must be perceived simultaneously. McGraw and colleagues slightly modify these conditions and postulate that humor is created by 1) a violation of a norm, that 2) is judged as benign, and 3) both conditions are perceived simultaneously. This benign violation theory, which has been extensively tested in a variety of settings (McGraw & Warren, 2010; McGraw et al., 2012; Warren & McGraw, 2016) has a high explanatory power when it comes to humorous communication. It shows why some people laugh about what others do not find funny (differences in subjective valuations of norms) and it explains how humor can fail when it is too tame (no perceived violation), when it is too aggressive (violation not perceived as benign), and even when it is too complicated (violation and benignity not perceived simultaneously). Finally, it allows for the inclusion of a variety of dimensions of emotional distance that allow us to distinguish between levels of subjective benignity, which describe what makes statements funny. As prime candidate for this last task we have previously suggested Campbell's (1963) Seven Circumstances: probability, plausibility, importance, proximity of time, connection of place, relation to the persons concerned, and interest in the consequences (Noland & Hoppmann, 2020). Looking through the lens of the BVT and these dimensions will be our main instrument for the analysis of the communicative situation below.

APPLICATION

What counts as benign – for the purpose of benign violations – is highly context dependent: In our particular scenario, the perception of benignity is quite a bit lower than in most communicative settings, because of the usually high expectations of professionalism and deference in doctor-patient communication; and expectation that is often to the detriment of the clarity of the communication (Neeman et al., 2012; Post, 2000). Accordingly, what would be a below-benign violation in most everyday communication settings, and may thereby be perceived as slightly odd, but not funny, is a benign violation in a formal doctor-patient interaction; and what would be a humorous benign violation in other communication settings, is perceived as a non-benign violation in doctor-patient communication and thereby also non-funny. As a result, the analyzed sample's violations will seem relatively tame, compared to most other instances of everyday humor.

Seen through the lens of the BVT, we observe four communicative settings in our short sample, each with a different set of norms and violations. The first of these involves the way in which the doctor communicates to and with her patient. The second setting is its counterpart: the communication of the patient to the doctor (which follows different norms and expectations, even though it happens almost simultaneously). The third setting involves a group of communications between the doctor and the patient on one side (as they retell the anecdote), and their families and friends on the other. The fourth and final setting involves the very retelling and analyzing that happens in this anthology, where we, the analysts and you, the reader are the audience for the doctor.

1) Doctor to Patient Communication

Doctors are expected to maintain a high level of professionalism and carefully check that this is represented in all forms of communication, including non-verbal aspects such as their attire and appearance.

By (unintentionally) violating part of that expectation, namely a careful dress code in the morning and then later (negligently) missing to double-check her appearance the doctor violated that expectation and sends a funny non-verbal message. She thereby is the counterpoint – similar in type, but opposite in quantity – to the event clown who dresses in comically large shoes. Given the opposite qualities of the settings (medical consultation vs. party) she achieves the same effect with a small fraction of the violation. What would otherwise be an almost meaningless mistake, thus creates a crack in the perfect front of professionalism, just enough to amuse the patient.

2) Patient to Doctor Communication

Patients are traditionally expected to portray great deference and respect to doctors. This relates to what the doctors say, but also to criticism of their personal appearance. By pointing out the doctor's mistake, our patient breaks this expectation of deference. Because the mistake is relatively minor (related to fashion and attire as opposed to medical matters) the violation remains benign.

An additional aspect should be noted here as well. While the benign violations 1) and 2) above do not occur simultaneously, they are revealed at the same time. The fact that they are of similar (non-) importance and opposite orientations (one violation of the doctor to the patient, the other of the patient against the doctor) may contribute to the safety and the feeling of comradery that the doctor reports about the incident. The dress code snafu alone might not have been funny, and perhaps neither the slight transgression of the patient, but taken together they balance each other out and create a safe and cooperative space for laughter. To put this in a larger, more general, frame: If the basic assumptions of the BVT hold true, then communicative settings, such as doctor-patient communication, that require a high level of professionalism and demand a large amount of deference will pose a serious problem for the use of humor. While it is very easy to *violate* norms in these formal settings, tuning these violations to a *benign* level is very challenging. The patient as the true protagonist of this story achieves this delicate task by intuitively tapping into two resources: 1) she points out a minor violation by the doctor that occurred previously (thus balancing her violation with the doctor's) and 2) she clearly communicates sympathy, understanding and goodwill to the doctor (as opposed to saying e.g., "I really would appreciate if you checked your attire more carefully before seeing patients!"), thereby minimizing the danger of her statement to the doctor's face.

3) Both to Family Communication

Violations 1 and 2 are part of the original encounter, violation 3 occurs during the perpetuation of the story ("*She would introduce each new family member to me by telling them the story of that day. If I came in with a medical student or resident, which I often did, she would make sure that they knew exactly why she was asking her doctor to see her shoes. I can't count the number of times we shared this story. Sometimes, she would tell it. Sometimes, I would tell it. Each new introduction brought a retelling. We would bond, laugh, and connect again.*") The expectation of a standard professional doctor-patient communication would include silence about previous mistakes or snafus to avoid threatening the face of the doctor. There is also an expectation of privacy. By choosing to ignore these expectations and retelling the event, both the doctor and the patient risk making the doctor look less than professional. This violation appears benign because a) once again – as in the original situation – the mistake was foreign to the core domain (fashion vs medicine) and b) the original mistake lead to a bonding experience thereby producing more good than harm. Had the lack of professionalism instead led to a formal reprimand of a supervisor, then we may speculate, retelling the story might be less funny, because the results would have been less benign.

4) Doctor to Peers (and us) Communication

Finally, the very act of including this anecdote in this anthology creates a violation not entirely unlike violation 3. The doctor risks appearing overworked or unprofessional – at first glance negative attributes for a professional. Yet by also revealing the positive bonding experience through the shared experience, and the continued narrative, that endures even through the terminal care for the patience, this potential face threat is more than healed and we enjoy a hearty chuckle about the situation. Many readers might experience the situation as less funny reading this report, than it was for the protagonists of the story, because the additional distance (no emotional relationship to doctor or patient) and the certainty of the positive outcome (no risk) might actually make the violation that was reported and experienced too benign to be funny for the third party. Where the violations were in the goldilocks-zone between threatening and meaningless for doctor and patient (primary violations), and perhaps for those with a closer emotional and temporal connection to both (secondary violations), they are now more distant to us (tertiary violations).

TAKE AWAY

Dr. Ratner framed much of her life-long doctor-patient relationship with Ms. S around the humorous encounter that they shared a few years after they established their relationship. The fact that Ms. S. felt comfortable enough with Dr. Ratner to initiate the humous encounter speaks to the years of rapport-building both participants put into the relationship prior to the encounter. Further, the fact that the medical doctor only became aware that she was wearing different shoes at the *end* of the day and this patient was the only person to comment on it cements the uniqueness of the encounter. It helps to form the special bond that they shared. Would this have been as funny if the Ms. S was her first patient of the day? No, it would not have been funny because the lead up to the joke was "*long day*?" (unless it was *long day, already?*). Also, it would negate the fact that Ms. S was the only one to notice (presumably) or comment on Dr. Ratner's misstep, adding to the unique nature of their doctor-patient relationship.

The interaction was also framed by the fact that Ms. S was savvy enough to use humor to broach the dress code violation. The tactful, face-saving approach by Ms. S. enabled the moment to morph into laughter: Consider Ms. S.'s language choices: "*Doctor, have you had a hard day?*" ... "*Look down.*" Ms. S. approached Dr. Ratner in a gentle, understanding manner. Surely, Dr. Ratner, in her own words felt "*refreshed*," by the exchange, but also probably felt acknowledged and cared for by her patient. Instead of seeing her patients, she was seen by her patient as more than a medical doctor, but as a human being. Acknowledged, woman-to-woman, that being a working professional is tough. And that Dr. Ratner is so busy she didn't even notice she put on different shoes, so dedicated to job that she did not take a minute to look at her feet all day. More than anything this exchange highlights the importance of building interpersonal connections, humor, and optimism at work.

A vast number of researchers from a variety of fields have studied grit, resilience, and the ability to succeed or even simply persevere against suffering, tragedy, trauma, personal and professional setbacks, chaotic systems and uncertainty. Happiness researchers overwhelmingly conclude that positive, close personal relationships are the most important factor for happiness (if basic needs are met). Other essential components to achieving happiness and combating burnout are optimism and humor, two closely related concepts. Humor in medicine has been long contemplated, as seen by a recent JAMA Revisited article from 1970.

Humor, like love, is indefinable and yet is found to be important for establishing good relationships with patients— particularly the old and the young. Patients appreciate the personal relationship that a private joke with their physician creates. Is the joke a regular part of your medical armamentarium? The joke could serve to put the patient at his ease, establish rapport, and allow for the introduction of questions which might otherwise develop anxiety (Reiling, 2020, p. 2435).

This verbatim reprint of the 50-year-old article provides insights into the role of sense of humor in ensuring the success of the physician when it comes to establishing good relationships with patients. The narrative "4:30 on Friday" shared by Dr. Ratner demonstrates the essential role and importance of humor to help medical professionals combat fatigue and burnout by enabling them to gain a sense of connection with patients. One of the most significant common complaints that medical providers share is that under current practices most have few opportunities to connect with patients and spent too much time completing paperwork or interacting with the electronic health record during the patient visit (Montori, 2017). Over time, patient care has become increasingly impersonal (Zulman et al., 2020) leading both physicians and patients to feel frustrated and alienated (Sanders et al., 2020), which in turn affects patient outcomes. The benefits of quality communication and a deep patient-physician connection cannot be overstated. Evidence demonstrates that a high-quality connection improves diagnosis (Stewart, 1995), adherence to prescribed regimens[REMOVED HYPERLINK FIELD] (Harmon, 2006) and outcomes (Stewart et al., 2000). Humor is a vehicle to establish connections with patients, as demonstrated in this narrative. Can we say that Ms. S. had a better health-care experience because of her relationship with Dr. Ratner, even during her terminal stages? Probably. The fact that each one brought it up during every encounter and retold it shows that they both sought to reconnect at that level, remember the good laugh they shared and enjoyed the experience of connecting with another human, especially in the context of the doctor-patient dyad.

One final observation, and perhaps the most important message that we can take away from this story is perhaps a counterintuitive one: The doctor-patient lasting bonding or even friendship was based on their long established professional, respectful and polite interactions, but it was boosted not by professionalism, respect and politeness, but by violations of these standards. The less than professional dress code of the doctor, the less than respectful hint of the patient, and the potentially face threatening (i.e., impolite) retelling of the story to others, allowed Dr. Ratner and Ms. S. to reach a new level of intimacy and trust that would otherwise have been less likely. We might generally be tempted to err on the side of careful adherence to communicative standards in doctor-patient communication, but this story illustrates that doing so, might take away opportunities that Dr. Ratner and Ms. S seized.

Ultimately, the analysis of humor in the doctor-patient interaction can demonstrate the importance of private human interaction and of making room for space in medical encounters to allow physicians to attain both the instrumental and inspirational goals that initially drew many of them to medicine.

REFERENCES

Campbell, G. (1963). *The philosophy of rhetoric*. Southern Illinois University Press.

Centers for Disease Control and Prevention (CDC). (2008). *Workplace health promotion*. Retrieved from https://www.cdc.gov/workplacehealthpromotion/tools-resources/workplace-health/stress.html

Gawande, A. (2007). *Better*. Picador Books.

Harmon, G., Lefante, J., & Krousel-Wood, M. (2006). Overcoming barriers: The role of providers in improving patient adherence to antihypertensive medications. *Current Opinion in Cardiology*, *21*(4), 310–315. doi:10.1097/01.hco.0000231400.10104.e2 PMID:16755199

Hulin, C., & Judge, T. (2003). Job attitudes. In W. C. Borman, D. R. Ilgen, & R. J. Klimoski (Eds.), *The handbook of psychology: Industrial and organizational psychology* (Vol. 12, pp. 255–276). Wiley. doi:10.1002/0471264385.wei1211

Jauhar, S. (2014). *Doctored: The disillusionment of an American physician*. Farrar, Straus & Giroux.

Keidel, G. C. (2016). Burnout and compassion fatigue among hospice caregivers. *The American Journal of Hospice & Palliative Care*, *19*(3), 200–205. doi:10.1177/104990910201900312 PMID:12026044

Lawton, R., Johnson, J., Janes, G., Foy, R., & Simms-Ellis, R. (2019). Supporting doctors who make mistakes. *British Medical Journal*, *365*, L2161. doi:10.1136/bmj.l2161 PMID:31101605

Locke, E. A. (1976). The nature and causes of job satisfaction. In M. D. Dunnette (Ed.), *The Handbook of industrial and organizational psychology* (pp. 1297–1343). Rand McNaly.

Maslach, C. (2001). Psychology of Burnout. In *International Encyclopedia of the Social and Behavioral Sciences 2001*. ScienceDirect. Downloaded from https://www-sciencedirect-com.ezproxy.neu.edu/topics/psychology/burnout

McGraw, A. P., & Warren, C. (2010). Benign violations: Making immoral behavior funny. *Psychological Science*, *21*(8), 1141–1149. doi:10.1177/0956797610376073 PMID:20587696

McGraw, P., & Warren, C. (2014). Benign violation theory. In S. Attardo (Ed.), *Encyclopedia of Humor Studies* (pp. 75–77). Sage.

McGraw, P., Warren, C., Williams, L., & Leonard, B. (2012). Too close for comfort, or too far to care? Finding humor in distant tragedies and close mishaps. *Psychological Science*, *23*(10), 1215–1223. doi:10.1177/0956797612443831 PMID:22941877

Montori, V. (2017). *Why we revolt: A patient revolution for careful and kind care*. Patient Revolution.

Morreall, J. (2020). Philosophy of humor. In *The Stanford Encyclopedia of Philosophy* (Fall 2020 Edition). Stanford University. https://plato.stanford.edu/archives/fall2020/entries/humor/

Neeman, N., Isaac, T., Leveille, S., Dimonda, C., Shin, J., Aronson, M., & Freedman, S. (2012). Improving doctor-patient communication in the outpatient setting using a facilitation tool: A preliminary study. *International Journal for Quality in Health Care*, *24*(4), 357–364. doi:10.1093/intqhc/mzr081 PMID:22190587

Noland, C., & Carl, W. J. (2006). It's not our ass: Medical resident sense-making regarding lawsuits. *Health Communication, 20*(1), 81–91. doi:10.120715327027hc2001_8 PMID:16813491

Noland, C., & Hoppmann, M. (2020). Stop! You're killing me: Food addiction and comedy. In P. Oplinger & E. Shouse (Eds.), *The dark side of stand-up comedy* (pp. 129–149). Palgrave MacMillian. doi:10.1007/978-3-030-37214-9_7

Petrilli, C., Saint, S., Jennings, J., Caruso, A., Kuhn, L., Snyder, A., & Chopra, V. (2018). Understanding patient preference for physician attire: A cross-sectional observational study of 10 academic medical centres in the USA. *BMJ Open, 8*(5), E021239. doi:10.1136/bmjopen-2017-021239 PMID:29844101

Post, D. (2000). The effects of communication skills training on patients' participation during medical interviews. *Patient Education and Counseling, 41*(2), 209–222. doi:10.1016/S0738-3991(00)00093-8 PMID:12024545

Reiling, J. (2020). The "sense" of humor—Art & science. *Journal of the American Medical Association, 323*(23), 2435. doi:10.1001/jama.2019.13477 PMID:32543676

Sanders, L., Fortin, A., & Schiff, G. (2020). Connecting with patients—The missing links. *Journal of the American Medical Association, 323*(1), 33–34. doi:10.1001/jama.2019.20153 PMID:31910264

Stewart, M., Brown, J., Donner, A., McWhinney, I., Oates, J., Weston, W., & Jordan, J. (2000). The impact of patient-centered care on outcomes. *The Journal of Family Practice, 49*(9), 796–804. PMID:11032203

Stewart, M. A. (1995). Effective physician-patient communication and health outcomes: A review. *Canadian Medical Association Journal, 152*(9), 1423–1433. PMID:7728691

Veatch, T. C. (1998). A theory of humor. *Humor: International Journal of Humor Research, 11*(2), 161–215. doi:10.1515/humr.1998.11.2.161

Warren, C., & McGraw, A. P. (2016). Differentiating what is humorous from what is not. *Journal of Personality and Social Psychology, 110*(3), 407–430. doi:10.1037/pspi0000041 PMID:26692355

Zulman, D., Haverfield, M., Shaw, J., Brown-Johnson, C., Schwartz, R., Tierney, A., Zionts, D. L., Safaeinili, N., Fischer, M., Israni, S. T., Asch, S. M., & Verghese, A. (2020). Practices to foster physician presence and connection with patients in the clinical encounter. *Journal of the American Medical Association, 323*(1), 70–81. doi:10.1001/jama.2019.19003 PMID:31910284

Chapter 39
"A Ph.D. Doesn't Count!"

Annette Folwell
University of Idaho, USA

Midterm grades were due by noon on Monday so, even though I was lethargic, achy, and felt a burning sensation when I took a deep breath, I went into the office to finish grading. A colleague remarked that I looked terrible. After I listed out my complaints, she told me it sounded like bronchitis. She urged me to go to our town's urgent care facility that addresses non-life-threatening issues. When I saw a doctor on Monday afternoon, I mentioned my friend's opinion about bronchitis. The doctor scoffed at that idea. He told me that I had the flu and didn't need antibiotics. He recommended to stay in bed and get a lot of rest.

By 6:30 on Tuesday night, I could not feel my right leg. As a person who lives by herself, I debated on whether I should go back to the urgent care facility or directly to the emergency room at the local hospital. I made the decision to go with the ER based on two facts: first, urgent care was located across town and only open until 7 pm; and second, I did not feel like the doctor believed me about my symptoms. Apprehensively, I entered the ER and gave my information to the intake receptionist. I did not have to wait long until I was brought back into an exam room. The nurse took my vitals and asked about my symptoms; I mentioned I was seen yesterday at their urgent care facility so they could access information from that appointment. The doctor briskly entered the exam room, spent very little time talking with me, and told me they needed to do an ultrasound of my leg.

The physician led me down a hallway to another room with an older female ultrasound technician. She was kind enough to talk with me while administering the test. We made small talk for the first few minutes but when I asked about my leg, all she would say is that she only administers the test and could not interpret the results. After the test concluded, she looked into my eyes and said, "I really shouldn't be telling you, but you have blockages in your veins. After the doctor views these results, he'll tell you more." She squeezed my hand as she left the room.

I was stunned. I never had been to the ER before, never had a serious health concern, and never been hospitalized. Before this information could register in my brain, I was taken to another room for a CT scan. Another technician was explaining the CT process when the ER doctor came into the room and said, "You have deep vein thrombosis—blood clots in your right leg. This CT scan will reveal any pulmonary embolisms. We are deciding if you should be life flighted to a larger hospital."

DOI: 10.4018/978-1-7998-4528-7.ch039

Wait! What? Life-flighted? Wasn't that only for dying patients?!? I started to cry. I told the ER doctor that I wanted to stay locally as my parents, who lived only 20 minutes away, would have a difficult time making the two-hour trip to the larger hospital. He smiled and quipped back, "I don't think you get to make that call." Without hesitating, I said, "But I am a doctor, too!" He threw his head back and laughed out loud. He put his hand on my shoulder and said, "A Ph.D. doesn't count!" I laughed through my tears.

The doctor continued to keep his hand on my shoulder while telling me that he was going to take good care of me. I felt my whole body relax. He explained the CT scan would reveal if one or both of my lungs contained embolisms. Also, he would prescribe a blood thinner and, depending on my body's reaction to this medication, he would then make the call about the life flight.

After the CT scan, I was taken back to the original exam room and given an intravenous blood thinner. By this time, it was after 10pm and the ER was dead, so the doctor chatted with me. He asked me what I taught at the university, to which I replied, "communication." He joked around and said, "Tell me your opinion, ***Doctor*** Folwell, how am I doing?" I laughed whole-heartedly and said, "Oh, so now I am a doctor, huh?" I told him that he was a hell of a lot better than the doctor who saw me yesterday at their urgent care facility. He asked about that appointment. I recounted the experience, telling him I felt dismissed by the other doctor who gave me the impression he thought I was fishing for antibiotics. I also shared with the ER doctor that I spent two years of my doctoral program as a research assistant at a Veterans Affairs healthcare clinic as well as at a college of family medicine. I told him about different research projects and my interactions with attending physicians, residents, nurses, and other healthcare workers. I believe my past experiences in healthcare settings gave me credibility with him—like he listened a little better and valued my opinion more.

He left the exam room about an hour later and returned with my most recent blood work results. "You're responding well to the blood thinner. You got your way—I am not life flighting you out, but you're being admitted to this hospital for a few days." I felt my entire body relax—my heart rate decreased, and I felt like I could breathe again—even though it still hurt to take a deep breath. The ER doctor smiled at my reaction. "You know, for a comm professor, you sure are stubborn! Maybe you should consider getting an M.D. and becoming a real doctor!" laughing as he left the room. For the next three days, I was hospitalized to make sure the blood clots in my leg and lungs did not break off and travel to my heart or brain.

I am incredibly grateful for this ER doctor. His humor allowed me to relax while lying on the CT exam table. His humor brought a sense of levity that made this life-threatening situation bearable. His humor allowed me to be comfortable with disclosing about my situation and life. Those instances when we laughed together opened avenues to other conversation topics, like my work history in the healthcare field. Most importantly, those humorous moments allowed me to be heard, which is not always the case in medical interactions. I believe every patient wants to be treated as an individual who has value. His willingness to joke with me made me feel like a person, not just a patient.

Chapter 40
Response: "'A Ph.D. Doesn't Count!'"

Clair Morrissey
Occidental College, USA

Kayla Heinze
Occidental College, USA

PERSONS AND PLAYFULNESS

Philosophers use the term dignity to refer to the special moral value of persons. According to Immanuel Kant's (1997) well-known articulation of this value,

everything has either a price or a dignity. What has a price can be replaced by something else as its equivalent; what, on the other hand, is raised above all price and therefore admits of no equivalent has a dignity. (p. 42)

This implies that things with dignity have both infinite and irreplaceable value. Persons have infinite value in not being equivalent to any number of things that have a price. Persons have irreplaceable value in that their value is not comparable to that of anything else, including other things with dignity (Zagzebski, 2001). In clinical practice in the United States, the obligation to respect persons' dignity has primarily been interpreted as the obligation of institutions and individuals to respect patients' autonomous decision-making. To fulfill this obligation, clinical institutions primarily focus on promoting and protecting what individuals need to make informed decisions about their own lives and bodies, including providing access to and ensuring understanding of relevant information, obtaining consent for interventions and treatments, and enforcing prohibitions on overriding the autonomously made decisions of individuals.

Some bioethicists have taken issue with this interpretation of respect for persons as coextensive with respect for autonomy, on the grounds that it is overly narrow or reductive with respect to what recognition of human dignity requires (Killmister, 2010; Morrissey, 2016). There are at least two ways we can

DOI: 10.4018/978-1-7998-4528-7.ch040

interpret the obligation to treat people "as" persons (Spelman, 1978). In the first sense, treating someone as a person is a matter of recognizing her as a being with a certain status. In this case, recognizing her as an autonomous decision-maker, a rights-bearer, or, most generally, a rational agent. In the second sense, treating someone as a person is a matter of recognizing her as "the person she is." Instead of recognizing someone as an instance of a particular kind, we recognize her by acknowledging, attending to, taking up, or considering her individual interests, perspective, history, and traits. When we demand this kind of treatment or respect from others, we are not asking them to recognize that we instantiate a quality that grants us a particular moral status. We are calling on them, instead, to "respect me, for who I am." That is, to recognize us as the unique, individual selves that we are, and, in this way, non-fungible, even with respect to other things with dignity.

Both interpretations of respect for persons are relevant to clinical practice. With respect to treating patients as "a person," as discussed above, there are well known ethical concerns about protecting and promoting patients' autonomous decision-making. Though less frequently discussed, treating patients as "the person they are" is also relevant to contemporary healthcare. Our clinical institutions are often large and anonymous. They serve, govern, and employ a number of different people with different levels of responsibility for care of patients. To function, these systems require rules and policies to make clear which healthcare providers (including physicians, nurses, administrators, etc.) are responsible for what kinds of decisions, and to make decision-making consistent across different levels and domains of the institution. This, in turn, often requires specific, clear procedures and metrics for measuring outcomes suited to relatively quick, consistent, and transparent decision-making, for example, the use of QALYs (Quality-adjusted life year) in allocation of scarce resources. The requirements of operating this kind of bureaucratic institution, thus, require abstracting away from the specific individuals at issue, to view patients either in aggregate or as substantially indistinguishable from one another. These bureaucratic necessities risk failing to respect patients as "the persons they are."

Recognition of someone as "the person they are" rather than "a person" requires demonstrating our attentiveness to them as an individual. Playfulness is one way of doing so. Lugones (1987) describes playfulness as an attitude that we exercise in being with other people creatively. We are playful when we spend time with or approach others in a manner not wedded to any particular way of doing things. In this way, playfulness exercises an ability to operate without relying on heuristics for social interaction or rote rule-governed responses and behaviors, while, at the same time, engaging in cooperative intentional activity. It requires flexibility, openness, and being "game."

There are few games as truly playful as Calvin and Hobbes' Calvinball (GoComics Team, 2018). The players make it up they go, and the only rule is that it cannot be played the same way twice. Calvinball requires players to be in the moment (e.g. - Look a stick! It is a goalpost…); they must pay close attention to one another (e.g. – Run to the goalpost…, now run backwards…, now grapevine…); they must all be willing to move in a new direction together, and to feel out and create that direction (e.g. – New rule! See how many other sticks we can find of the same length…); they must be mutually receptive to how well it is going and be willing to adapt to make the game more fun for everyone (e.g. – One person is much faster than the other. New rule! Now we use the sticks we collected for a round of poohsticks in the stream…) (Evans, 2015).

These features of the game of Calvinball also characterize a way of being with other people in more everyday contexts that recognizes them as the people they are. When we engage others playfully we are sensitive to them (we attend carefully to them, we care to promote their welfare) and flexible (we are present in this moment, we are open to following their lead and are not tied to tightly to "how we do things"). Being playful with others is not required, or even appropriate, in every relationship or in every interaction within any particular relationship. Sometimes, we need and want others to recognize us as "this person" who needs to be serious right now. At the same time, precisely because it is not the default mode of communication and engagement, playfulness can indicate a willingness to connect with other persons in a way that is "extra" (i.e., not required) and beyond the norm. It shows a special kind of attentiveness between people and can lead to a sense of connection or intimacy. Insofar as its success requires acknowledging, attending to, taking up, or considering the other individual as an individual, it is one way of valuing someone as "the person they are."

One dimension of playfulness is spontaneous humor. That is, humor which arises in real time, from real-life experience, and from the imagination of the teller(s) (Morreall, 2009). This kind of joking, like play generally, requires sensitivity to the individuals one is with (i.e., what would they find funny, how does this story build on the jokes we have been telling) and flexibility (i.e., going with flow of the banter and riffing and finding out, together, where it is taking you).

Spontaneous humor's success depends on this sensitivity in part because jokes are conditional. Getting a joke, both understanding it as a joke and finding it funny, requires some degree of shared background knowledge, understanding, and sensibility (Cohen, 1999). For example:

What do you call it when you drop a piano on a guy working in the mines?

(A flat miner/A-flat minor)

Significant background knowledge is required to "get" this joke. In addition to the basic understanding of gravity, the set-up itself -- "what do you call it…" -- indicates that a particular kind of punchline is coming. Namely, a silly pun, a Dad-joke, a groaner. Second, to get this play on words, you need at least minimal familiarity with music theory (i.e., that there are various scales, one of which is A-flat minor) and the ability to recognize linguistic ambiguity in the sound "a" between an indefinite article and as part of a proper name for this scale. In this way, as Noël Carroll (2014) characterizes it, jokes have an "inside" and an "outside," and can thereby be used in "the construction and maintenance of what we may call an *Us,* a type of community" (p. 77).

RESPECTFUL PLAY IN "A PHD DOESN'T COUNT"

Given our interest in dignity, persons, and playfulness, here we focus primarily on how Folwell's interactions with her ER doctor exemplify the sort of joking around that respects the irreplaceable value of persons. In drawing out the connection between our characterization of playfulness and respect we hope to make clear how the playfulness in the Folwell case is a valuable kind of interaction between patient and provider.

The case starts with an emphasis on the isolation Folwell feels. In her telling of the events, she emphasizes both the fact she was living alone when she started feeling ill, and that she felt unheard by the medical professionals with whom she interacted at the local urgent care facility. She said of the first doctor she saw there, "I did not feel like the doctor believed me about my symptoms." Moreover, when she arrived at the emergency room the next night, the doctor she first saw, "briskly entered the exam room, spent very little time talking with me, and told me they needed to do an ultrasound of my leg." From her description of these initial interactions, we can tell Folwell felt unseen by the providers, which may have exacerbated her anxiety about and loneliness in dealing with her unknown illness. It is clear that she is unhappy with the care and attention she receives in these initial interactions, both with respect to the limited time the providers spend with her, and with respect to the lack of warmth, concern, or personal recognition in their interactions.

The contrast between these first interactions and the later connection Folwell builds with her ER doctor (to which we will turn in more depth below) makes apparent the importance of recognizing both aspects of respect for persons: recognizing someone both as "a person" and as "this person." Notice, neither of the first two providers failed to respect Folwell as "a person." She does not indicate that they failed to ask for her consent throughout their examinations, or that they undermined or otherwise directly set back her autonomous decision-making. However, the coldness, briefness, and perfunctory nature of their interactions with her may have contributed to her feeling as if her individuality as "this person" was not being adequately considered.

The first hint of personal connection between Folwell and a healthcare worker comes from the technician who takes an ultrasound of Folwell's leg. The ultrasound technician shows a heightened level of attention to Folwell as "this person" in a few ways. First, Folwell describes the technician's physical attentiveness, such as looking directly into her eyes and squeezing her hand. In a small way, Folwell seems to feel, quite literally, seen by the technician in a way that her previous providers failed to see her.

The second instance of personal attention from the technician is more complicated. During the procedure the technician says: "I really shouldn't be telling you, but you have blockages in your veins." Her lead in - "I really shouldn't be telling you…" - indicates she is breaking an institutional rule and signals to Folwell that she is receiving special information that would not normally be disclosed in this way, at this time, or by this person. However, this divergence from "the way things are done" appears to actually heighten Folwell's anxiety, rather than build a trust that her providers recognize and respect her. We suggest this is because the technician's disclosure in this case was insufficiently sensitive to how best to promote Folwell's welfare. Healthcare institutions have protocols regarding interpretation and disclosure of results because they believe they are in the best interests of promoting the patients' health. The breach of this protocol gave Folwell information, but not in a way that led to her understanding that information or enhancing her agency to act on it. Instead, it only seems to have amplified her feelings of alienation from the healthcare system and feelings of being alone in this serious decision-making.

The most poignant aspect of Folwell's case with respect to the relationship between dignity and playfulness, is the use of jokes to build the relationship between her and the ER doctor who is primarily responsible for her care. After he informs her about the blood clots in her leg and the possibility she will need to be life flighted to another hospital, the ER doctor eases the seriousness of the situation by beginning to joke around with Folwell. His body language of smiling, laughing, and touching Folwell's shoulder likely contribute to the relaxation Folwell feels in the midst of dealing with the difficult news of her diagnosis. Though, it seems to be his quips - "I don't think you get to make that call" and "A Ph.D. doesn't count!"- that makes Folwell feel the most at ease and seen during her time at the hospital. The playfulness of the joking leads her to laugh even as she cries; she shares that the attention and reassurance of the doctor in this moment made her whole body relax.

This value of playfulness is also clear later in the evening when the emergency room is less busy. The ER doctor who was joking around with her earlier returns to check in and chat. They talk about her scholarship and the doctor, "joked around and said, 'Tell me your opinion, *Doctor* Folwell, how am I doing?' I laughed whole-heartedly and said, 'Oh, so now I am a doctor, huh?'" Here, they are beginning to build a sort of inside joke, which further implies that the playfulness has successfully created an *Us* (even if just a small one that lasts for that evening, or the course of her treatment for her blood clots) between Folwell and the ER doctor.

A few components of this interaction make it a stellar exemplar of the kind of respectful playfulness we describe above. First, the specific joke the doctor makes to Folwell highlights the conditional nature of jokes that Cohen describes. Only people with shared background knowledge about graduate degrees and academia will understand the background context that makes the joke funny. Folwell's doctor brings to light this shared understanding by making the joke and Folwell affirms the commonality by responding and laughing. This starts to build the sort of personal connection that indicates the ER doctor's sensitivity to Folwell's individuality. The ER doctor is joking in a way that makes clear he sees Folwell for the specific person she is, which, for her, seems to centrally involve her profession and academic expertise. (This centrality to her identity is clear throughout Folwell's narrative - she even includes as salient that she was grading before going to the hospital!) He also makes clear that he sees her anxiety about her medical condition and feeling of responsibility for her own health. The joke both reassures her of his expertise, and invites her to trust that he will make decisions with her best interests at heart.

Second, the playfulness of the ER doctor shows an important sensitivity to context. He is attentive to Folwell's need to be able to rely on or trust the providers, and that humor and lightness could help her to cope in this moment. His joke is playful enough to ease the moment, but it does not go so far as to insult Folwell or inappropriately imply that the very serious circumstance is, itself, funny.

Finally, when the ER doctor jokes around with Folwell, he is unexpectedly and spontaneously introducing humor into a conversation, when that is not the norm. This interaction is not rote or mechanical, but dynamic. In this moment of playfulness, the ER doctor is communicating to Folwell that she is worth his time, and that he is not merely ticking boxes, or meeting minimal requirements of provider-patient interaction. Throughout the interaction, he demonstrates this by choosing to spend extra time sitting and joking around with her even though he certainly does not have to.

PRACTICAL WISDOM AND THE RESPECTFUL USE OF PLAY

As conceived above, humor and playfulness are, to a large extent, intrinsically opposed to heuristics and rule-following. Moreover, our analysis of Folwell's case suggests that the morally valuable use of humor in the clinical context will not be easily or neatly summed up in a set of guidelines. Thus, rather than articulating principles for the appropriate use of humor, in this section we describe and recommend character traits and attitudes to be cultivated and adopted by providers.

The appropriate use of humor between providers and their patients may be best understood as one aspect of the provider's practical wisdom about how to promote the welfare of patients and to demonstrate respect for them as the people they are. By practical wisdom we mean to highlight the sensitivity or insight that underlies clinical judgment, in contrast with that element of such judgment that relies directly on the deductive reasoning involved in applying particular principles or rules to cases. This judgment, following Montgomery (2006) "is neither a science nor a technical skill" (p. 5). Instead, it is a way of "seeing" a situation or context. Practical wisdom, in any domain, involves learning how to understand a situation in its full complexity, by honing one's ability to identify the salient and relevant particulars, in order to act well or "rightly" in that context. In medicine, practical wisdom involves not only a well-honed capacity for diagnosis, but sensitivity to the personhood of the patient, and to the complexity of the social context of clinical encounters. This facility or aptitude cannot be learned from a book, it must be developed over time through experience and reflection.

Nussbaum (1985) describes being someone "on whom nothing is lost" as a moral ideal. She praises one of William James' characters in the *Golden Bowl* for her moral vision and imagination in language that enriches our description above of how providers with practical wisdom may see their patients. Nussbaum describes the character's insight as:

subtle and high, rather than simple and coarse; precise rather than gross; richly colored rather than monochromatic; exuberant rather than reluctant, generous rather than stingy, suffused with loving emotion rather than mired in depression. (p. 521)

She attributes to James the view that this kind of moral knowledge is not simply an intellectual grasp of particular facts. Instead, as she writes: "It is seeing a complex concrete reality in a highly lucid and richly responsive way; it is taking in what is there, with imagination and feeling" (p. 521).

We have described the use of humor as one aspect of providers' ability to see a situation or context richly, lucidly, and with imagination. Most centrally, with respect to their responsibility to see and care for their patients as the people they are: to respect, to recognize, and to work with each patient as "this patient" and not only "a patient." Although we resist using these reflections to ground guidelines for humor's use in a medical setting, our emphasis on context-sensitivity suggests that there are some characteristic ways in which humor can miss the mark, and that the aim of playful respect provides a way to evaluate one's success in doing so. As we mention above, one important way in which the use of humor may miss the mark is for the provider to joke around and laugh when it is important to the patient to be serious. This failure to appropriately "read the room" is to misjudge the mood or sensibilities of the patient (and perhaps their loved ones). It reflects being insufficiently present or attuned to how one's joke will be received, which undermines rather than enhances the demonstration of respect for the personhood of the patient.

Jokes are not one size fits all, either with respect to patients, or with respect to contexts. For example, playfully saying something like "it was touch and go there for a minute" when a patient returns for a follow-up appointment, may work to strengthen the provider-patient relationship as a mutual acknowledgement of having been through a difficult experience together. The same joke may instead undermine that relationship if told by the provider immediately upon the patient waking up from anesthesia. Similarly, a joke about getting a patient out of the office by the time the game starts may signal to an ardent sports fan a commonality that puts them at ease; and to one who is not, truly misplaced priorities that causes a sense of foreboding.

Inevitably, given the importance of common background knowledge and shared sensibility to the success of jokes, using humor as a mode of connection for any provider will be easier with some patients than with others. Shared age, gender, race, ethnicity, religion, or cultural or socio-economic background (and other aspects of our identity that may be tied to the background knowledge and sensibility we bring into the medical setting) will be shared with some patients and not with others. Folwell's case highlights this, as the central joke about who is a "doctor" relies on a shared understanding that is deeply bound up with socio-economic and cultural status. The value of this commonality is further reflected in the subsequent discussions between her and the ER doctor, in which they are able to continue building a relationship in which Folwell feels seen as the person she is through sharing her professional expertise and experience related to healthcare.

This raises the legitimate concern that the use of humor in medicine may unwittingly further or amplify disparate health outcomes attributed to differences with respect to provider-patient communication. Researchers have found significant links between poor patient-provider communication, disparities in health care quality, providers' ability to appropriately respond to and discern minority patients' symptoms, and interpersonal dynamics (Balsa & McGuire, 2001, 2003; Balso et al., 2005; Cooper et al., 2006; Stewart et al., 2007, 1999). That humor's success is conditional on at least some shared understanding may then give us pause about recommending or celebrating its use as an appropriate mode of communicating respect for patients. Although humor is valuable as a way to communicate that one recognizes patients as the people they are, it is also potentially vulnerable to reifying or perpetuating existing social hierarchies. Thus, the practical wisdom providers develop with respect the appropriate use of humor will necessarily involve not only an understanding of when not to joke around, but also, the ability to find ways of communicating respect for the personhood of patients with whom they do not share easy or ready background sensibilities or experiences. In this way, it may involve providers learning how to see or find moments of connection or commonality with each and every one of their patients.

The aim of building a meaningful connection with a particular patient should be what guides a provider's playful joking. It must begin with the provider's best understanding of what would serve the needs and welfare of the patient, as opposed to, say, what makes the interaction most comfortable for the provider. Being playful with patients requires taking one's cue from them, which in turn requires keen observation of the emotional and physical responses of the patient to the presence of the provider and to the clinical environment itself. This sensitivity goes beyond recognition of symptoms of an illness, to include the ability to pick up on indications of the patient's personality, history, and broader welfare. Moreover, this kind of engagement requires attending carefully to patients' responses to how information is communicated, and not only to what information is communicated.

The valuable use of humor by providers with their patients is, importantly, creative. It requires the provider to actively generate moments in which the patient understands they are seen for who they are, and not merely as just another bundle of symptoms. Humor, then, is not merely an aspect of some providers' personalities. It is an intentional way of engaging with patients that can be cultivated and practiced that requires both humility and vulnerability: humility to put the personhood of the patient at the center of your interactions, and vulnerability to be the person you are with them, as well.

REFERENCES

Balsa, A. I., & McGuire, T. G. (2001). Statistical discrimination in health care. *Journal of Health Economics*, *20*(6), 881–907. doi:10.1016/S0167-6296(01)00101-1 PMID:11758051

Balsa, A. I., McGuire, T. G., & Meredith, L. S. (2005). Testing for statistical discrimination in health care. *Health Services Research*, *40*(1), 227–252. doi:10.1111/j.1475-6773.2005.00351.x PMID:15663711

Carroll, N. (2014). *Humour: A very short introduction*. Oxford University Press. doi:10.1093/actrade/9780199552221.001.0001

Cohen, T. (1999). *Jokes: Philosophical thoughts on joking matters*. University of Chicago Press. doi:10.7208/chicago/9780226112329.001.0001

Cooper, L. A., Beach, M. C., Johnson, R. L., & Inui, T. S. (2006). Delving below the surface: Understanding how race and ethnicity influence relationships in health care. *Journal of General Internal Medicine, 21*(S1), S21–S27. doi:10.1111/j.1525-1497.2006.00305.x PMID:16405705

Evans, M. (2015). *The poohsticks handbook: A poohstickopedia*. Egmont.

GoComics Team. (2018, August 16). *Calvin and Hobbes: Calvinball*. https://www.gocomics.com/comics/lists/1643217/calvin-and-hobbes-calvinball

Kant, I. (1997). *Groundwork for the metaphysics of morals* (M. Gregor, Ed. & Trans.). Cambridge University Press.

Killmister, S. (2010). Dignity: Not such a useless concept. *Journal of Medical Ethics, 36*(3), 160–164. doi:10.1136/jme.2009.031393 PMID:20211996

Lugones, M. (1987). Playfulness, "world"-travelling, and loving perception. *Hypatia, 2*(2), 3–19. doi:10.1111/j.1527-2001.1987.tb01062.x

Montgomery, K. (2006). *How doctors think: Clinical judgment and the practice of medicine*. Oxford University Press.

Morreall, J. (2009). *Comic relief: A comprehensive philosophy of humor*. Wiley-Blackwell. doi:10.1002/9781444307795

Morrissey, C. (2016). The value of dignity in and for bioethics: Rethinking the terms of the debate. *Theoretical Medicine and Bioethics, 37*(3), 173–192. doi:10.100711017-016-9368-6 PMID:27301253

Nussbaum, M. (1985). "Finely aware and richly responsible": Moral attention and the moral task of literature. *The Journal of Philosophy, 82*(10), 516–529. doi:10.5840/jphil1985821024

Spelman, E. V. (1978). On treating persons as persons. *Ethics, 88*(2), 150–161. doi:10.1086/292066

Stewart, A. L., Napoles-Springer, A., Gregorich, S. E., & Santoyo-Olsson, J. (2007). Interpersonal process of care survey: Patient-reported measures for diverse groups. *Health Services Research, 42*(3p1), 1235-56. doi:10.1111/j.1475-6773.2006.00637.x

Stewart, A. L., Napoles-Springer, A., Perez-Stable, E. J., Posner, S. F., Bindman, A. B., Pinderhughes, H. L., & Washington, A. E. (1999). Interpersonal processes of care in diverse populations. *The Milbank Quarterly, 77*(3), 305–339. doi:10.1111/1468-0009.00138 PMID:10526547

Zagzebski, L. (2001). The uniqueness of persons. *The Journal of Religious Ethics, 29*(3), 401–423. doi:10.1111/0384-9694.00090

Afterword

This anthology has been a pleasure to bring together. From the candor of the authors of the case studies to the insights and discussions of the issues provided by our response authors, there is plenty in this text to create a rich, engaging, and valuable set of readings. We expect this text will be helpful for anyone interested in the use of humor as it relates to the world of medical care. In fact, the lessons learned here can assuredly be applied in realms beyond healthcare. We want to again express our thanks to all our authors, reviewers, and others who contributed for their time and effort in bringing these chapters to life. As editors it is our hope that this edition is just the beginning.

One of the rewards of putting together this text together was seeing the themes develop across the various responses. This proved to be incredibly interesting because there were certain commonalities that began to emerge. As we close this anthology, we wanted to provide our impressions on some of the important themes and topics that emerged. We hope that this provides some basis for others to work and further the much needed exploration of the way humor works in medical care settings.

From the perspective of philosophy, a couple of important themes emerged. One of the first and possibly most important themes was the way that humor and its use often taps in our deep need to connect with people as individuals. While we are often told, whether by our faith or philosophical or political traditions, to value the other as simply an individual, humor allows us to more easily practice that directive. In Foresman's chapter, he stresses the importance of agape, or love of others as such, and how humor is an extension or practice of agapic love. This theme is explored in a different way by authors Morrisey and Heinz in that humor requires more than simply treating a person in a general sense. They stress that we can also relate to others in a more direct and specific sense, a sense important to many healthcare settings, through play. That is, when we play, or joke, or invite humor, we're not just treating the person as a generic person, but as a specific individual who is unique and special. This sort of relationship, one where the other is shown to be valued by these entreaties to play, is crucially important in a relationship that's primarily about care. As author Gimbel points out, the care relationship requires more than a simple customer client relationship. When we're receiving medical treatment we of course expect the best care. But as patients, we're also part of the group of folks who are responsible for the delivery of that care. We have opinions, and while we may not be experts, it's important that our voices are heard in any care regimen. Humor provides an outlet for those voices to be heard. Whether we're joking with our care providers about some butter falling out of a purse, or when a surgeon leaves a little joke in the way that the person was bandaged up, as in the case from author North, humor is a way to reach out even when the person isn't directly present. In a sense, it's a gift. These little asides, these invitations to play not only adhere to the respect directive we are told to follow, but also makes that respect less clinical and rooted in a more human and playful place.

Another more cautionary theme that emerged is the difficulty in interpreting humor. Often it's this worry, the worry that our jokes or humor may lead to offense, that makes people hesitant to use humor, especially in situations like those encountered in healthcare settings. The case of the playful tease about the bar fight by Dr. Tailor or the humor in Mr. Kauer's case are ones where humor might have had an adverse effect. One of the things to see as a result of the chapters here, is that humor isn't always about making someone laugh or providing humor to others. While we often attribute perceived humor as a thing designed to make us laugh, it's not always so. We need to be aware both as audience and provider of humor, that we may be misinterpreting what is actually being done. This isn't to say that being alarmed or offended isn't a legitimate response, but what is that alarm, offense, or indignation signaling? If I tend to use humor a lot, then I need to know more, and practice more carefully, my use of humor with these issues in mind. In the same way that we are asked to focus on individuals with levels of respect, the foregoing chapters also show that knowing what we know about humor, part of demonstrating that respect is being aware of how our humor could be taken, regardless of our intent.

There are surely more themes relevant to the philosophical issues that are present in the chapters you have read and we can't do justice to all those our authors have raised. We also need to work on describing some of the themes that arise from our communication studies authors. As with the responses from the philosophical perspective, there were a number of recurring themes from the communication perspective. Perhaps the two most crucial for readers to note are that of listening and stress management.

In many early response drafts, authors called for healthcare experts to "read the room" to know whether humor was well received after delivery or welcomed before delivery. When respondents were asked to unpack that idea, it was revealed that to "read the room" means, in part, to actively listen. As Garland explains, active listening is much more than simply taking meaning from the words someone says. It involves paying attention to *how* words are said and what nonverbal behaviors accompany them. It also means paying special attention to the nonverbal behaviors of patients when they are not speaking. Eldredge and colleagues explain that in Beach's case, Beach was able to note her client's discomfort from nonverbal communication and note that while humor was needed to break the tension, the sensitivity of the topic meant that the humor should be at the expense of Beach, not the client. In another response, Goke and Berndt explain that providers will likely be able to tell whether a patient is receptive to humor based on whether the patient tries to provide playful responses themselves. If responses are not playful, the patient may not be receptive to the humor and it should not be forced onto them, regardless of provider intention. Silence does not always mean acceptance.

A second theme throughout the communication responses is that of stress management. Health conditions create a lot of uncertainty for individuals. As many response authors explain, uncertainty can cause so much stress that patients shut down and are unable to process new information from their healthcare provider. Yet, humor can act as an intervention to help alleviate some patients from their stress, allowing them to process new information. For example, in the Thompson case as analyzed by Miller, Thompson realizes that laughter at the situation is alright because laughter more than anything else will signal to the patient how *not* dire the situation actually is. Yet, Baeriss also stresses that sometimes healthcare providers need to practice their facework, holding in their amusement of the situation until the patient is also ready to laugh. As Iannarino points out, attempting to reach patients on a psychological level is an expression of care, but sometimes withholding information or humor for a moment until that patient is ready to hear it, until they have managed their stress and are ready to process something more, is part of optimal patient care.

Certainly, there are many more themes that could be explored throughout the text. We will leave it to you, dear reader, to pull those themes out. If you feel a desire to ever discuss those themes with us, please do not hesitate to reach out.

FUTURE DIRECTIONS

Indeed, we hope that this edition is just the first. As we've noted before, it's been a great experience reaching out and gathering the cases, but also working with the respondents to craft their chapters. We've learned a great deal and see just how rich and rewarding an area of research this is. We also see now how much more will be done.

Given the scope of humor in healthcare settings there are certainly things that we missed. One issue with the text is that the cases reviewed tend towards the positive. That is, this text very much plays the part of humor apologist. Anyone reading this text would think that humor is a good tool, with few issues in its use. This is not true. Humor is helpful for both patient and practitioner, but not always. The difficulty is that it's tough to get either a patient or a practitioner to relate a case where humor failed or had untoward outcomes. Imagine a physician telling a story about the failure of a joke? In this day and age of social media, relating such a tale could come back to have negative consequences. As we think about future directions, exploring the failure of humor is every bit as illuminating as the successes.

One of our wishes for future directions is to have more cases from differing areas of medical care. While we have a relatively wide range of cases from mental health counseling, to surgery, to undiagnosed medical maladies, there are certainly areas we've missed. In future editions of this text we want to broaden the scope of entries. How is humor used in areas like convalescence, or terminal disease, or perhaps palliative care different than say the sorts of humor one sees in a counselor's office? What can we learn from these differences? What sorts of ways can humor be used to help both patient and care provider? Are there certain forms of humor that are in general more effective? Are there types of humor that are just out and out wrong? These are all tantalizing questions. While we feel we have advanced in important ways the research and discussion of the use of humor in the healthcare spaces, we know that there is, as we often hear from researchers, "more research to be done." This is what keeps us getting out of bed in the morning.

It would be a shame to leave the reader thinking that the editors didn't also learn something in putting together this text. It's enjoyable to be able to read perspectives other than your own. They show you aspects of situations you may have missed. As a philosopher, reading the communication studies literature was enlightening for the way that stages of communication and elements of the practice of communicating came to the fore. Even regarding the philosophical topics much was learned about what we do when we joke and use humor, how it's a sort of reaching out of one individual to another. As a communication scholar, it was useful to read the contributions of our philosophers as they took what might be considered "common-sense" ideas and showed the complexity and the larger extent to which those concepts reached. While we take it as accepted that we should treat others with respect, to see how that everyday rule can be aligned with how humor works was interesting.

As we close this anthology, we again thank all our contributing authors for their tireless work on getting submissions in and done. We also want to thank our reviewers for their contributions. Thanks to the publishers and IT staff of IGI Global for working with us on this unique anthology. Without any of them, this project would never have come to fruition. Of course, we also have to thank our family and friends for their tireless support of our academic work. And finally our thanks to the reader. We hope you enjoyed reading this as much as we did putting it together.

Michael K. Cundall, Jr.

Stephanie Kelly

Compilation of References

Abbott, R. (2014, April 22). Unconscious patient says doctors mocked him. *Courthouse News*. https://www.courthouse-news.com/unconscious-patient-says-doctors-mocked-him/

Abel, M. H. (2002). Humor, stress, and coping strategies. *Humor: International Journal of Humor Research, 15*(4). 365-381. doi:10.1515/humr.15.4.365

Abramson, A. (2019, August 26). The power of humor in healthcare. *Elemental*. https://elemental.medium.com/the-power-of-humor-in-healthcare-1bd412254daf

Abrams, T. E., Ogletree, R. J., Ratnapradipa, D., & Neumeister, M. W. (2016). Adult survivors' lived experience of burns and post-burn health: A qualitative analysis. *Burns, 42*(1), 152–162. doi:10.1016/j.burns.2015.09.011 PMID:26527372

Acitelli, L. K., & Badr, H. J. (2005). My illness or our illness? Attending to the relationship when one partner is ill. In T. A. Revenson, K. Kayser, & G. Bodenmann (Eds.), *Couples coping with stress: Emerging perspectives on dyadic coping* (pp. 121–156). American Psychological Association. doi:10.1037/11031-006

Adams, E. T. (2017). *Managing multiple goals in opioid prescription communication: Perspectives from trauma physicians* [Masters Thesis]. Communication, University of Kentucky. doi:10.13023/etd.2017.107

Adamson, M., Choi, K., Notaro, S., & Cotoc, C. (2018). The doctor-patient relationship and information-seeking behavior: Four orientations to cancer communication. *Journal of Palliative Care, 33*(2), 79–87. doi:10.1177/0825859718759881 PMID:29514545

Afifi, T. D., Hutchinson, S., & Krouse, S. (2006). Toward a theoretical model of communal coping in postdivorce families and other naturally occurring groups. *Communication Theory, 16*(3), 378–409. doi:10.1111/j.1468-2885.2006.00275.x

Albrecht, T. L., & Adelman, M. B. (1987). Communicating social support: A theoretical perspective. In T. L. Albrecht, M. B. Adelman, & ... (Eds.), *Communicating social support* (pp. 18–39). Sage.

Albrecht, T. L., & Goldsmith, D. J. (2003). Social support, social networks, and health. In T. L. Thompson, A. Dorsey, K. I. Miller, & R. Parrott (Eds.), *Handbook of health communication* (pp. 263–284). Lawrence Erlbaum.

Altman, I., & Taylor, D. (1973). *Social penetration: The development of interpersonal relationships*. Holt.

Amati, R., & Hannawa, A. F. (2014). Relational dialectics theory: Disentangling physician-perceived tensions of end-of-life communication. *Health Communication, 29*(10), 962–973. doi:10.1080/10410236.2013.815533 PMID:24345181

Anderson, G. (2015). Humor in treatment is no joke. *ASHA Leader, 20*(7). Advance online publication. doi:10.1044/leader.HYTT.20072015.np

Andeweg, B., Gagestein, S., de Jong, J., & Wackers, M. (2011). *'Poke fun at yourself': The problem of self-deprecating humor*. First World Engineering Education Flash Week.

Anonymous. (2008, June 11). Joking with patients seen as risky. *Nursing Standard*, *22*(40), 7. doi:10.7748/ns.22.40.7.s6

Antonovsky, A. (1979). *Health, stress, and coping*. Jossey-Bass.

Antonovsky, A. (1987). *Unraveling the mystery of health – How people manage stress and stay well*. Jossey-Bass.

Antonovsky, A. (1993). Complexity, conflict, chaos, coherence, coercion and civility. *Social Science & Medicine*, *37*(8), 969–981. doi:10.1016/0277-9536(93)90427-6 PMID:8235741

Antonovsky, A. (1996). The salutogenic model as a theory to guide health promotion. *Health Promotion International*, *11*(1), 11–18. doi:10.1093/heapro/11.1.11

Archer, B., Azios, J. H., & Moody, S. (2019). Humour in clinical–educational interactions between graduate student clinicians and people with aphasia. *International Journal of Language & Communication Disorders*, *54*(4), 580–595. doi:10.1111/1460-6984.12461 PMID:30779411

Aristotle. (1934). *Nicomachean ethics* (H. Rackham Trans). Harvard University Press, Perseus Digital Library. (Original work published 350 B.C.E.)

Aultman, J. M. (2009). When humor in the hospital is no laughing matter. *The Journal of Clinical Ethics*, *20*(3), 227–234. PMID:19845193

Austin, J. L. (1962). *How to do things with words*. Oxford University Press.

Babrow, A. S. (2001). Uncertainty, value, communication and problematic integration. *Journal of Communication*, *51*(3), 553–573. doi:10.1111/j.1460-2466.2001.tb02896.x

Babrow, A. S., Hines, S. C., & Kasch, C. R. (2000). Managing uncertainty in illness explanation: An application of problematic integration theory. In B. B. Whaley (Ed.), *Explaining illness: Research, theory, and strategies* (pp. 41–67). Lawrence Erlbaum.

Babrow, A. S., Kasch, C. R., & Ford, L. A. (1998). The many meanings of uncertainty in illness: Toward a systematic accounting. *Health Communication*, *10*(1), 1–23. doi:10.120715327027hc1001_1 PMID:16370987

Baisley, M. C., & Grunberg, N. E. (2019). Bringing humor theory into practice: An interdisciplinary approach to online humor training. *New Ideas in Psychology*, *55*, 24–34. doi:10.1016/j.newideapsych.2019.04.006

Balsa, A. I., & McGuire, T. G. (2001). Statistical discrimination in health care. *Journal of Health Economics*, *20*(6), 881–907. doi:10.1016/S0167-6296(01)00101-1 PMID:11758051

Balsa, A. I., McGuire, T. G., & Meredith, L. S. (2005). Testing for statistical discrimination in health care. *Health Services Research*, *40*(1), 227–252. doi:10.1111/j.1475-6773.2005.00351.x PMID:15663711

Barnlud, D. C. (1970). Transactional model of communication. In K. K. Sereno & C. D. Mortensen (Eds.), *Foundations of communication theory* (pp. 83–102). Harper & Row.

Bast, E. S., & Berry, E. M. (2014). Laugh away the fat? Therapeutic humor in the control of stress-induced emotional eating. *Rambam Maimonides Medical Journal*, *5*(1), e0007. doi:10.5041/RMMJ.10141 PMID:24498514

Bateson, G. (1972). *Steps to an ecology of mind*. Ballantine.

Bauer, M., Lee, S., Tossone, K., Lazebnik, R., & Lazebnik, N. (2017). Patterns of social support and compliance with ultrasound study in teen pregnancy. *Journal of Pediatric and Adolescent Gynecology*, *30*(2), 299–331. doi:10.1016/j.jpag.2017.03.113

Beach, W. A., & Dixson, C. N. (2001). Revealing moments: Formulating understandings of adverse experiences in a health appraisal interview. *Social Science & Medicine*, *52*(1), 25–44. doi:10.1016/S0277-9536(00)00118-0 PMID:11144915

Beach, W. A., Easter, D. W., Good, J. S., & Pigeron, E. (2005). Disclosing and responding to cancer "fears" during oncology interviews. *Social Science & Medicine*, *60*(4), 893–910. doi:10.1016/j.socscimed.2004.06.031 PMID:15571904

Beach, W. A., & Prickett, E. (2017). Laughter, humor, and cancer: Delicate moments and poignant interactional circumstances. *Health Communication*, *32*(7), 791–802. doi:10.1080/10410236.2016.1172291 PMID:27420294

Becker, M. H., & Rosenstock, I. M. (1984). Compliance with medical advice. In A. Steptoe & A. Matthews (Eds.), *Health care and human behavior* (pp. 175–208). Academic Press.

Bell, E. (2008). *Theories of Performance*. Sage Publications, Inc.

Belous, C. K., & Bauman, M. L. (2017). What's in a name? Exploring pansexuality online. *Journal of Bisexuality*, *17*(1), 58–72. doi:10.1080/15299716.2016.1224212

Bennett, H. J. (2003). Humor in medicine. *Southern Medical Journal*, *96*(12), 1257–1261. doi:10.1097/01.SMJ.0000066657.70073.14 PMID:14696878

Bensing, J., van Dulmen, S., & Tates, K. (2003). Communication in context: New directions in communication research. *Patient Education and Counseling*, *50*(1), 27–32. doi:10.1016/S0738-3991(03)00076-4 PMID:12767581

Berger, A. A. (1976). Anatomy of the joke. *Journal of Communication*, *26*(3), 113–115. doi:10.1111/j.1460-2466.1976.tb01913.x

Berger, C. R. (1979). Beyond initial interaction: Uncertainty, understanding, and the development of interpersonal relationships. In H. Giles & R. N. St. Clair (Eds.), *Language and sociology* (pp. 122–144). Basil-Blackwell.

Berger, C. R. (1987). Communicating under uncertainty. In M. E. Roloff & G. R. Miller (Eds.), *Interpersonal processes* (pp. 39–62). Sage.

Berger, C. R., & Bradac, J. J. (1982). *Language and social knowledge: Uncertainty in interpersonal relationships*. Arnold.

Berger, C. R., & Calabrese, R. J. (1975). Some explorations in initial interaction and beyond: Toward a developmental theory of interpersonal communication. *Human Communication Research*, *1*(2), 99–112. doi:10.1111/j.1468-2958.1975.tb00258.x

Berger, J., Coulehan, J., & Belling, C. (2004). Humor in the physician-patient encounter. *Archives of Internal Medicine*, *164*(8), 825–830. doi:10.1001/archinte.164.8.825 PMID:15111367

Berger, J., Wilson, D., Potts, L., & Polivka, B. (2014). Wacky Wednesday: Use of distraction through humor to reduce preoperative anxiety in children and their parents. *Journal of Perianesthesia Nursing*, *29*(4), 285–291. doi:10.1016/j.jopan.2013.06.003 PMID:25062572

Bergum, V., & Dossetor, J. (2005). *Relational ethics: The full meaning of respect*. University Publishing Group.

Berk, R. (2009). Derogathory and cynical humor in clinical teaching and the workplace: The need for professionalism. *Medical Education, 43*(1), 7-9. .1365-2923.2008.03239.x doi:10.1111/j

Berlyne, D. E. (1972). Humor and its kin. In J. H. Goldstein & P. E. McGhee (Eds.), *The psychology of humor: Theoretical perspectives and empirical issues* (pp. 43–60). Academic Press. doi:10.1016/B978-0-12-288950-9.50008-0

Besnier, N. (2016). Humour and humility: Narratives of modernity on Nukulaelae Atoll. *Etnofoor*, *28*(1), 75–95.

Bethea, L. S., Travis, S. S., & Pecchioni, L. (2000). Family caregivers' use of humor in conveying information about caring for dependent older adults. *Health Communication, 12*(4), 361–376. doi:10.1207/S15327027HC1204_3 PMID:11063286

Bingham, S. C., & Green, S. E. (2016). *Seriously funny: Disability and the paradoxical power of humor*. Lynne Rienner Publishers.

Binhammer, K. (2017). The story within the story of sentimental fiction. *Narrative, 25*(1), 45–64. doi:10.1353/nar.2017.0003

Bisel, R. S., Messersmith, A. S., & Kelley, K. M. (2012). Supervisor-subordinate communication hierarchical mum effect meets organizational learning. *Journal of Business Communication, 49*(2), 128–147. doi:10.1177/0021943612436972

Bitterly, T. B., Brooks, A. W., & Schweitzer, M. E. (2017). Risky business: When humor increases and decreases status. *Journal of Personality and Social Psychology, 112*(3), 431–455. doi:10.1037/pspi0000079 PMID:27831701

Bitterly, T. B., & Schweitzer, M. E. (2019). The impression management benefits of humorous self-disclosures: How humor influences perceptions of veracity. *Organizational Behavior and Human Decision Processes, 151*, 73–89. doi:10.1016/j.obhdp.2019.01.005

Black, S. P. (2012). Laughing to death: Joking as support amid stigma for Zulu-speaking South Africans living with HIV. *Journal of Linguistic Anthropology, 22*(1), 87–108. doi:10.1111/j.1548-1395.2012.01140.x

Booth-Butterfield, M., Booth-Butterfield, S., & Wanzer, M. (2007). Funny students cope better: Patterns of humor enactment and coping effectiveness. *Communication Quarterly, 55*(3), 299–315. doi:10.1080/01463370701490232

Booth-Butterfield, M., Wanzer, M. B., Weil, N., & Krezmien, E. (2014). Communication of humor during bereavement: Intrapersonal and interpersonal emotion management strategies. *Communication Quarterly, 62*(4), 436–454. doi:10.1080/01463373.2014.922487

Booth-Butterfield, S., & Booth-Butterfield, M. (1991). Individual differences in the communication of humorous messages. *The Southern Communication Journal, 56*(3), 32–40. doi:10.1080/10417949109372831

Borchert, D. M. (1999). *Philosophy and ethics*. Macmillan Library Reference.

Bradac, J. J. (2001). Theory comparison: Uncertainty reduction, problematic integration, uncertainty management, and other curious constructs. *Journal of Communication, 51*(3), 456–476. doi:10.1111/j.1460-2466.2001.tb02891.x

Brashers, D. E. (2001). Communication and uncertainty management. *Journal of Communication, 51*(3), 477–497. doi:10.1111/j.1460-2466.2001.tb02892.x

Brashers, D. E., Goldsmith, D. J., & Hsieh, E. (2002). Information seeking and avoiding in health contexts. *Human Communication Research, 28*(2), 258–271. doi:10.1111/j.1468-2958.2002.tb00807.x

Bridges, N. A. (2001). Therapist's self-disclosure: Expanding the comfort zone. *Psychotherapy (Chicago, Ill.), 38*(1), 21–30. doi:10.1037/0033-3204.38.1.21

Brinkmann, J. T. (2019). Humor in clinical encounters: It's not about being funny. *The O&P Edge*. Retrieved from https://opedge.com/Articles/ViewArticle/2019-07-01/humor-in-clinical-encountersits-not-about-being-funny

Brownell, J. (1985). A model for listening instruction: Management applications. *The ABCA Bulletin, 48*(3), 39–44. doi:10.1177/108056998504800312

Brown, P., & Levinson, S. (1987). *Politeness: Some universals of language use*. Cambridge University Press. doi:10.1017/CBO9780511813085

Burgoon, J. K., Dillman, L., & Stem, L. A. (1993). Adaption in dyadic interaction: Defining and operationalizing patterns of reciprocity and compensation. *Communication Theory*, *3*(4), 295–316. doi:10.1111/j.1468-2885.1993.tb00076.x

Burgoon, J. K., & Hale, J. L. (1988). Nonverbal expectancy violations: Model elaboration and application to immediacy behaviors. *Communication Monographs*, *55*(1), 58–79. doi:10.1080/03637758809376158

Burke, K. (1961). *The rhetoric of religion: Studies in logology*. University of California Press.

Burke, K. (1969). *A grammar of motives*. University of California Press. doi:10.1525/9780520341715

Burton, L. L. (2012). Defacement: Indigenous patients' experiences in Baja Verapaz, Guatemala. *The Howard Journal of Communications*, *23*(2), 119–135. doi:10.1080/10646175.2012.667723

Buxman, K. (2000). Humor in critical care: No joke. *AACN Clinical Issues*, *11*(1), 120–127. doi:10.1097/00044067-200002000-00013 PMID:11040558

Byrd, A., Iheagwara, K., McMahon, P., Bolton, M., & Roy, M. (2020). Using multisource feedback to assess resident communication skills: Adding a new dimension to milestone data. *The Ochsner Journal*, *20*(3), 255–260. doi:10.31486/toj.19.0054 PMID:33071656

Cabridge University Press. (n.d.). Joke. In *Cambridge English dictionary*. https://dictionary.cambridge.org/us/dictionary/english/joke

Cain, C. L. (2012). Integrating dark humor and compassion: Identities and presentations of self in the front and back regions of hospice. *Journal of Contemporary Ethnography*, *41*(6), 668–694. doi:10.1177/0891241612458122

Cambridge University Press. (n.d.). Deadpan. In *Cambridge English dictionary*. https://dictionary.cambridge.org/us/dictionary/english/deadpan

Campbell, G. (1963). *The philosophy of rhetoric*. Southern Illinois University Press.

Canha, B. (2016). Using humor in treatment of substance use disorders: Worthy of further investigation. *The Open Nursing Journal*, *10*(1), 37–44. doi:10.2174/1874434601610010037 PMID:27347254

Cant, B. (2006). Exploring the implications for health professionals of men coming out as gay in healthcare settings. *Health & Social Care in the Community*, *14*(1), 9–16. doi:10.1111/j.1365-2524.2005.00583.x PMID:16324183

Carroll, N. (2014). *Humour: A very short introduction*. Oxford University Press. doi:10.1093/actrade/9780199552221.001.0001

Carson, V. B. (1989). *Spiritual dimensions of nursing practice*. Saunders.

Carver, C. S., Harris, S. D., Noriega, V., Pozo, C., Robinson, D. S., & Ketcham, A. S. (1993). How coping mediates the effect of optimism on distress: A study of women with early stage breast cancer. *Journal of Personality and Social Psychology*, *65*(2), 375–390. doi:10.1037/0022-3514.65.2.375 PMID:8366426

Centers for Disease Control and Prevention (CDC). (2008). *Workplace health promotion*. Retrieved from https://www.cdc.gov/workplacehealthpromotion/tools-resources/workplace-health/stress.html

Chapple, A., & Ziebland, S. (2004). The role of humor for men with testicular cancer. *Qualitative Health Research*, *14*(8), 1123–1139. doi:10.1177/1049732304267455 PMID:15359047

Charon, R. (2001). Narrative medicine: A model for empathy, reflection, profession, and trust. *Journal of the American Medical Association*, *286*(15), 1897-1902. doi:10.1001/jama.286.15.1897

Charon, R. (2006). *Narrative medicine: Honoring the stories of illness*. Oxford University Press.

Charon, R. (2005). Narrative medicine: Attention, representation, and affiliation. *Narrative*, *13*(3), 261–270. doi:10.1353/nar.2005.0017

Charon, R., DasGupta, S., Hermann, N., Irvine, C., Marcus, E. R., Colón, E. R., Spencer, D., & Spiegel, M. (2016). *The principles and practice of narrative medicine* [Kindle Version]. doi:10.1093/med/9780199360192.001.0001

Cheng, D., & Wang, L. (2015). Examining the energizing effects of humor: The influence of humor on persistence behavior. *Journal of Business and Psychology*, *30*(4), 759–772. doi:10.100710869-014-9396-z

Chen, L. (2016). Laughter, smiling and their pragmatic/interpersonal functions: An interactional linguistic account. *Concentric: Studies in Linguistics*, *42*(2). Advance online publication. doi:10.6241/concentric.ling.42.2.05

Cheung, C.-K., & Yue, X. D. (2012). Sojourn students' humor styles as buffers to achieve resilience. *International Journal of Intercultural Relations*, *36*(3), 353–364. doi:10.1016/j.ijintrel.2011.10.001

Chiodo, C. P., Broughton, K. K., & Michalski, M. P. (2020). Caution: Wit and humor during the COVID-19 pandemic. *Foot & Ankle International*, *41*(6), 763–764. https://doi-org.pitt.idm.oclc.org/10.1177/1071100720923651. doi:10.1177/1071100720923651 PMID:32338052

Cho, M. K., & Sillars, A. (2015). Face threat and facework strategies when family (health) secrets are revealed: A comparison of South Korea and the United States. *Journal of Communication*, *65*(3), 535–557. doi:10.1111/jcom.12161

Christoff, M., & Dauphin, B. (2017). Freud's theory of humor. In V. Zeigler-Hill & T. Shackelford (Eds.), Encyclopedia of personality and individual differences (living edition). Springer. doi:10.1007/978-3-319-28099-8_588-1

Claramita, M., Prabandari, Y. S., Graber, A., & Scherpbier, A. J. J. (2020). Challenges of communication skills transfer of medical students in the cultural context of Indonesia. *The Interdisciplinary Journal of Problem-Based Learning*, *14*(1). Advance online publication. doi:10.14434/ijpbl.v14i1.28594

Clark, C., Nicholas, J., Gordon, E., Golden, H., Cohen, M., Woodward, F., Macpherson, K., Slattery, C., Mummery, C., Schott, J., Rohrer, J., & Warren, J. (2016). Altered sense of humor in dementia. *Journal of Alzheimer's Disease*, *49*(1), 111–119. doi:10.3233/JAD-150413 PMID:26444779

Clarke, A. (2008). *The pattern recognition theory of humour*. Pyrrhic House.

Clark, R. A., & Delia, J. G. (1979). TOPOI and rhetorical competence. *The Quarterly Journal of Speech*, *65*(2), 187–206. doi:10.1080/00335637909383470

Claxton-Oldfield, S., & Bhatt, A. (2017). Is there a place for humor in hospice palliative care? Volunteers say "yes"! *The American Journal of Hospice & Palliative Care*, *34*(5), 417–422. doi:10.1177/1049909116632214 PMID:26917788

Cobb, S. (1974). Physiological changes in men whose jobs were abolished. *Journal of Psychosomatic Research*, *18*(4), 245–258. doi:10.1016/0022-3999(74)90005-1 PMID:4459457

Cobb, S. (1976). Social support as a moderator of life stress. *Psychosomatic Medicine*, *38*(5), 300–314. doi:10.1097/00006842-197609000-00003 PMID:981490

Cody, W. K. (2003). Paternalism in nursing and healthcare: Central issues and their relation to theory. *Nursing Quebec*, *16*(4), 288–296. doi:10.1177/0894318403257170 PMID:14596114

Cohen, S., & Wills, T. A. (1985). Stress, social support, and the buffering hypothesis. *Psychological Bulletin*, *98*(2), 310–357. doi:10.1037/0033-2909.98.2.310 PMID:3901065

Cohen, T. (1978). Metaphor and the cultivation of intimacy. *Critical Inquiry*, *5*(1), 3–12. doi:10.1086/447969

Cohen, T. (1999). *Jokes: Philosophical thoughts on joking matters.* University of Chicago Press. doi:10.7208/chicago/9780226112329.001.0001

Collins, R. F., Bekker, H. L., & Dodwell, D. J. (2004). Follow-up care of patients treated for breast cancer: A structured review. *Cancer Treatment Reviews*, *30*(1), 19–35. doi:10.1016/S0305-7372(03)00141-5 PMID:14766124

Cooper, L. A., Beach, M. C., Johnson, R. L., & Inui, T. S. (2006). Delving below the surface: Understanding how race and ethnicity influence relationships in health care. *Journal of General Internal Medicine*, *21*(S1), S21–S27. doi:10.1111/j.1525-1497.2006.00305.x PMID:16405705

Coser, R. L. (1959). Some social functions of laughter: A study of humor in a hospital setting. *Human Relations*, *12*(2), 171–182. doi:10.1177/001872675901200205

Coyne, J. C., & Fiske, V. (1992). Couples coping with chronic illness and catastrophic illness. In A. P. Stephens & J. Crowther (Eds.), *Family health psychology* (pp. 129–149). Hemisphere. doi:10.4324/9781315800837-9

Coyne, J. C., & Smith, D. A. F. (1991). Couples coping with a myocardial infarction: A contextual perspective on wives' distress. *Journal of Personality and Social Psychology*, *61*(3), 404–412. doi:10.1037/0022-3514.61.3.404 PMID:1941511

Creative Commons. (2016, November 8). *5.1 why conduct an audience analysis.* https://open.lib.umn.edu/publicspeaking/chapter/5-1-why-conduct-an-audience-analysis/

Cundall, M. K. Jr. (2007). Humor and the limits of incongruity. *Creativity Research Journal*, *19*(2–3), 203–211. doi:10.1080/10400410701397263

Cutrona, C. E., & Suhr, J. A. (1992). Controllability of stressful events and satisfaction with spouse support behaviors. *Communication Research*, *19*(2), 154–174. doi:10.1177/009365092019002002

Dalton, E. D., Pjesivac, I., Eldredge, S., & Miller, L. (2020). From vulnerability to disclosure: A normative approach to understanding trust in obstetric and intrapartum nurse-patient communication. *Health Communication*, *0*(0), 1–14. doi:10.1080/10410236.2020.1733225 PMID:32122160

Davidhizar, R., & Shearer, R. (1996). Using humor to cope with stress in home care. *Home Healthcare Nurse*, *14*(10), 825–830. doi:10.1097/00004045-199610000-00012 PMID:9052068

Davidson, L. G. (2016). Would you like a map? *Departures in Critical Qualitative Research*, *5*(1), 23–36. doi:10.1525/dcqr.2016.5.1.23

de Botton, A. (2000). *The consolations of philosophy.* Pantheon Books.

Dean, R. A. K., & Gregory, D. M. (2005). More than trivial: Strategies for using humor in palliative care. *Cancer Nursing*, *28*(4), 292–300. doi:10.1097/00002820-200507000-00009 PMID:16046892

Dean, R. A. K., & Major, J. E. (2008). From critical care to comfort care: The sustaining value of humour. *Journal of Clinical Nursing*, *17*(8), 1088–1095. doi:10.1111/j.1365-2702.2007.02090.x PMID:18321272

Deckers, L., & Devine, J. (1981). Humor by violating an existing expectancy. *The Journal of Psychology*, *108*(1), 107–110. doi:10.1080/00223980.1981.9915251

Demjén, Z. (2016). Laughing at cancer: Humour, empowerment, solidarity and coping online. *Journal of Pragmatics*, *101*, 18–30. doi:10.1016/j.pragma.2016.05.010

Deshields, T., Tibbs, T., Fan, M. Y., Bayer, L., Taylor, M., & Fisher, E. (2005). Ending treatment: The course of emotional adjustment and quality of life among breast cancer survivors immediately following radiation therapy. *Supportive Care in Cancer*, *13*(12), 1018–1026. doi:10.100700520-005-0801-z PMID:15800768

Dieser, R. B., Edginton, C. R., & Ziemer, R. (2017). Decreasing patient stress and physician/medical workforce burnout through health care environments: Uncovering the serious leisure perspective at Mayo Clinic's campus in Rochester, Minnesota. *Mayo Clinic Proceedings*, *92*(7), 1080–1087. doi:10.1016/j.mayocp.2017.03.017 PMID:28624118

Dillard, J. P. (1990). A goal-driven model of interpersonal influence. In J. P. Dillard (Ed.), *Seeking compliance: The production of interpersonal influence messages* (pp. 41–56). Gorsuch Scarisbrick.

Dillard, J. P., Segrin, C., & Harden, J. M. (1989). Primary and secondary goals in the production of interpersonal influence messages. *Communication Monographs*, *56*(1), 19–38. doi:10.1080/03637758909390247

Drew, S. K., Mills, M. B., & Gassaway, B. M. (2007). *Dirty work*. Baylor University Press.

du Pre, A., & Foster, E. (2016). Transactional communication. In E. Wittenberg & B. R. Ferrell (Eds.), Textbook of palliative care communication (pp. 14-21). Oxford University Press.

du Pre, A. (1998). *Humor and the healing arts: A multimethod analysis of humor use in health care*. Lawrence Erlbaum Associates.

Duke Health. (2019a). *Reiki: Level one*. Available at: https://dukeintegrativemedicine.org/programs-training/professionals/reiki-level-one/

Duke Health. (2019b). *Reiki: Level two*. Available at: https://dukeintegrativemedicine.org/programs-training/professionals/reiki-level-two/

Dunbar, R. I. M., & Mehu, M. (2008). Naturalistic observations of smiling and laughter in human group interactions. *Behaviour*, *145*(12), 1747–1780. doi:10.1163/156853908786279619

Dziegielewski, S. F., Jacinto, G. A., Laudadio, A., & Legg-Rodriguez, L. (2003). Humor: An essential communication tool in therapy. *International Journal of Mental Health*, *32*(3), 74–90. doi:10.1080/00207411.2003.11449592

Ebeling, P. R. (2008). Osteoporsis in men. *The New England Journal of Medicine*, *358*(14), 1474–1482. doi:10.1056/NEJMcp0707217 PMID:18385499

Ekman, P., & Friesen, W. V. (1971). Constants across cultures in the face and emotion. *Journal of Personality and Social Psychology*, *17*(2), 124–129. doi:10.1037/h0030377 PMID:5542557

Elal-Lawrence, G., & Celikoglu, P. (1995). Social support and psychological well-being in breast cancer patients. *Health & Social Care in the Community*, *3*(1), 1–7. doi:10.1111/j.1365-2524.1995.tb00001.x

Ellithorpe, M., Esralew, S., & Holbert, L. (2014). Putting the "self" in self-deprecation: When deprecating humor about minorities is acceptable. *Humor: International Journal of Humor Research*, *27*(3), 401–422. doi:10.1515/humor-2014-0070

Epictetus. (2008). *Discourses and selected writings* (R. Dobbin, Trans.). Penguin Classics. (Original work published in 108)

Epstein, R., & Joker, V. R. (2007). A threshold theory of the humor response. *The Behavior Analyst*, *30*(1), 49–58. doi:10.1007/BF03392145 PMID:22478488

Eriksson, M., & Lindström, B. (2008). A salutogenic interpretation of the Ottawa Charter. *Health Promotion International*, *23*(2), 190–199. doi:10.1093/heapro/dan014 PMID:18356285

Eriksson, M., & Lindström, B. (2011). Life is more than survival: Exploring links between Antonovsky's salutogenic theory and the concept of resilience. In K. M. Gow & M. J. Celinski (Eds.), *Wayfinding through life's challenges: Coping and survival* (pp. 31–46). Nova Publishers.

Ervin-Tripp, S., & Lampert, M. (2009). The occasioning of self-disclosure in humor. In N. R. Norrick & D. Chiaro (Eds.), *Humor in interaction* (pp. 3–27). John Benjamins Publishing. doi:10.1075/pbns.182.01erv

Evans, M. (2015). *The poohsticks handbook: A poohstickopedia*. Egmont.

Fadenrecht, K. M. (2015). *The influence of medical dramas on patient expectations of physician communication* (Master's thesis). University of Montana.

Falkenberg, I., Jarmuzek, J., Bartels, M., & Wild, B. (2011). Do depressed patients lose their sense of humor? *Psychopathology*, *44*(2), 98–105. doi:10.1159/000317778 PMID:21196810

Fallowfield, L., & Jenkins, V. (2004). Communicating sad, bad, and difficult news in medicine. *Lancet*, *363*(9405), 312–319. doi:10.1016/S0140-6736(03)15392-5 PMID:14751707

Feinberg, L. (1978). *The secret of humor*. Rodopi.

Ferguson, S. (2015, January 14). Labels: Empowering, harmful, or both? *Everyday Feminism*. Retrieved from https://everydayfeminism.com/2015/01/labels-empowering-harmful/

Fine, S. B. (1991). Resilience and human adaptability: Who rises above adversity? *The American Journal of Occupational Therapy*, *45*(6), 493–503. doi:10.5014/ajot.45.6.493 PMID:2063939

Folkman, S., & Lazarus, R. S. (1988). Coping as a mediator or emotion. *Journal of Personality and Social Psychology*, *54*(3), 466–475. doi:10.1037/0022-3514.54.3.466 PMID:3361419

Folkman, S., Lazarus, R. S., Dunkel-Schetter, C., DeLongis, A., & Gruen, R. J. (1986). Dynamics of a stressful encounter: Cognitive appraisal, coping, and encounter outcomes. *Journal of Personality and Social Psychology*, *50*(5), 992–1003. doi:10.1037/0022-3514.50.5.992 PMID:3712234

Forabosco, G. (1998). The ill side of humor: Pathological conditions and sense of humor. In W. Ruch (Ed.), *Humor research. The sense of humor. Explorations of a personality characteristic* (pp. 271–292). De Gruyter Mouton. doi:10.1515/9783110804607.271

Forabosco, G. (2009). Cognitive aspects of the humor process: The concept of incongruity. *Humor: International Journal of Humor Research*, *5*(1), 45–68. doi:10.1515/humr.1992.5.1-2.45

Francis, L. E. (1994). Laughter, the best medication: Humor as emotion management in interaction. *Symbolic Interaction*, *17*(2), 147–163. doi:10.1525i.1994.17.2.147

Francis, L., Monahan, K., & Berger, C. (1999). A laughing matter? The uses of humor in medical interactions. *Motivation and Emotion*, *23*(2), 155–174. doi:10.1023/A:1021381129517

Freud, S. (1961). The ego and the id. In *The standard edition of the complete psychological works of Sigmund Freud* (Vol. 19, J. Strachey, Ed. & Trans., pp. 3–66). Hogarth Press. (Original work published 1923)

Freud, S. (1990). *Jokes and their relations to the unconscious* (J. Strachey, Trans.). W.W. Norton & Company.

Gadsby, H. (Writer), & Olb, J. & Parry, M. (Directors), & Bruzzese, F. (Prod.). (2018). Nanette [Netflix Special]. Los Gatos, CA: Netflix.

Garrison, S. (2018). On the limits of "Trans enough": Authenticating trans identity narratives. *Gender & Society*, *32*(5), 613–637. doi:10.1177/0891243218780299

Gawande, A. (2007). *Better*. Picador Books.

Giles, H. (2016). Communication accommodation theory. In K. B. Jensen, E. W. Rothenbuhrler, J. D. Pooley, & R. T. Craig (Eds.), *The international encyclopedia of communication theory and philosophy* (pp. 1–7). Wiley Blackwell. doi:10.1002/9781118766804.wbiect056

Gilligan, C. (1982). *In a different voice: psychological theory and women's development.* Harvard.

Gimbel, S. (2017). *Isn't that clever: A philosophy of humor and comedy.* Routledge. doi:10.4324/9781315112633

Gimbel, S. (2018). *Isn't that clever.* Routledge.

Glenright, M., Tapley, B., Rano, J. K. S., & Pexma, P. M. (2017). Developing appreciation for sarcasm and sarcastic gossip: It depends on perspective. *Journal of Speech, Language, and Hearing Research: JSLHR, 60*(11), 3295–3309. doi:10.1044/2017_JSLHR-L-17-0058 PMID:29098274

GoComics Team. (2018, August 16). *Calvin and Hobbes: Calvinball.* https://www.gocomics.com/comics/lists/1643217/calvin-and-hobbes-calvinball

Goffman E. (2003). On face-work: An analysis of ritual elements in social interaction. *Reflections, 4*(3), 7-13. (Original work published 1967) doi:10.1162/15241730360580159

Goffman, E. (1963). *Stigma: Notes on the management of spoiled identity.* Prentice Hall.

Goldsmith, D. J., & Albrecht. (2011). Social support, social networks, and health: A guiding framework. In T. L. Thompson, R. Parrott, & J. F. Nussbaum (Eds.), *The Routledge handbook of health communication* (2nd ed., pp. 335-348). Routledge.

Goldsmith, D. J. (2001). A normative approach to the study of uncertainty and communication. *Journal of Communication, 51*(3), 514–533. doi:10.1111/j.1460-2466.2001.tb02894.x

Goldsmith, D. J. (2004). *Communicating social support.* Cambridge University Press. doi:10.1017/CBO9780511606984

Goldsmith, D. J. (2009). Uncertainty and communication in couples coping with serious illness. In T. D. Afifi & W. A. Afifi (Eds.), *Uncertainty, information management, and disclosure decisions: Theories and applications* (pp. 203–225). Routledge.

Goldsmith, D. J. (2019). Normative rhetorical theory. In S. Wilson & S. Smith (Eds.), *Reflections on interpersonal communication research* (pp. 211–230). Sage.

Goldsmith, D. J., Miller, L. E., & Caughlin, J. P. (2008). Openness and avoidance in couples communicating about cancer. *Communication Yearbook, 31*(1), 62–115. doi:10.1080/23808985.2007.11679065

Goodenough, B., & Ford, J. (2005). Self-reported use of humor by hospitalized pre-adolescent children to cope with pain-related distress from a medical intervention. *Humor: International Journal of Humor Research, 18*(3), 279–298. doi:10.1515/humr.2005.18.3.279

Goold, S. D., & Lipkin, M. Jr. (1999). The doctor-patient relationship: Challenges, opportunities, and strategies. *Journal of General Internal Medicine, 14*(1), S26–S33. doi:10.1046/j.1525-1497.1999.00267.x PMID:9933492

Graham, R., Berkowitz, B., Blum, R., Bockting, W., Bradford, J., de Vries, B., & Makadon, H. (2011). The health of lesbian, gay, bisexual, and transgender people: Building a foundation for better understanding. Washington, DC: Institute of Medicine.

Graham, E. E., Papa, M. J., & Brooks, G. P. (1992). Functions of humor in conversation: Conceptualization and measurement. *Western Journal of Communication, 56*(2), 161–183. doi:10.1080/10570319209374409

Gramling, D., & Gramling, R. (2012). Laughing at the dark: Tactical humor for autonomous decision making in serious illness. *Journal of Palliative Medicine*, *15*(11), 1170–1172. doi:10.1089/jpm.2012.0279 PMID:23116272

Granek-Catarivas, M., Goldstein-Ferber, S., Azuri, Y., Vinker, S., & Kahan, E. (2005). Use of humour in primary care: Different perceptions among patients and physicians. *Postgraduate Medical Journal*, *81*(952), 126–130. doi:10.1136/pgmj.2004.019406 PMID:15701747

Greene, K. (2009). An integrated model of health disclosure decision-making. In T. D. Afifi & W. A. Afifi (Eds.), *Uncertainty and information regulation in interpersonal contexts: Theories and applications* (pp. 226–253). Routledge.

Grice, H. P. (1975). Logic and conversation. In P. Cole & J. Morgan (Eds.), Syntax and semantics (Vol. 3, pp. 41–58). Academic Press.

Gruner, C. R. (1997). *The game of humor: A comprehensive theory of why we laugh.* Transaction Publishers.

Grunloh, C., Myreteg, G., Cajander, A., & Rexhepi, H. (2018). "Why do they need to check me?" Patient participation through ehealth and the doctor-patient relationship: Qualitative study. *Journal of Medical Internet Research*, *20*(1), 1–14. doi:10.2196/jmir.8444 PMID:29335237

Gunnery, R., & Ruben, M. A. (2015). Perceptions of Duchenne and non-Duchenne smiles: A meta-analysis. *Cognition and Emotion*, *30*(3), 501–515. doi:10.1080/02699931.2015.1018817 PMID:25787714

Haakana, M. (2002). Laughter in medical interactions: From quantification to analysis, and back. *Journal of Sociolinguistics*, *6*(2), 207–235. doi:10.1111/1467-9481.00185

Haidet, P. (2007). Jazz and the 'art' of medicine: Improvisation in the medical encounter. *Annals of Family Medicine*, *5*(2), 164–169. doi:10.1370/afm.624 PMID:17389542

Ha, J. F., & Longnecker, N. (2010). Doctor-patient communication: A review. *The Ochsner Journal*, *10*(1), 38–43. PMID:21603354

Hall, J. A., Roter, D. L., & Rand, C. S. (1981). Communication of affect between patient and physician. *Journal of Health and Social Behavior*, *22*(1), 18–30. doi:10.2307/2136365 PMID:7240703

Hampes, W. P. (2001). Relation between humor and empathic concern. *Psychological Reports*, *88*(1), 241–244. doi:10.2466/pr0.2001.88.1.241 PMID:11293036

Hardy, C. (2020). Humor and sympathy in medical practice. *Medicine, Health Care and Philosophy, 23*(2), 179-190. doi:10.100711019-019-09928-0

Harmon, G., Lefante, J., & Krousel-Wood, M. (2006). Overcoming barriers: The role of providers in improving patient adherence to antihypertensive medications. *Current Opinion in Cardiology*, *21*(4), 310–315. doi:10.1097/01.hco.0000231400.10104.e2 PMID:16755199

Hasan, H., & Hasan, T. F. (2009). Laugh yourself into a healthier person: A cross cultural analysis of the effects of varying levels of laughter on health. *International Journal of Medical Sciences*, *6*(4), 200–211. doi:10.7150/ijms.6.200 PMID:19652724

Haydon, G., van der Reit, P., & Browne, G. (2015). A narrative inquiry: Humour and gender differences in the therapeutic relationship between nurses and their patients. *Contemporary Nurse*, *50*(2-3), 214–226. doi:10.1080/10376178.2015.1021436 PMID:26073613

Haydon, G., & van der Riet, P. (2014). A narrative inquiry: How do nurses respond to patients' use of humour? *Contemporary Nurse*, *46*(2), 197–205. doi:10.5172/conu.2014.46.2.197 PMID:24787253

Hayes-Bautista, D. E. (1976). Termination of the patient-practitioner relationship: Divorce, patient style. *Journal of Health and Social Behavior*, *17*(1), 12–21. doi:10.2307/2136463 PMID:1270781

Haynes, R. B., Taylor, D. W., & Sackett, D. L. (1979). *Compliance in health care*. John Hopkins University Press.

Heaney, C. A., & Isreal, B. A. (2008). Social networks and social support. In K. Glanz, B. K. Rimer, & K. Viswanath (Eds.), *Health behavior and health education: Theory, research, and practice* (4th ed., pp. 189–210). Jossey-Bass.

Hehl, F.-J., & Ruch, W. (1985). The location of sense of humor within comprehensive personality spaces: An exploratory study. *Personality and Individual Differences*, *6*(6), 703–715. doi:10.1016/0191-8869(85)90081-9

Heiss, S. N., & Carmack, H. J. (2012). Knock, knock; Who's there? Making sense of organizational entrance through humor. *Management Communication Quarterly*, *26*(1), 106–132. doi:10.1177/0893318911414914

Held, V. (2006). *The ethics of care: Personal, political, and global*. Oxford University Press.

HelmB. (2017, August 11). *Love*. https://plato.stanford.edu/entries/love/

Hodson, G., Rush, J., & MacInnis, C. C. (2010). A joke is just a joke (except when it isn't): Cavalier humor beliefs facilitate the expression of group dominance motives. *Journal of Personality and Social Psychology*, *99*(4), 660–682. doi:10.1037/a0019627 PMID:20919777

Hoerger, M., Epstein, R. M., Winters, P. C., Fiscella, K., Duberstein, P. R., Gramling, R., Butow, P. N., Mohile, S. G., Kaesber, P. R., Tang, W., Plumb, S., Walczak, A., Back, A. L., Tancredi, D., Venuti, A., Cipri, C., Escalera, G., Ferro, C., Gaudion, D., ... Kravitz, R. L. (2013). Values and options in cancer care (VOICE): Study design and rationale for a patient-centered communication and decision-making intervention for physicians, patients with advanced cancer, and their caregivers. *BMC Cancer*, *13*(188), 1–14. doi:10.1186/1471-2407-13-188 PMID:23570278

Holahan, C. J., Moos, R. H., & Schaefer, J. A. (1996). Coping, stress resistance, and growth: Conceptualizing adaptive functioning. In M. Zeidner & N. S. Endler (Eds.), *Handbook of Coping: Theory, research, applications* (pp. 24–43). Wiley.

Howland, M., & Simpson, J. A. (2014). Attachment orientations and reactivity to humor in a social support context. *Journal of Social and Personal Relationships*, *31*(1), 114–137. doi:10.1177/0265407513488016

Hudon, C., Fortin, M., Haggerty, J., Loignon, C., Lambert, M., & Poitras, M. E. (2012). Patient-centered care in chronic disease management: A thematic analysis of the literature in family medicine. *Patient Education and Counseling*, *88*(2), 170–176. doi:10.1016/j.pec.2012.01.009 PMID:22360841

Hulin, C., & Judge, T. (2003). Job attitudes. In W. C. Borman, D. R. Ilgen, & R. J. Klimoski (Eds.), *The handbook of psychology: Industrial and organizational psychology* (Vol. 12, pp. 255–276). Wiley. doi:10.1002/0471264385.wei1211

Iannarino, N. T. (2018). "My insides feel like Keith Richards' face": A narrative analysis of humor and biographical disruption in young adults' cancer blogs. *Health Communication*, *33*(10), 1233–1242. doi:10.1080/10410236.2017.1350909 PMID:28825504

Idan, O., Eriksson, M., & Al-Yagon, M. (2017). The salutogenic model: The role of generalized resistance resources. In M. B. Mittelmark, S. Sagy, M. Eriksson, G. F. Bauer, J. M. Pelikan, B. Lindström, & G. A. Espnes (Eds.), *The handbook of sautogenesis* (pp. 57–69). Springer. doi:10.1007/978-3-319-04600-6_7

Jablin, F. M. (1982). Organizational communication: An assimilation approach. In M. E. Roloff & C. R. Berger (Eds.), *Social cognition and communication* (pp. 255–286). Sage Publications.

Jablin, F. M. (1987). Organizational entry, assimilation, and exit. In F. M. Jablin, L. L. Putnam, K. H. Roberts, & L. W. Porter (Eds.), *Handbook of organizational communication: An interdisciplinary perspective* (pp. 679–740). Sage Publications.

Jablin, F. M. (2001). Organizational entry, assimilation, and disengagement/exit. In F. Jablin & L. Putnam (Eds.), *The new handbook of organizational communication: Advances in theory, research, and methods* (pp. 732–818). Sage. doi:10.4135/9781412986243.n19

Jackson, S. W. (1994). Catharsis and abreaction in the history of psychological healing. *The Psychiatric Clinics of North America, 17*(3), 471–491. doi:10.1016/S0193-953X(18)30094-7 PMID:7824376

Jadad, A. R., Rizo, C. A., & Enkin, M. W. (2003). I am a good patient, believe it or not. *BMJ (Clinical Research Ed.), 326*(7402), 1293–1295. doi:10.1136/bmj.326.7402.1293 PMID:12805157

Jaffee, B.-J. (1996). Using laughter as a cathartic process in grief counseling. In J. D. Morgan (Ed.), *Ethical issues in the care of the dying and bereaved aged* (pp. 283–296). Routledge.

Jauhar, S. (2014). *Doctored: The disillusionment of an American physician.* Farrar, Straus & Giroux.

Jensen, P. R. (2018). Undignified dignity: Using humor to manage the stigma of mental illness and homelessness. *Communication Quarterly, 66*(1), 20–37. doi:10.1080/01463373.2017.1325384

Jiang, S. (2019). Pathways linking patient-centered communication to health improvement: A longitudinal study in China. *Journal of Health Communication, 24*(2), 156–164. doi:10.1080/10810730.2019.1587110 PMID:30849289

Johnson, P. (2002). The use of humor and its influences on spirituality and coping in breast cancer survivors. *Oncology Nursing Forum, 29*(4), 691–695. doi:10.1188/02.ONF.691-695 PMID:12011915

Joseph, S., & Sagy, S. (2017). Positive psychology in the context of salutogenesis. In M. B. Mittelmark, S. Sagy, M. Eriksson, G. F. Bauer, J. M. Pelikan, B. Lindström, & G. A. Espnes (Eds.), *The handbook of sautogenesis* (pp. 83–88). Springer. doi:10.1007/978-3-319-04600-6_10

Joshua, A. M., Cotroneo, A., & Clarke, S. (2005). Humor and oncology. *Journal of Clinical Oncology, 23*(3), 645–648. doi:10.1200/JCO.2005.09.064 PMID:15659513

Kaebnick, G. E. (2011, September-October). From the editor: Laughter in the best medicine. *The Hastings Center Report, 41*(5), 2. Retrieved from https://www.jstor.org/stable/41241295

Kant, I. (1996). *Groundwork of the metaphysics of morals* (M. Gregor, Trans.). Cambridge at the University Press.

Kant, I. (1997). *Groundwork for the metaphysics of morals* (M. Gregor, Ed. & Trans.). Cambridge University Press.

Kärtner, J. (2015). The autonomous developmental pathway: The primacy of subjective mental states for human behavior and experience. *Child Development, 86*(4), 1298–1309. doi:10.1111/cdev.12377 PMID:25930102

Kayser, K., Sormanti, M. E., & Strainchamps, E. (1999). Women coping with cancer: The influence of relationship factors on psychosocial adjustment. *Psychology of Women Quarterly, 23*(4), 725–739. doi:10.1111/j.1471-6402.1999.tb00394.x

Keidel, G. C. (2016). Burnout and compassion fatigue among hospice caregivers. *The American Journal of Hospice & Palliative Care, 19*(3), 200–205. doi:10.1177/104990910201900312 PMID:12026044

Keller, A. (2017). *Performing narrative medicine: Understanding familial chronic illness through performance* [Doctoral Dissertation, University of South Florida]. University of South Florida Scholar Commons. https://scholarcommons.usf.edu/etd/6876

Killmister, S. (2010). Dignity: Not such a useless concept. *Journal of Medical Ethics, 36*(3), 160–164. doi:10.1136/jme.2009.031393 PMID:20211996

Kim, J. (2015, February 26). Should health care providers joke about patients? Medical gallows humor can help providers cope, but at what cost? *Psychology Today*. https://www.psychologytoday.com/us/blog/culture-shrink/201502/should-health-care-providers-joke-about-patients

Klitzman, R. L., & Greenberg, J. D. (2002). Patterns of communication between gay and lesbian patients and their health care providers. *Journal of Homosexuality, 42*(4), 65–75. doi:10.1300/J082v42n04_04 PMID:12243485

Knapp, M. L. (1978). *Social intercourse: From greeting to goodbye*. Allyn and Bacon.

Knox, S., & Hill, C. E. (2003). Therapist self-disclosure: Research-based suggestions for practitioners. *Journal of Clinical Psychology, 59*(5), 529–539. doi:10.1002/jclp.10157 PMID:12696129

Konaszewski, K., Kolemba, M., & Niesiobędzka, M. (2019). Resilience, sense of coherence and self-efficacy as predictors of stress coping style among university students. *Current Psychology*, 1–11. doi:10.100712144-019-00363-1

Kramer, M. (2004). *Managing uncertainty in organizational communication*. Erlbaum.

Kuiper, B., & Borowicz-Sibenik, M. (2005). A good sense of humor doesn't always help: Agency and communion as moderators of psychological well-being. *Personality and Individual Differences, 38*(2), 365–377. doi:10.1016/j.paid.2004.04.015

Kuiper, N. A. (2012). Humor and resiliency: Towards a process model of coping and growth. *Europe's Journal of Psychology, 8*(3), 475–491. doi:10.5964/ejop.v8i3.464

Kuiper, N., Grimshaw, M., Leite, C., & Kirsh, G. (2004). Humor is not always the best medicine: Specific components of sense of humor and psychological well-being. *Humor: International Journal of Humor Research, 17*(1), 135–168. doi:10.1515/humr.2004.002

Kurtz, L. E., & Algoe, S. B. (2017). When sharing a laugh means sharing more: Testing the role of shared laughter on short-term interpersonal consequences. *Journal of Nonverbal Behavior, 41*(1), 45–65. doi:10.100710919-016-0245-9

Lancaster, J. (2020). *Welcome to the United States of anxiety: Observations from a reforming neurotic*. Little A.

Larson, G. (1990). *Weiner dog art: A Far Side collection* (Vol. 15). FarWorks.

Lawton, R., Johnson, J., Janes, G., Foy, R., & Simms-Ellis, R. (2019). Supporting doctors who make mistakes. *British Medical Journal, 365*, L2161. doi:10.1136/bmj.l2161 PMID:31101605

Lazarus, R. S., & Folkman, S. (1984). *Stress, appraisal, and coping*. Springer.

Lazarus, R. S., & Folkman, S. (1991). The concept of coping. In A. Monat & R. S. Lazarus (Eds.), *Stress and coping: An anthology* (pp. 189–206). Columbia University Press.

Lee, C. Y., Chiang, Y. C., Li, A., Li, X., Wu, Y. T., Lin, Y. J., Zhao, Y., & Zhang, X. (2020). Influence of humor expression on suicidal ideation among adolescents: Mediating effects of depressive emotion and positive emotion. *BMC Psychiatry, 20*(1), 421. doi:10.118612888-020-02814-7 PMID:32842996

Lee, J. Y., Slater, M. D., & Tchernev, J. (2015). Self-deprecating humor versus other-deprecating humor in health messages. *Journal of Health Communication, 20*(10), 1185–1195. doi:10.1080/10810730.2015.1018591 PMID:26020507

Lefcourt, H. M., & Martin, R. A. (1986). *Humor and life stress: Antidote to adversity*. SpringerVerlag. doi:10.1007/978-1-4612-4900-9

Lefcourt, H. M., & Thomas, S. (1998). Humor and stress revisited. In W. Ruch (Ed.), *The sense of humor: Explorations of a personality characteristic* (pp. 179–202). De Gruyter Mouton. doi:10.1515/9783110804607.179

Leiber, D. B. (1986). Laughter and humor in critical care. *Dimensions of Critical Care Nursing*, *5*(3), 162–170. doi:10.1097/00003465-198605000-00006 PMID:3635471

Lett, H. S., Blumenthal, J. A., Babyak, M. A., Catellier, D. J., Carney, R. M., Berkman, L. F., Burg, J. A., Mitchell, P., Jaffe, A. S., & Schneiderman, N. (2009). Dimensions of social support and depression in patients at increased psychosocial risk recovering from myocardial infarction. *International Journal of Behavioral Medicine*, *16*(3), 248–258. doi:10.100712529-009-9040-x PMID:19288205

Levinson, W., Roter, D., Mullooly, J., Dull, V., & Frankel, R. (1997). Physician-patient communication: The relationship with malpractice claims among primary care physicians and surgeons. *Journal of the American Medical Association*, *277*(7), 533–559. doi:10.1001/jama.1997.03540310051034 PMID:9032162

Lewis, C. S. (2017). *The four loves*. HarperOne.

Lingard, L. (2013). Language matters: Towards an understanding of silence and humour in medical education. *Medical Education*, *47*(1), 40–48. doi:10.1111/medu.12098 PMID:23278824

Lintott, S. (2016). Superiority in humor theory. *The Journal of Aesthetics and Art Criticism*, *74*(4), 347–358. doi:10.1111/jaac.12321

Literary Devices Editors. (2020, November 12). *Sarcasm - definition and examples of sarcasm*. https://literarydevices.net/sarcasm/

Little, M., Jordens, C. F. C., Paul, K., Sayers, E., & Sriskandarajah, D. (2000). Face, honor and dignity in the context of colon cancer. *The Journal of Medical Humanities*, *21*(4), 229–243. doi:10.1023/A:1009077209274

Liu, Y. P., Sun, L., Wu, X. F., Yang, Y., Zhang, C. T., Zhou, H. L., & Quan, X. Q. (2017). Use of humour in medical education: A survey of students and teachers at a medical school in China. *BMJ Open*, *7*(11), e018853. doi:10.1136/bmjopen-2017-018853 PMID:29187417

LoBue, V. (2019). *9 months in, 9 months out: A scientist's tale of pregnancy and parenthood*. Oxford University Press. doi:10.1093/oso/9780190863388.001.0001

Locke, E. A. (1976). The nature and causes of job satisfaction. In M. D. Dunnette (Ed.), *The Handbook of industrial and organizational psychology* (pp. 1297–1343). Rand McNaly.

Lockwood, N. L., & Yoshimura, S. M. (2014). The heart of the matter: The effects of humor on well-being during recovery from cardiovascular disease. *Health Communication*, *29*(4), 410–420. doi:10.1080/10410236.2012.762748 PMID:23829386

Low, L., Goodenough, B., Fletcher, J., Xu, K., Casey, A., Chenoweth, L., Fleming, R., Spitzer, P., Bell, J., & Brodaty, H. (2014). The effects of humor therapy on nursing home residents measured using observational methods: The SMILE cluster randomized trial. *Journal of the American Medical Directors Association*, *15*(8), 564–569. doi:10.1016/j.jamda.2014.03.017 PMID:24814320

Lugones, M. (1987). Playfulness, "world"-travelling, and loving perception. *Hypatia*, *2*(2), 3–19. doi:10.1111/j.1527-2001.1987.tb01062.x

Lynch, O. H. (2002). Humorous communication: Finding a place for humor in communication research. *Communication Theory*, *12*(4), 423–445. doi:10.1111/j.1468-2885.2002.tb00277.x

Lyons, R. F., Mickelson, K. D., Sullivan, M. J. L., & Coyne, J. C. (1998). Coping as a communal process. *Journal of Social and Personal Relationships, 15*(5), 579–605. doi:10.1177/0265407598155001

Maccarone, E. M. (2010). Ethical responsibilities to subjects and documentary filmmaking. *Journal of Mass Media Ethics, 25*(3), 192–206. doi:10.1080/08900523.2010.497025

Mahvar, T., Mohammadi, N., Seyedfatem, N., & Vedadhir, A. (2020). Interpersonal communication among critical care nurses: An ethnographic study. *Journal of Caring Sciences, 9*(1), 57–64. doi:10.34172/jcs.2020.009 PMID:32296660

Martin, R. A., & Ford, T. (2018). The psychology of humor: An integrative approach (2nd ed.). Elsevier Science & Technology.

Martin, C. J. H. (2011). Transactional analysis: A method of analysing communication. *British Journal of Midwifery, 19*(9), 587–593. doi:10.12968/bjom.2011.19.9.587

Martin, R. A. (1996). The situational humor response questionnaire (SHRQ) and coping humor scale (CHS): A decade of research findings. *Humor: International Journal of Humor Research, 9*(3-4), 251–272. doi:10.1515/humr.1996.9.3-4.251

Martin, R. A. (2008). Humor and health. In V. Raskin (Ed.), *The primer of humor research* (pp. 479–521). Mouton de Gruyter. doi:10.1515/9783110198492.479

Martin, R. A. (2019). Humor. In M. W. Gallagher & S. J. Lopez (Eds.), *Positive psychological assessment: A handbook of models and measures* (pp. 305–316). American Psychological Association. doi:10.1037/0000138-019

Martin, R. A., Puhlik-Doris, P., Larsen, G., Gray, J., & Weir, K. (2003). Individual differences in uses of humor and their relation to psychological well-being: Development of the Humor Styles Questionnaire. *Journal of Research in Personality, 37*(1), 48–75. doi:10.1016/S0092-6566(02)00534-2

Marx, K. (1844). *Economic and philosophical manuscripts of 1844.* Prometheus.

Maslach, C. (2001). Psychology of Burnout. In *International Encyclopedia of the Social and Behavioral Sciences 2001.* ScienceDirect. Downloaded from https://www-sciencedirect-com.ezproxy.neu.edu/topics/psychology/burnout

Maxwell, W. (2003). The use of gallows humor and dark humor during crisis situations. *International Journal of Emergency Mental Health, 5*(2), 93–98. PMID:12882095

McCornack, S. (2016). *Reflect & relate: An introduction to interpersonal communication.* Bedford/St. Martin's.

McCreaddie, M. (2008, April 23-29). You must be joking. *Nursing Standard, 22*(33), 22–23. doi:10.7748/ns.22.33.22.s26 PMID:18540555

McCreaddie, M., & Payne, S. (2014). Humour in health-care interactions: A risk worth taking. *Health Expectations, 17*(3), 332–344. doi:10.1111/j.1369-7625.2011.00758.x PMID:22212380

McGhee, P. E. (1979). *Humor: Its origin and development.* W. H. Freeman.

McGraw, P. (n.d.). *Humor research lab (HuRl).* http://humorresearchlab.org

McGraw, A. P., & Warren, C. (2010). Benign violations: Making immoral behavior funny. *Psychological Science, 21*(8), 1141–1149. doi:10.1177/0956797610376073 PMID:20587696

McGraw, P., & Warren, C. (2014). Benign violation theory. In S. Attardo (Ed.), *Encyclopedia of Humor Studies* (pp. 75–77). Sage.

McGraw, P., Warren, C., Williams, L., & Leonard, B. (2012). Too close for comfort, or too far to care? Finding humor in distant tragedies and close mishaps. *Psychological Science*, *23*(10), 1215–1223. doi:10.1177/0956797612443831 PMID:22941877

Mead, N., & Bower, P. (2000). Measuring patient-centeredness: A comparison of three observation- based instruments. *Patient Education and Counseling*, *39*(1), 71–80. https://doi.org/10.1016/S0738-3991(99)00092-0

Meisenbach, R. J. (2010). Stigma management communication: A theory and agenda for applied research on how individuals manage moments of stigmatized identity. *Journal of Applied Communication Research*, *38*(3), 268–292. doi:10.1080/00909882.2010.490841

Meluch, A. L. (2018). "Above and beyond": An exploratory study of breast cancer patient accounts of healthcare provider information-giving practices and informational support. *Qualitative Research in Medicine & Healthcare, 2*(2), 113-120. doi:10.4081/qrmh.2018.7387

Meyer, J. (2017). *Understanding humor through communication: Why be funny, anyway?* Lexington Books.

Meyer, J. C. (2000). Humor as a double-edged sword: Four functions of humor in communication. *Communication Theory*, *10*(3), 310–331. doi:10.1111/j.1468-2885.2000.tb00194.x

Millard, W. B. (2015). Gallows humor, fearmongering continue to spread. *Annals of Emergency Medicine*, *65*(2), 21A–22A. doi:10.1016/j.annemergmed.2014.12.022 PMID:25756100

Miller, L. E. (2009). *Cancer survivorship: Couples' communication and adjustment after treatment is complete* [Doctoral Dissertation, University of Illinois at Urbana-Champaign]. IDEALS Dissertation Publishing. http://hdl.handle.net/2142/87548

Miller, L. E. (2014a). Communication dilemmas in the context of cancer: Survivors' and partners' strategies for communicating throughout survivorship. *Issues in Mental Health Nursing*, *35*(12), 914–923. doi:10.3109/01612840.2014.934939 PMID:25426747

Miller, L. E. (2014b). Uncertainty and information seeking in cancer survivorship. *Health Communication*, *29*(3), 233–243. doi:10.1080/10410236.2012.739949 PMID:23682727

Mills, M. E., & Sullivan, K. (1999). The importance of information giving for patients newly diagnosed with cancer: A review of literature. *Journal of Clinical Nursing*, *8*(6), 631–642. https://doi.org/10.1046/j.1365-2702.1999.00296.x

Montgomery, K. (2006). *How doctors think: Clinical judgment and the practice of medicine*. Oxford University Press.

Montori, V. (2017). *Why we revolt: A patient revolution for careful and kind care*. Patient Revolution.

Mordechai, G. (2014). Friendship, intimacy and humor. *Educational Philosophy and Theory*, *46*(2), 162–174. doi:10.1080/00131857.2012.721732

Morreall, J. (1983). *Taking laughter seriously*. State University of New York Press.

Morreall, J. (1986). *The philosophy of laughter and humor (SUNY Series in Philosophy)*. State University of New York Press.

Morreall, J. (2009). *Comic relief*. Wiley Blackwell. doi:10.1002/9781444307795

Morreall, J. (2020). Philosophy of humor. In *The Stanford Encyclopedia of Philosophy* (Fall 2020 Edition). Stanford University. https://plato.stanford.edu/archives/fall2020/entries/humor/

Morreall, J. (2020). Philosophy of humor. In E. N. Zalta (Ed.), *The Stanford encyclopedia of philosophy (online)*. The Metaphysics Research Lab.

Morrissey, C. (2016). The value of dignity in and for bioethics: Rethinking the terms of the debate. *Theoretical Medicine and Bioethics*, *37*(3), 173–192. doi:10.100711017-016-9368-6 PMID:27301253

Neeman, N., Isaac, T., Leveille, S., Dimonda, C., Shin, J., Aronson, M., & Freedman, S. (2012). Improving doctor-patient communication in the outpatient setting using a facilitation tool: A preliminary study. *International Journal for Quality in Health Care*, *24*(4), 357–364. doi:10.1093/intqhc/mzr081 PMID:22190587

Neuling, S. J., & Winefield, H. R. (1988). Social support and recovery after surgery for breast cancer: Frequency and correlates of supportive behaviors by family, friends and surgeon. *Social Science & Medicine*, *27*(4), 385–392. https://doi.org/10.1016/0277-9536(88)90273-0

Nikopoulos, J. (2017). The stability of laughter. *Humor: International Journal of Humor Research*, *30*(1), 1–21. doi:10.1515/humor-2016-0062

Nipp, R. D., El-Jawahri, A., Fishbeing, J. N., Eusebio, J., Stagl, J. M., Gallagher, E. R., Park, E. R., Jackson, V. A., Pirl, W. F., Greer, J. A., & Temel, J. S. (2016). The relationship between coping strategies, quality of life, and mood in patients with incurable cancer. *Cancer*, *122*(13), 2110–2116. doi:10.1002/cncr.30025 PMID:27089045

Noddings, N. (1984). *Caring: A feminine approach to ethics and moral obligation*. University of California Press.

Noland, C., & Carl, W. J. (2006). It's not our ass: Medical resident sense-making regarding lawsuits. *Health Communication*, *20*(1), 81–91. doi:10.120715327027hc2001_8 PMID:16813491

Noland, C., & Hoppmann, M. (2020). Stop! You're killing me: Food addiction and comedy. In P. Opplinger & E. Shouse (Eds.), *The dark side of stand-up comedy* (pp. 129–149). Palgrave MacMillian. doi:10.1007/978-3-030-37214-9_7

Noltensmeyer, C. J., & Meisenbach, R. J. (2016). Emerging patterns of stigma management communication among burn survivors and relational partners. *The American Behavioral Scientist*, *60*(11), 1378–1397. doi:10.1177/0002764216657384

Nussbaum, M. (1985). "Finely aware and richly responsible": Moral attention and the moral task of literature. *The Journal of Philosophy*, *82*(10), 516–529. doi:10.5840/jphil1985821024

Ogden, S. N., Scheffey, K. L., Blosnich, J. R., & Dichter, M. E. (2020). "Do I feel safe revealing this information to you?": Patient perspectives on disclosing sexual orientation and gender identity in healthcare. *Journal of American College Health*, *68*(6), 617–623. doi:10.1080/07448481.2019.1583663 PMID:32897171

Olson, M. L., Hugelshofer, D. S., Kwon, P., & Reff, R. C. (2005). Rumination and dysphoria: The buffering role of adaptive forms of humor. *Personality and Individual Differences*, *39*(8), 1419–1428. doi:10.1016/j.paid.2005.05.006

Osincup, P. (2020). How to use humor in clinical settings. *AMA Journal of Ethics*, *22*(7), 588–595. doi:10.1001/amajethics.2020.588 PMID:32744227

Papousek, I., Schulter, G., Lackner, H. K., Samson, A., & Freudenthaler, H. H. (2014). Experimentally observed responses to humor are related to individual differences in emotion perception and regulation in everyday life. *Humor: International Journal of Humor Research*, *27*(2), 271–286. doi:10.1515/humor-2014-0018

Parkes, C. M. (1972). *Bereavement: Studies of grief in adult life*. International Universities Press.

Parks, M. R., & Adelman, M. B. (1983). Communication networks and the development of romantic relationships: An expansion of uncertainty reduction theory. *Human Communication Research*, *10*(1), 85–107. doi:10.1111/j.1468-2958.1983.tb00004.x

Parsons, N. G., Kinsman, S. B., Bosk, C. L., Sankar, P., & Ubel, P. A. (2001). Between two worlds: Medical student perceptions of humor and slang in the hospital setting. *Journal of General Internal Medicine*, *16*(8), 544–549. doi:10.1046/j.1525-1497.2001.016008544.x PMID:11556931

Pennebaker, J. W., & Harber, K. D. (1993). A social stage model of collective coping: The Loma Prieta earthquake and the Persian Gulf War. *The Journal of Social Issues*, *49*(4), 125–145. doi:10.1111/j.1540-4560.1993.tb01184.x

Penson, R. T., Partridge, R. A., Rudd, P., Seiden, M. V., Nelson, J. E., Chabner, B. A., & Lynch, T. J. Jr. (2005). Laughter: The best medicine? *The Oncologists*, *10*(8), 651–660. doi:10.1634/theoncologist.10-8-651 PMID:16177290

Perseus Greek Word Study Tool. (n.d.). Retrieved January 15, 2021, from http://www.perseus.tufts.edu/hopper/morph?l=%E1%BC%90%CF%80%CE%AF%CE%BA%CF%84%CE%B7%CF%84%CE%BF%CF%82&la=greek#lexicon

Petrilli, C., Saint, S., Jennings, J., Caruso, A., Kuhn, L., Snyder, A., & Chopra, V. (2018). Understanding patient preference for physician attire: A cross-sectional observational study of 10 academic medical centres in the USA. *BMJ Open*, *8*(5), E021239. doi:10.1136/bmjopen-2017-021239 PMID:29844101

Phillips, K. A., Ospina, N. S., Rodriguez-Gutierrez, R., Castaneda-Guarderas, A., Gionfriddo, M. R., Branda, M., & Montori, V. (2018). Humor during clinical practice: Analysis of recorded clinical encounters. *Journal of the American Board of Family Medicine*, *31*(2), 270–278. doi:10.3122/jabfm.2018.02.170313 PMID:29535244

Phua, D., Tang, H., & Tham, K. (2005). Coping responses of emergency physicians and nurses to the 2003 severe acute respiratory syndrome outbreak. *Academic Emergency Medicine*, *12*(4), 322–328. doi:10.1197/j.aem.2004.11.015 PMID:15805323

Piemonte, N. M. (2015). Last laughs: Gallows humor and medical education. *The Journal of Medical Humanities*, *36*(4), 375–390. doi:10.100710912-015-9338-4 PMID:26062447

Pigliucci, M. (n.d.). Stoicism. *Internet encyclopedia of philosophy*. https://iep.utm.edu/stoicism/

Pigliucci, M. (2017). *How to be a stoic*. Basic Books.

Pinna, M. Á. C., Mahtani-Chugani, V., Sánchez Correas, M. Á., & Sanz Rubiales, A. (2018). The use of humor in palliative care: A systematic literature review. *The American Journal of Hospice & Palliative Care*, *35*(10), 1342–1354. doi:10.1177/1049909118764414 PMID:29587520

Platt, F. W., & Keating, K. N. (2007). Differences in physician and patient perceptions of uncomplicated UTI symptom severity: Understanding the communication gap. *International Journal of Clinical Practice*, *61*(2), 303–308. doi:10.1111/j.1742-1241.2006.01277.x PMID:17263717

Politi, M., & Street, R. L. (2011). Patient-centered communication during collaborative decision making. In T. L. Thompson, R. Parrott, & J. F. Nussbaum (Eds.), *The Routledge handbook of health communication* (2nd ed., pp. 399–414). Routledge.

Porteous, J. (1988). Humor as a process of defense: The evolution of laughing. *Humor: International Journal of Humor Research*, *1*(1), 63–80. doi:10.1515/humr.1988.1.1.63

Post, D. (2000). The effects of communication skills training on patients' participation during medical interviews. *Patient Education and Counseling*, *41*(2), 209–222. doi:10.1016/S0738-3991(00)00093-8 PMID:12024545

Priego-Valverde, B. (2009). Failed humor in conversation. In N. R. Norrick & D. Chiaro (Eds.), *Humor in interaction* (pp. 165–186). John Bejamins Publishing Company. doi:10.1075/pbns.182.08pri

Ramirez, A. Jr, Walther, J. B., Burgoon, J. K., & Sunnafrank, M. (2002). Information-seeking strategies, uncertainty, and computer-mediated communication: Toward a conceptual model. *Human Communication Research*, *28*(2), 213–228. doi:10.1111/j.1468-2958.2002.tb00804.x

Randall, T. C., & Wearn, A. M. (2005). Receiving bad news: Patients with haematological cancer reflect upon their experience. *Palliative Medicine*, *19*(8), 594–601. doi:10.1191/0269216305pm1080oa PMID:16450876

Reiling, J. (2020). The "sense" of humor—Art & science. *Journal of the American Medical Association*, *323*(23), 2435. doi:10.1001/jama.2019.13477 PMID:32543676

Repede, E. (2008). All that holds: A story of healing. *Journal of Holistic Nursing*, *26*(3), 226–232. doi:10.1177/0898010108323012 PMID:18755883

Revenson, T. A., Kayser, K., & Bodenmann, G. (2005). Introduction. In T. A. Revenson, K. Kayser, & G. Bodenmann (Eds.), *Couples coping with stress: Emerging perspectives on dyadic coping* (pp. 3–10). American Psychological Association. doi:10.1037/11031-000

Rhys, C. S., & Schmidt-Renfree, N. (2000). Facework, social politeness and the Alzheimer's patient. *Clinical Linguistics & Phonetics*, *14*(7), 533–543. doi:10.1080/026992000750020350

Richards, R. (2013). *A philosopher looks at the sense of humor*. Healing Time Books.

Riessman, C. K. (1993). *Narrative analysis*. Sage Publications.

Robinson, J. D., Turner, J. W., Levine, B., & Tian, Y. (2011). Expanding the walls of the health care encounter: Support outcomes of patients online. *Health Communication*, *26*(2), 125–134. https://doi.org/10.1080/10410236.2010.541990

Romundstad, S., Svebak, S., Holen, A., & Holmen, J. (2016). A 15-year follow-up study of sense of hand causes of mortality: The Nord-Trondelag Health Study. *Psychosomatic Medicine*, *78*(3), 345–353. doi:10.1097/PSY.0000000000000275 PMID:26569539

Rossman, K., Salamanca, P., & Macapagal, K. (2017). A qualitative study examining young adults' experiences of disclosure and nondisclosure of LGBTQ identity to health care providers. *Journal of Homosexuality*, *64*(10), 1390–1410. doi:10.1080/00918369.2017.1321379 PMID:28459379

Roter, D. L., & Hall, J. A. (2011). How medical interaction shapes and reflects the physician–patient relationship. In T. L. Thompson, R. Parrott, & J. F. Nussbaum (Eds.), *The Routledge handbook of health communication* (pp. 83–96). Routledge.

Ruch, W., & Köhler, G. (2007). A temperamental approach to humour. In W. Ruch (Ed.), *The sense of humor: Explorations of a personality characteristic* (pp. 203–228). De Gruyter Mouton. doi:10.1515/9783110804607-011

Rushton, C. H., Reina, M. L., & Reina, D. S. (2007). Building trustworthy relationships with critically ill patients and families. *AACN Advanced Critical Care*, *18*(1), 19–30. doi:10.4037/15597768-2007-1004 PMID:17284945

Sala, R., Krupet, E., & Roter, D. (2002). Satisfaction and the use of humor by physicians and patients. *Psychology & Health*, *17*(3), 269–280. doi:10.1080/08870440290029520

Sanders, L., Fortin, A., & Schiff, G. (2020). Connecting with patients—The missing links. *Journal of the American Medical Association*, *323*(1), 33–34. doi:10.1001/jama.2019.20153 PMID:31910264

Santos, V., Paes, F., Pereira, V., Arias-Carrion, O., Silva, A. C., Carta, M. G., Nardi, A. E., & Machado, S. (2013). The role of positive emotion and contributions of positive psychology in depression treatment: Systematic review. *Clinical Practice and Epidemiology in Mental Health*, *9*(1), 221–237. doi:10.2174/1745017901309010221 PMID:24358052

Sarason, B. R., Sarason, I. G., & Pierce, G. R. (1990). Traditional views of social support and their impact on assessment. In B. R. Sarason, I. G. Sarason, & G. R. Pierce (Eds.), *Social support: An interactional view* (pp. 9–25). Wiley.

Sastre, M. T. M., Sorum, P. C., & Mullet, E. (2011). Breaking bad news: The patient's viewpoint. *Health Communication, 26*(7), 649–655. doi:10.1080/10410236.2011.561919 PMID:21598151

Saunders, P. A. (1998). "You're out of your mind!": Humor as a face-saving strategy during neuropsychological examinations. *Health Communication, 10*(4), 357–372. doi:10.120715327027hc1004_4 PMID:16370980

Scheff, T. J., & Bushnell, D. D. (1984). A theory of catharsis. *Journal of Research in Personality, 18*(2), 238–264. doi:10.1016/0092-6566(84)90032-1

Scholl, J. C. (2007). The use of humor to promote patient-centered care. *Journal of Applied Communication Research, 35*(2), 156–176. doi:10.1080/00909880701262658

Scholl, J. C., & Ragan, S. L. (2003). The use of humor in promoting positive provider-patient interactions in a hospital rehabilitation unit. *Health Communication, 15*(3), 319–330. https://doi.org/10.1207/S15327027HC1503_4

Schöpf, A. C., Martin, G. S., & Keating, M. A. (2016). Humor as a communication strategy in provider-patient communication in a chronic care setting. *Qualitative Health Research, 27*(3), 1–17. 10.1177%2F1049732315620773 PMID:26717942

Schöpf, A. C., Martin, G. S., & Keating, M. A. (2017). Humor as a communication strategy in provider–patient communication in a chronic care setting. *Qualitative Health Research, 27*(3), 374–390. doi:10.1177/1049732315620773 PMID:26717942

Schultes, L. S. (1997). Humor with hospice clients: You're putting me on. *Home Healthcare Nurse, 15*(8), 561–566. https://doi.org/10.1097/00004045-199708000-00013

Schweikart, S. J. (2020). Could humor in health care become malpractice? *AMA Journal of Ethics, 22*(7), 596–601. doi:10.1001/amajethics.2020.596 PMID:32744228

Scott, A. M., Harrington, N. G., & Spencer, E. (2020). Primary care physicians' strategic pursuit of multiple goals in cost-of-care conversations with patients. *Health Communication, 0*(0), 1–13. doi:10.1080/10410236.2020.1723051 PMID:32019346

Seale, C. (2003). Health and media: An overview. *Sociology of Health & Illness, 25*(6), 513–531. doi:10.1111/1467-9566.t01-1-00356 PMID:12919443

Seneca, L. A. (1882). *On the happy life* (R. L'Estrange Trans). Independently Published. (Original work published in 58)

Seneca, L. A. (1910). *Minor dialogs together with the dialog "On Clemency"* (A. Stewart, Trans.). George Bell and Sons. (Original work published in 40)

Shannon, C. E., & Weaver, W. (1949). *The mathematical theory of communication.* University of Illinois Press.

Sherif, C. W., Sherif, M., & Nebergall, R. E. (1965). *Attitudes and attitude change: The social judgment-involvement approach.* W. B. Saunders.

Sherif, M. (1936). *The psychology of social norms.* Harper.

Sidelinger, R. J. (2014). Using relevant humor to moderate inappropriate conversations: Maintaining student communication satisfaction in the classroom. *Communication Research Reports, 31*(3), 292–301. doi:10.1080/08824096.2014.924339

Sliter, M., Kale, A., & Yuan, Z. (2014). Is humor the best medicine? The buffering effect of coping humor on traumatic stressors in firefighters. *Journal of Organizational Behavior, 35*(2), 257–272. doi:10.1002/job.1868

Sloan, A. G., & Knowles, A. (2013). Improving communication between healthcare providers and cancer patients: A pilot study. *Journal of Communication in Healthcare*, *6*(4), 208–215. https://doi.org/10.1179/1753807613Y.0000000040

Smith, P. S., Parton, D. (Writers) & Fleming, A. (Director). (2019). Jolene [Netflix series episode]. In S. Haskell (Producer), Dolly Parton's Heartstrings. Los Gatos, CA: Netflix Studios.

Smith, C. M., & Powell, L. (1988). The use of disparaging humor by group leaders. *The Southern Speech Communication Journal*, *53*(3), 279–292. doi:10.1080/10417948809372729

Smith, R. A., & Applegate, A. (2018). Mental health stigma and communication and their intersections with education. *Communication Education*, *67*(3), 382–393. doi:10.1080/03634523.2018.1465988 PMID:31354181

Smuts, A. (2009). Do moral flaws enhance amusement? *American Philosophical Quarterly*, *46*(2), 151–162.

Sobel, R. K. (2006). Does laughter make good medicine? *The New England Journal of Medicine*, *354*(11), 1114–1115. doi:10.1056/NEJMp058089 PMID:16540611

Sokol, D. K. (2012). No laughing matter. *British Journal of Medicine*, *344*(e2119), 1–2. doi:10.1136/bmj.e2119 PMID:22438391

Sousa, L., Marques-Vieira, C., Antunes, A. V., Frade, M., Severino, S., & Valentim, O. S. (2019). Humor intervention in the nurse-patient interaction. *Revista Brasileira de Enfermagem*, *72*(4), 1078–1085. doi:10.1590/0034-7167-2018-0609 PMID:31432968

Sparks, L., Travis, S. S., & Thompson, S. R. (2005). Listening for the communicative signals of humor, narratives, and self-disclosure in the family caregiver interview. *Health & Social Work*, *30*(4), 340–343. doi:10.1093/hsw/30.4.340 PMID:16323726

Spelman, E. V. (1978). On treating persons as persons. *Ethics*, *88*(2), 150–161. doi:10.1086/292066

Spencer, H. (1911). On the physiology of laughter. Essays on education, etc. *Dent, Contemporary Dentistry*.

Spradley, E. L. (2020). Storying clinical interactions: Narrative medicine as an artistic intervention in medical training and education. In K. Afary & A. M. Fritz (Eds.), *More than words: Communication research on expressive arts and narrative as forms of healing* (pp. 241–262). Lexington Books.

Steele, B. (2020). "A catharsis for anxieties": Insights from Goffman on the politics of humor. *Global Society*, 1-15. doi:10.1080/13600826.2020.1828296

Stewart, A. L., Napoles-Springer, A., Gregorich, S. E., & Santoyo-Olsson, J. (2007). Interpersonal process of care survey: Patient-reported measures for diverse groups. *Health Services Research*, *42*(3p1), 1235-56. doi:10.1111/j.1475-6773.2006.00637.x

Stewart, A. L., Napoles-Springer, A., Perez-Stable, E. J., Posner, S. F., Bindman, A. B., Pinderhughes, H. L., & Washington, A. E. (1999). Interpersonal processes of care in diverse populations. *The Milbank Quarterly*, *77*(3), 305–339. doi:10.1111/1468-0009.00138 PMID:10526547

Stewart, M. (2001). Towards a global definition of patient centred care. *British Medical Journal*, *322*, 444–445. https://doi.org/10.1136/bmj.322.7284.444

Stewart, M. A. (1995). Effective physician-patient communication and health outcomes: A review. *Canadian Medical Association Journal*, *152*(9), 1423–1433. PMID:7728691

Stewart, M., Brown, J., Donner, A., McWhinney, I., Oates, J., Weston, W., & Jordan, J. (2000). The impact of patient-centered care on outcomes. *The Journal of Family Practice*, *49*(9), 796–804. PMID:11032203

Strick, M., Holland, R. W., Van Baaren, R. B., & Van Knippenberg, A. D. (2009). Finding comfort in a joke: Consolatory effects of humor through cognitive distraction. *Emotion (Washington, D.C.)*, *9*(4), 574–578. doi:10.1037/a0015951 PMID:19653782

Strick, M., Holland, R. W., Van Baaren, R. B., & Van Knippenberg, A. D. (2010). The puzzle of joking: Disentangling the cognitive and affective components of humorous distraction. *European Journal of Social Psychology*, *40*(1), 43–51. doi:10.1002/ejsp.720

Tajfel, H. (1981). *Human groups and social categories: Studies in social psychology*. Cambridge University Press.

Tanay, M. A. L., Roberts, J., & Ream, E. (2013). Humour in adult cancer care: A concept analysis. *Journal of Advanced Nursing*, *69*(9), 2131–2140. doi:10.1111/jan.12059 PMID:23215893

Tanto-Beck, W. (1997). Humor in nursing practice: A phenomenological study. *International Journal of Nursing Studies*, *34*(5), 346–352. doi:10.1016/S0020-7489(97)00026-6 PMID:9559383

Tanveer, F., Shahid, S., & Hafiz, M. M. (2018). Impact of doctor's interpersonal communication skill on patient's satisfaction level. *ISRA Medical Journal*, *10*(5), 306–309.

Taylor, K. (2009). Paternalism, participation and partnership—The evolution of patient centeredness in the consultation. *Patient Education and Counseling*, *74*(2), 150–155. doi:10.1016/j.pec.2008.08.017 PMID:18930624

The Johns Hopkins Hospital. (n.d.). *Reiki*. Available at: https://www.hopkinsmedicine.org/integrative_medicine_digestive_center/services/reiki.html

Thoits, P. A. (1995). Stress, coping, and social support processes: Where are we? What next? *Journal of Health and Social Behavior,* 53-79. doi:10.2307/2626957

Thom, D. H. (2001). Physician behaviors that predict patient trust. *The Journal of Family Practice*, *50*(4), 323–323. PMID:11300984

Thom, D. H., & Campbell, B. (1997). Patient-physician trust: An exploratory study. *The Journal of Family Practice*, *44*(2), 169–176. PMID:9040520

Tomlinson, T. (2015 Sept. 29). Humor in medicine: Nasty, dark, and shades of gray. *Michigan State University's Bioethics in the News.* Retrieved from https://msubioethics.com/2015/09/29/humor-in-medicine/

Tomlinson, T. (2012, May-June). Uncomfortable humor. *The Hastings Center Report*, *42*(3), 9. https://www.jstor.org/stable/23883181 PMID:22670292

Tremblay, M. (2017). Humor in teams: Multilevel relationships between humor climate, inclusion, trust, and citizenship behaviors. *Journal of Business and Psychology*, *32*(4), 363–378. doi:10.100710869-016-9445-x

Tse, M. M., Lo, A. P., Cheng, T. L., Chan, E. K., Chan, A. H., & Chung, H. S. (2010). Humor therapy: Relieving chronic pain and enhancing happiness for older adults. *Journal of Aging Research*, *2010*, 1–9. Advance online publication. doi:10.4061/2010/343574 PMID:21151506

Vallade, J. I., Booth-Butterfield, M., & Vela, L. E. (2013). Taking back power: Using superiority theory to predict humor use following relational transgression. *Western Journal of Communication*, *77*(2), 231–248. doi:10.1080/10570314.2012.669018

Vandenberghe, C., Bentein, K., & Panaccio, A. (2017). Affective commitment to organizations and supervisors and turnover: A role theory perspective. *Journal of Management*, *43*(7), 2090–2117. doi:10.1177/0149206314559779

Veatch, T. C. (1998). A theory of humor. *Humor: International Journal of Humor Research*, *11*(2), 161–215. doi:10.1515/humr.1998.11.2.161

Venetis, M., Chernichky-Karcher, S., & Lillie, H. (2019). Communicating resilience: Predictors and outcomes of dyadic communication resilience processes among both cancer patients and cancer partners. *Journal of Applied Communication Research*, *48*(1), 49–69. doi:10.1080/00909882.2019.1706098

Vergeer, G., & MacRae, A. (1993). Therapeutic use of humor in occupational therapy. *The American Journal of Occupational Therapy*, *47*(8), 678–683. doi:10.5014/ajot.47.8.678 PMID:8352326

Villagran, M., Goldsmith, J., Wittenberg-Lyles, E., & Baldwin, P. (2010). Creating COMFORT: A communication-based model for breaking bad news. *Communication Education*, *59*(3), 220–234. doi:10.1080/03634521003624031

VoxTalk. (2014). *George Carlin near miss*. YouTube. https://www.youtube.com/watch?v=zDKdvTecYAM

Wanzer, M., Booth-Butterfield, M., & Booth-Butterfield, S. (2005). "If we didn't use humor, we'd cry": Humorous coping communication in health care settings. *Journal of Health Communication*, *10*(2), 105–125. doi:10.1080/10810730590915092 PMID:15804903

Warner, S. L. (1991). Humor: A coping response for student nurses. *Archives of Psychiatric Nursing*, *5*(1), 10–16. doi:10.1016/0883-9417(91)90004-O PMID:2039275

Warren, C., & McGraw, A. P. (2015). Differentiating what is humorous from what is not. *Journal of Personality and Social Psychology*, *110*(3), 407–430. doi:10.1037/pspi0000041 PMID:26692355

Watson, K. (2011). Gallows humor in medicine. *The Hastings Center Report*, *41*(5), 37–45. doi:10.1002/j.1552-146X.2011.tb00139.x PMID:21980898

Wear, D., Aultman, J., Zarconi, J., & Varley, J. (2008). Derogatory and cynical humour directed towards patients: Views of residents and attending doctors. *Medical Education*, *43*(1), 34–41. doi:10.1111/j.1365-2923.2008.03171.x PMID:19148979

Weisenberg, M., Tepper, I., & Schwarzwald, J. (1995). Humor as a cognitive technique for increasing pain tolerance. *Pain*, *63*(2), 207–212. doi:10.1016/0304-3959(95)00046-U PMID:8628586

WisemanR. (n.d.). *LaughLab*. https://richardwiseman.wordpress.com/2018/04/17/laughlab/

Wortman, C. B. (1984). Social support and the cancer patient: Conceptual issues and methodological issues. *Cancer*, *53*(10), 2339–2360. doi:10.1002/cncr.1984.53.s10.2339 PMID:6367944

Wrench, J. S., & Booth-Butterfield, M. (2003). Increasing patient satisfaction and compliance: An examination of physician humor orientation, compliance-gaining strategies, and perceived credibility. *Communication Quarterly*, *51*(4), 482–503. doi:10.1080/01463370309370169

Xu, Y., & Burleson, B. R. (2001). Effects of sex, culture, and support type, on perceptions of spousal social support: An assessment of the "Support Gap" hypothesis in early marriage. *Human Communication Research*, *27*(4), 535–566. https://doi.org/10.1111/j.1468-2958.2001.tb00792.x

Yovetich, N. A., Dale, J. A., & Hudak, M. A. (1990). Benefits of humor in reduction of threat-induced anxiety. *Psychological Reports*, *66*(1), 51–58. doi:10.2466/pr0.1990.66.1.51 PMID:2326429

Yue, X. D., Liu, K. W.-Y., Jiang, F., & Hiranandani, N. A. (2014). Humor styles, self-esteem, and subjective happiness. *Psychological Reports*, *115*(2), 517–525. doi:10.2466/07.02.PR0.115c18z6 PMID:25153846

Zagzebski, L. (2001). The uniqueness of persons. *The Journal of Religious Ethics*, *29*(3), 401–423. doi:10.1111/0384-9694.00090

Zautra, A. J., Hall, J. S., & Murray, K. E. (2010). Resilience: A new definition of health for people and communities. In J. R. Reich, A. J. Zautra, & J. S. Hall (Eds.), *Handbook of adult resilience* (pp. 3–30). Guilford Press.

Zillmann, D., Rockwell, S., Schweitzer, K., & Sundar, S. S. (1993). Does humor facilitate coping with physical discomfort? *Motivation and Emotion*, *17*(1), 1–21. doi:10.1007/BF00995204

Zulman, D., Haverfield, M., Shaw, J., Brown-Johnson, C., Schwartz, R., Tierney, A., Zionts, D. L., Safaeinili, N., Fischer, M., Israni, S. T., Asch, S. M., & Verghese, A. (2020). Practices to foster physician presence and connection with patients in the clinical encounter. *Journal of the American Medical Association*, *323*(1), 70–81. doi:10.1001/jama.2019.19003 PMID:31910284

Zweyer, K., Velker, B., & Ruch, W. (2004). Do cheerfulness, exhilaration, and humor production moderate pain tolerance? A FACS study. *Humor: International Journal of Humor Research*, *17*(1), 85–119. doi:10.1515/humr.2004.009

About the Contributors

Michael K. Cundall, Jr. Ph.D., Associate Professor of Philosophy. He has been researching humor for nearly two decades and published on topics ranging from the cognition of humor, racist and ethnic humor, and humor in the workplace. His company, Mirth Management (www.mirthmanagement.co) works with organizations to improve morale, engagement, using humor to empower people to be more creative and engaged in their work. When not teaching or doing research, he can be found woodworking, or doing some less than ready for primetime comedy routines.

Stephanie Kelly, Ph.D., Associate Professor of Communication. She is a presence scholar, meaning she studies the nebulous things that happen in people's minds between a message being sent and received. This means her work spans contexts, but she usually researches interactions that take place in instruction, business, or health. Outside of research, she spends a lot of time reading things that have no contribution to her research whatsoever, preferably with a good monster, vampire, or face character.

***

Susan Avanzino, Ph.D., Associate Professor, California State University, Chico. As a volunteer researcher with EMC for a decade, she has been studying PCC Transformations from a Health and Organizational Communication perspective.

Warren ("Wren") Bareiss researches and teaches about relationships among communication, culture, and health. He is particularly interested in stories that people tell about health and illness. He also regularly leads workshops for nursing students about communication with patients whose first language is other than English. His most recent work explores connections between Buddhist philosophy and health communication.

Regina Beach, MA, Centerstone. She focuses her practice on community mental health.

Maranda Berndt, doctoral student, the Pennsylvania State University. Maranda received her master's degree from North Dakota State University. Her interests include media psychology, body image, mental health, and sexual health.

Carrie H. Cox, Ph.D. (University of Missouri), is an Assistant Professor of Fashion Merchandising at Western Kentucky University where she teaches fashion history, perspectives of dress, clothing and human behavior, textile and apparel quality analysis, and apparel design production. Carrie's research explores 1920s women's dress, Shaker textiles, 1920s women's retail, and the meanings of contemporary, everyday dress. She has also conducted research and curated exhibits on Mrs. A.H. (Carrie) Taylor, a Victorian/Edwardian-era modiste and entrepreneur from Bowling Green, KY.

Stephen A. Cox, Ph.D. (University of Missouri), is an Associate Professor of Organizational Communication and Leadership in Murray State University's Arthur J. Bauernfeind College of Business. Steve's primary research interests include communication processes of organizational innovation, creativity, and employee exit. In addition to publishing in regional, national, and international journals, he has provided training and consulting to healthcare, governmental, educational, and manufacturing organizations.

Elizabeth ("Betsy") Dalton is a health communication researcher and Assistant Professor at Middle Tennessee State University. Some of her recent publications include Dalton, E.D. & Gruber, K. (2021). Being PAL: Uncertainty and coping in r/PregnancyAfterLoss. Health Communication (in press). Dalton, E.D., Pjesivac, I., Eldredge, S., & Miller, L. (2020). From vulnerability to disclosure: A normative approach to understanding trust in obstetric and intrapartum nurse-patient communication. Health Communication, 2, 1-14. Miller, L., Eldredge, S., & Dalton, E.D. (2016). "Pain is what the patient says it is": Nurse-patient communication, information seeking, and pain management. American Journal of Hospice and Palliative Medicine, 34(10), 966-976.

Scott A. Eldredge is an Associate Professor of Communication at Western Carolina University. His research interests include patient-provider interaction and uncertainty management among LGBTQ+ relational partners. Some relevant publications include: Eldredge, S. A., (Forthcoming). Intimacy uncertainty in a post-AIDS culture: HIV and the role it plays as an uninvited third party in serodiscordant relationships. In A. Basu, P. J. Dillon, & A. R. Spieldenner (Eds.), Post-AIDS Discourse in Health Communication: Sociocultural Interpretations Routledge: New York. Dalton, E.D., Pjesivac, I., Eldredge, S. A., & Miller, L. (2020). From vulnerability to disclosure: A normative approach to understanding trust in obstetric and intrapartum nurse-patient communication. Health Communication, 2, 1-14. Eldredge, S. A., Dalton, E. D., & Miller, L. E. (2014). Pain Management as Triadic Interaction: Shifting Alliances in Nurse-Patient-Family-Member Communication. Southern Communication Journal. 79(5), 448-467.

Isaac Evans, MA, NCC, Temp. LPC/MHSP, Tennessee Technological University.

Florian Fischer, Ph.D. He is an expert in public health and researcher at the Institute of Gerontological Health Services and Nursing Research at Ravensburg-Weingarten University of Applied Sciences, Germany. Furthermore, he is affiliated with the Institute of Public Health at Charité – Universitätsmedizin Berlin, Germany. He is interested in studying the effects of humor in health communication.

Annette Folwell, Ph.D., Associate Professor of Communication, University of Idaho. Her current research investigates the lived experiences of first responders; her other publications are in interpersonal communication research, with studies examining deception, family communication, and communication and culture.

Galen Foresman, Ph.D., Professor of Philosophy at North Carolina A&T State University. He's not as funny as he thinks, but he means well.

Brigitte Fosque, Baptist Christian, Pastor, Social Worker, Spiritual Life Coach, Certified Medium and Holy Fire III Karuna Reiki Master Affiliated with Triad Essence Energy and Wellness, Light Energy Workers and Association and The International Center for Reiki Training.

Robert Fosque, Methodist Christian, Pastor, Civil Engineer, Healer, Certified Holy Fire III Karuna Reiki Master, Sound Energy, Certified Holistic Hand and Foot Reflexologist. Affiliated with Triad Essence Energy and Wellness, Light Energy Workers Association and The International Center for Reiki Training.

Elena Gabor, Ph.D., Associate Professor of Communication at Bradley University, Peoria, IL. Her research has focused on issues of organizational communication, migration, identity and careers in groups such as wildland firefighters, immigrant women engineers, and classical musicians.

Octavian Gabor is Professor of Philosophy at Methodist College. Recent essays include: "Responses to Divine Communication: Oedipus and Socrates" (Philosophy and Theology, 2020), "Taming the Beast: Constantin Noica and Doing Philosophy in Critical Political Contexts" (Dialogos, 2019), "Justice between Mercy and Revenge in Sophocles' Antigone and Plato's Crito" (Lexicon Philosophicum: International Journal for the History of Texts and Ideas, 2019) and "Constantin Noica's Becoming Within Being and Meno's Paradox" (Companion to Classical Reception in Eastern and Central Europe, eds. Zara Torlone & Dana Munteanu. Blackwell, 2017).

Michelle Garland, Ph.D., Directory of Interdisciplinary Studies and Assistant Professor of Communication Studies, University of South Carolina Upstate. She primarily studies Instructional Communication with a secondary area of Assessment and Evaluation. She has interest in teacher-student communication, particularly as it relates to the impact of teacher messages on student learning and affective outcomes.

Kaylie George is an LPN in Missouri, where she graduated from the Cape Girardeau Career and Technology Center in September 2019.

Steven Gimbel is a Professor of Philosophy at Gettysburg College and author of seven books including Einstein's Jewish Science: Physics at the Intersection of Politics and Religion (Johns Hopkins, 2014), Einstein: His Space and Times (Yale, 2016), Exploring the Scientific Method: Cases and Questions (Chicago, 2011), and Isn't that Clever: A Philosophical Account of Humor and Comedy (Routledge, 2017).

Ryan Goke is a PhD student at North Dakota State University. He received his master's degree from Murray State University in 2019. His research interests include workplace relationships, conflict mediation and negotiation, and organizational dynamics.

Kayla Heinze, Undergraduate Student, Class of 2022, Occidental College Philosophy major, biology minor.

Michael Hoppmann is Associate Teaching Professor and Public Speaking Director in the Department of Communication Studies at Northeastern University (Boston). Previous to joining Northeastern University Dr. Hoppmann worked at the University of Tübingen, designing the curriculum for a Masters program for rhetoric trainers, and teaching classes in Classical Rhetoric and modern Argumentation Theory. Dr. Hoppmann is author or co-author of five books, including A Synoptic History of Classical Rhetoric, Handbook of Rhetorical Training (Trainingsbuch Rhetorik), Argumentative Competence (Schlüsselkompetenz Argumentation) and Argumentative Defense (Argumentative Verteidigung). Dr. Hoppmann sees his main tasks as a rhetorician in carefully observing verbal conflicts, analyzing the structures of its underlying reasoning (Argumentation Theory), learning from the most experienced rhetorical grand masters about human persuasion (Classical Rhetoric) and developing tools for the effective teaching and training of rhetorical skills (Rhetorical Training).

Nicholas T. Iannarino, Ph.D., Associate Professor of Health Communication, University of Michigan-Dearborn. He studies how people in close relationships manage the social experience of severe and chronic illness.

Trevor Kauer, Interpersonal, Family, & Health Communication Doctoral Student, University of Nebraska-Lincoln. He studies the sensemaking, coping, and supportive communication that emerges at the intersection of one's work/life. He has studied the experience of first responders, helicopter parenting and teaching, and military post-deployment and reintegration. Here is some of his work: Folwell, A., & Kauer, T. (2018). "You see a baby die and you're not fine": A case study of stress and coping strategies in volunteer EMTs. Journal of Applied Communication Research, 46(6), 723-743. https://doi.org/10.1080/00909882.2018.1549745 Farris, K., Houser, M., Kauer, T., & Carpenter, L. (2021). The road to hel(l)icopter teaching: How do instructors make sense of their helicopter teaching behaviors and student effects?. Qualitative Research Reports in Communication. Online. https://doi.org/10.1080/17459435.2020.1853209 Segrin, C., Burke, T., & Kauer, T. (2020). Overparenting is associated with perfectionism in parents of young adults. Couple and Family Psychology: Research and Practice, 9(3), 181–190. https://doi.org/10.1037/cfp0000143.

Alyse Keller, Ph.D., Assistant Professor of Communication Studies, CUNY Kingsborough Community College. Her research looks at the intersection of performance and narrative medicine, and specifically focuses on her family's experience with maternal multiple sclerosis. She believes humor is the best form of medicine, and as such will continue advocating for and infusing her own research with humor.

Andrea L. Meluch, Ph.D., is an Assistant Professor of Business and Organizational Communication in the School of Communication and Department of Management at The University of Akron. Her research focuses on the intersections of health, organizational, and instructional communication. Specifically, she is interested in issues of organizational culture, mental health, and social support. She has published in *Communication Studies, Communication Education, Southern Communication Journal, Qualitative Research in Medicine & Healthcare, Journal of Communication in Healthcare,* and the *Journal of Communication Pedagogy*. She has also authored/co-authored more than a dozen book chapters and encyclopedia entries.

Laura E. Miller, Associate Professor of Communication Studies, University of Tennessee, Knoxville. Dr. Miller's research explores health communication among families and close relational partners. Exemplars of her work may be read here: Miller, L. E. (2015). Young breast cancer survivors' experiences of uncertainty. *Journal of Applied Communication Research, 43*(4), 429-449. Crowley, J. L. & Miller, L. E. (2020). "Who's going to love a junkie? But he does": Exploring couples' identity negotiations and dyadic coping in the context of opioid use disorder. *Journal of Social and Personal Relationships, 37*(5), 1634-1652.

Clair Morrissey specializes in practical ethics and political philosophy, including the relationship between aesthetics and ethics. Her work includes: A. Sherman and C. Morrissey (2017) "What is Art Good For? The Socio-Epistemic Value of Art," Frontiers in Human Neuroscience 11: 411. C. Morrissey (2016) "The Value of Dignity in and for Bioethics: Rethinking the Terms of the Debate," Theoretical Medicine and Bioethics 37(3): 173-192. C. Morrissey and R. L. Walker (2018) "The Ethics of General Population Preventive Genomic Sequencing: Rights and Social Justice," Journal of Medicine and Philosophy 43: 22-43.

Carey Noland (Ph.D., Ohio University) is an award winning researcher and professor with over 25 years experience. She is currently an Associate Professor of Communication Studies at Northeastern University, Boston. Her most recent publications include Contemporary Studies of Sexuality & Communication: Theoretical and Applied Perspectives with Jimmie Manning by Kendall-Hunt and articles in Patient Education and Counseling, Health Communication and Qualitative Health Research. Of note, her last publication exploring the intersection of humor and communication won Top Paper at the National Communication Association Annual Meeting in 2019. Hoppmann, M. & Noland, C. (2020). Stop! You're Killing Me: Food Addiction and Comedy. In P. Opplinger & E. Shouse (Eds). The Dark Side of Stand-Up Comedy. Palgrave Macmillan.

Candy J. Noltensmeyer, Ph.D., Associate Professor of Communication, Western Carolina University. Research interests include the scholarship of teaching and learning (SoTL) and the relational aspects of stigma and sexuality.

Christine North, Professor, Oklahoma City County Health Department. Dr. North teaches for several institutions and works in public health. Her work focuses on health literacy, health communication and social determinants of health. Recent publications include North, C. L., Henriksen, B., Beckett, R.D, Etheridge, K. M., & Smith, W. T (2018). Impact of training and student self-identification on frequency, constructiveness, and professionalism of pharmacy student evaluations of teaching. Currents in Pharmacy Teaching and Learning, 10(9), 1175-1183. doi: 10.1016/j.cptl.2018.06.016 North, C. L. (2017). Practicing medicine with CLAS. In R. W. Davis & A. Patterson-Matsuko (Eds.) (pp. 424-440). Communication for global engagement across cultural boundaries (2nd ed). Dubuque, IA: Kendall-Hunt.

Allison Noyes, Assistant Professor of Communication Studies, Loyola Marymount University. Dr. Noyes studies collaboration in health organizations. Her work has examined topics like language access for limited English proficient patients and power relationships among members of collaborative care teams.

Suzy Prentiss, PhD, Human Ecology- Family Studies, The University of Tennessee MA, Communication Studies, Emerson College BA, Speech Communication, University of Maine Phi Beta Kappa, Phi Kappa Phi.

Shana Ratner, MD, Clinical Associate Professor of Medicine, Division of General Internal Medicine and Clinical Epidemiology at University of North Carolina at Chapel Hill. She is Associate Director UNC Institute for Healthcare Quality Improvement. She teaches Medical Students and Residents, leads multiple quality improvement initiatives, and strives to provide patient and family-centered care to her primary care patients.

Kenneth T. Rocker, Doctoral Student (Communication), Massey University (Wellington, NZ). Kenneth is entering his second semester at Massey University. He has interests in organizational communication with a focus in organizational dissent.

Elizabeth Spradley, Ph.D., Assistant Professor at Stephen F. Austin State University. She currently teaches basic courses and coordinates the undergraduate communication studies program.

Robert Spradley, Ph.D., Associate Professor of Communication at Stephen F. Austin State University. He was awarded the 2013-2014 and 2014-2015 Jim Towns Endowed Mentoring Professorship. He researches organizational communication, specifically high reliability organizations, risk and crisis communication, and mentoring. He is published in The *International Encyclopedia of Organizational Communication, Sage Research Methods Cases, Journal of Human Services, International Research Journal of Health Education*, and the *International Research Journal of Public Health.*

Ian Stark is a Ph.D. student in Technical Communication and Rhetoric at Texas Tech University. With an interdisciplinary background in healthcare management and medical humanities, they conduct research on the administrative systems and rhetorical practices of mental health communication.

Monalisa Tailor, MD, is a graduate of the University of Louisville School of Medicine, through which she also completed her residency in Internal Medicine and then served as faculty for three years. Today, she practices with Norton Community Medical Associates: Barret. She currently serves as the President of the Greater Louisville Medical Society, the Kentucky Medical Association Vice Speaker, and a member of the KMAC Museum Board. She served on the Louisville Metro Public Health and Wellness Board of Health for 2 years.

Joy Todd, RN, MS, CPXP, Manager Patient Centered Care (PCC), Enloe Medical Center (EMC), Chico, CA. Joy has been a national speaker about PCC Transformations, Managing PCC during Major Crises, and is the liaison with Planetree where EMC has earned the Gold Designation.

Joshua Tovey, Phlebotomist, specializing in whole blood donations, double packed red cell apheresis, and autologous donations ordered by surgeons.

Elizabeth Victor, Associate Professor of Philosophy & Liberal Studies, William Paterson University. In addition to her work in humor studies, Dr. Victor has published on the concept of vulnerability,

LGBTQIA healthcare inequities, implicit bias in clinical contexts, personal identity, relational autonomy and duties to future generations, and research ethics. Here is some of her recent work: Victor, E. and L. Guidry-Grimes (eds.) (forthcoming, 2021). Applying nonideal theory to bioethics: Living and dying in a nonideal world. Springer: Philosophy & Medicine Series. Victor, E. (2019). Vulnerability and incarceration: Evaluating protections for prisoners in research. Lexington Books. Victor, E. and L. Guidry-Grimes (2019). Relational autonomy in action: Rethinking dementia and sexuality in care facilities. Nursing Ethics 26 (6): 1654-1664.

Vanessa Voss is an Associate Professor of Philosophy at Lone Star College, University Park. She has an MA in Philosophy from the University of Houston and an MA in Central Eurasian and Iranian Studies from Indiana University. She writes on the philosophy of humor and comparative philosophy. She has published work on feminism, evolution, and humor in the collection, "Who's Laughing Now: Feminist Perspectives on Humour and Laughter" and on Relief Theory in "It's Funny Cause It's True: The Lighthearted Philosophers' Society Introduction to Philosophy through Humor".

Susan M. Wieczorek, Associate Professor of Communication at University of Pittsburgh at Johnstown and Medical Interviewing Preceptor at University of Pittsburgh Medical School, studies effective practitioner/patient shared decision-making. Wieczorek, S. M. (2020). eMessaging and the physician/patient dynamic: Practices in transition. Lexington. Wieczorek, S.M. (2019). The midlife experience: Thirty years in the making. In L. Peterson and C. Kiesinger (Eds.), Narrating midlife: Crisis, transition, and transformation. Lexington. pp. 191-204. Wieczorek, S.M. (2018). Patient engagement in co-authored medical records. The Journal of the American Osteopathic Association. 18. 361-362. Wieczorek, S.M. (2017). Now and at the hour of death. Journal of Patient Experience. 5(1). pp. 4-5.

Eugene Zaldivar, Ph.D., Associate Professor of Philosophy, Santa Fe College. As a member of the Cuban diaspora, he has a keen interest in intersectional ethics and social justice. A longtime member of the Lighthearted Philosophers Association, he is pleased as punch to sponsor its undergraduate writing award.

Index

www.ingramcontent.com/pod-product-compliance
Lightning Source LLC
LaVergne TN
LVHW062155300926
849161LV00010B/2672